313
Current Topics in Microbiology and Immunology

Editors

R.W. Compans, Atlanta/Georgia
M.D. Cooper, Birmingham/Alabama
T. Honjo, Kyoto · H. Koprowski, Philadelphia/Pennsylvania
F. Melchers, Basel · M.B.A. Oldstone, La Jolla/California
S. Olsnes, Oslo · C. Svanborg, Lund
P.K. Vogt, La Jolla/California · H. Wagner, Munich

P. P. Pandolfi and P. K. Vogt (Eds.)

Acute Promyelocytic Leukemia

Molecular Genetics, Mouse Models
and Targeted Therapy

With 16 Figures and 12 Tables

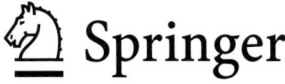

Pier Paolo Pandolfi, MD, Ph.D.
Sloan-Kettering-Institute
Memorial Sloan-Kettering Cancer Center
1275 York Avenue
New York, New York 10021
USA

e-mail: p-pandolfi@ski.mskcc.org

Peter K. Vogt, Ph.D.
The Scripps Research Institute
10550 North Torreye Pines Road
La Jolla, CA 92037
USA

e-mail: pkvogt@scripps.edu

Cover Illustration:
APL: a journey of discovery from gene identification to cure. The understanding of the molecular genetics underlying the disease and faithful modeling of the disease in the mouse has been instrumental in developing and optimizing effective treatment modalities in preclinical trials. As a result, this form of leukemia is now considered curable.

Library of Congress Catalog Number 72-152360

ISSN 0070-217X
ISBN-10 3-540-34592-2 Springer Berlin Heidelberg New York
ISBN-13 978-3-540-34592-3 Springer Berlin Heidelberg New York

This work is subject to copyright. All rights reserved, whether the whole or part of the material is concerned, specifically the rights of translation, reprinting, reuse of illustrations, recitation, broadcasting, reproduction on microfilm or in any other way, and storage in data banks. Duplication of this publication or parts thereof is permitted only under the provisions of the German Copyright Law of September, 9, 1965, in its current version, and permission for use must always be obtained from Springer-Verlag. Violations are liable for prosecution under the German Copyright Law.

Springer is a part of Springer Science+Business Media
springer.com
© Springer-Verlag Berlin Heidelberg 2007

The use of general descriptive names, registered names, trademarks, etc. in this publication does not imply, even in the absence of a specific statement, that such names are exempt from the relevant protective laws and regulations and therefore free for general use.
Product liability: The publisher cannot guarantee the accuracy of any information about dosage and application contained in this book. In every individual case the user must check such information by consulting the relevant literature.

Editor: Simon Rallison, Heidelberg
Desk editor: Anne Clauss, Heidelberg
Production editor: Nadja Kroke, Leipzig
Cover design: WMX Design, Heidelberg
Typesetting: LE-TEX Jelonek, Schmidt & Vöckler GbR, Leipzig
Printed on acid-free paper   SPIN 11735670   27/3150/YL – 5 4 3 2 1 0

List of Contents

APL as a Paradigm in Biomedical Research: A Journey Toward the Cure 1
   P. P. Pandolfi

Mouse Models of Acute Promyelocytic Leukemia 3
   S. C. Kogan

The PLZF Gene of t(11;17)-Associated APL 31
   M. J. McConnell and J. D. Licht

SUMO, the Three Rs and Cancer 49
   J.-S. Seeler, O. Bischof, K. Nacerddine, and A. Dejean

Emerging Role for MicroRNAs in Acute Promyelocytic Leukemia 73
   C. Nervi, F. Fazi, A. Rosa, A. Fatica, and I. Bozzoni

The Theory of APL Revisited 85
   P. P. Scaglioni and P. P. Pandolfi

Treatment of Acute Promyelocytic Leukemia by Retinoids 101
   P. Fenaux, Z. Z. Wang, and L. Degos

Arsenic Trioxide and Acute Promyelocytic Leukemia: Clinical and Biological . . . 129
   Z. Chen, W.-L. Zhao, Z.-X. Shen, J.-M. Li, S.-J. Chen, J. Zhu,
   V. Lallemand-Breittenbach, J. Zhou, M.-C. Guillemin, D. Vitoux, and H. de Thé

Front Line Clinical Trials and Minimal Residual Disease Monitoring
in Acute Promyelocytic Leukemia 145
   F. Lo-Coco and E. Ammatuna

Histone Deacetylase Inhibitors in APL and Beyond 157
   K. Petrie, N. Prodromou, and A. Zelent

Monoclonal Antibody Therapy of APL 205
   P. G. Maslak, J. G. Jurcic, and D. A. Scheinberg

Targeting APL Fusion Proteins by Peptide Interference 221
   A. Melnick

The Design of Selective and Non-selective Combination Therapy
for Acute Promyelocytic Leukemia 245
   Y. Jing and S. Waxman

Subject Index 271

List of Contributors

(Addresses stated at the beginning of respective chapters)

Ammatuna, E.   145

Bischof, O.   49
Bozzoni, I.   73

Chen, S.-J.   129
Chen, Z.   129

de Thé, H.   129
Degos, L.   101
Dejean, A.   49

Fatica, A.   73
Fazi, F.   73
Fenaux, P.   101

Guillemin, M.-C.   129

Jing, Y.   245
Jurcic, J. G.   205

Kogan, S. C.   3

Lallemand-Breittenbach, V.   129
Li, J.-M.   129
Licht, J. D.   31
Lo-Coco, F.   145

Maslak, P. G.   205
McConnell, M. J.   31
Melnick, A.   221

Nacerddine, K.   49
Nervi, C.   73

Pandolfi, P. P.   1, 85
Petrie, K.   157
Prodromou, N.   157

Rosa, A.   73

Scaglioni, P. P.   85
Scheinberg, D. A.   205
Seeler, J.-S.   49
Shen, Z.-X.   129

Vitoux, D.   129

Wang, Z. Z.   101
Waxman, S.   245

Zelent, A.   157
Zhao, W.-L.   129
Zhou, J.   129
Zhu, J.   129

APL as a Paradigm in Biomedical Research: A Journey Toward the Cure

P. P. Pandolfi

Cancer Biology and Genetics Program, Department of Pathology,
Memorial Sloan-Kettering Cancer Center, Sloan-Kettering Institute,
1275 York Avenue, New York, NY 10021, USA
p-pandolfi@ski.mskcc.org

This volume is meant to summarize some of the most recent progress made in elucidating the pathogenesis of acute promyelocytic leukemia (APL) and in the treatment of this form of leukemia.

It is also meant to celebrate one of the most successful accomplishments in cancer research and contemporary biomedical research.

APL was in fact regarded as an almost invariably fatal disease just a decade ago, while it is now considered a curable leukemia—if not cured—in many advanced cancer centers in the world. The story of APL represents perhaps the most compelling example to date of what could be done and will be done in the years to come in the combat and defeat of the cancer plague if appropriate resources are made available to the scientific community.

This tremendous progress in APL research and treatment has been made possible through a number of seminal discoveries and by the concerted efforts of many labs worldwide that have raced and competed with each other, but also interacted and cooperated, to reach this remarkable goal. Many of these groups and investigators have contributed to this dedicated volume.

The story of APL in the last decade has become a paradigmatic example with many "firsts" and, importantly, a compelling illustration of the efficacy of a discovery journey from bed- to bench-side, and back to the bedside toward disease cure and eradication. It is a journey of discovery that heavily relied on the use of in vivo approaches in the mouse and on animal modeling not only for mechanistic analyses, but also for preclinical efforts; a journey of discovery that will serve as a trail-blazing guide in cancer research in the years to come.

Indeed, the story of APL offers many firsts, and each first has contributed substantially toward the cure:

1. For the *first* time in the case of APL, the knowledge of the genetic basis of the disease (the presence of the APL-specific chromosomal translocations)

has had an impact on the management of the disease. A simple RT-PCR test to amplify the breakpoint of the fusion transcript made it possible to diagnose APL at a molecular level as well as predict which patients would remain in remission and which would relapse upon therapy (i.e., RT-PCR-positive patients would relapse and need additional therapy, while RT-PCR-negative ones would remain in long-term remission and could be spared additional therapy).

2. APL treatment with retinoic acid (RA) represents the *first* example of "targeted therapy," way ahead of Gleevec. This makes it the *first* example of "transcription therapy" (whereby the drug specifically targets an oncogenic transcription factor and its aberrant action) and the *first* example of "differentiation therapy" where the drug reprograms the leukemic cell for terminal differentiation and normal function rather than killing it as conventional chemotherapy would do.

3. APL has served as a unique example of the utility of the knockout (KO) and transgenic approaches in the comprehensive deconstruction of the molecular genetics of human cancer.

4. Mouse modeling of APL has formally demonstrated for the *first* time that faithful transgenic and KO mouse models of human cancer behave as human patients in terms of response to treatment and can therefore be utilized to test novel treatment modalities.

5. In the case of APL, preclinical testing in mouse models has been for the *first* time instrumental in changing the current way in which we treat a human malignancy. It is in fact on the basis of experiments performed in APL mouse models that combinatorial treatment with RA and As_2O_3 or histone deacetylase inhibitors (HDACIs) is currently being tested in human APL.

6. The story of APL as a whole has also proved another fundamental principle in cancer research and therapy: the need to have at hand not one but a number of molecular-targeted weapons to be used sequentially or combinatorially toward the cure.

7. Finally, the APL saga has developed entirely in the realm of academia worldwide, which formally demonstrates that cancer can be defeated in universities and other academic institutions as an international effort through governmental and philanthropic support.

All these critical aspects will be the focus of the following chapters, written by many of the key investigators that made this possible.

Mouse Models of Acute Promyelocytic Leukemia

S. C. Kogan

Department of Laboratory Medicine and Comprehensive Cancer Center,
University of California, San Francisco, Room S-864, 513 Parnassus Avenue,
San Francisco, CA 94143-0100, USA
Scott.Kogan@ucsf.edu

1	Models	4
1.1	X-RARα Fusions	8
1.2	Mechanisms of Leukemogenesis	9
1.3	Role of Reciprocal Fusions	10
1.4	Targeting, Expression Level, Strain Effects	10
2	Cooperating Events	11
2.1	Hypothesis Testing	11
2.2	Non-engineered Cooperating Events	12
2.3	Restrictive and Permissive Factors	14
3	Pathogenesis, Conclusions	14
4	Immune Modulation of APL	15
5	Therapies	16
5.1	Mechanism of ATRA Response	17
5.2	Preclinical Studies	18
6	Arsenic Trioxide	18
7	Histone Deacetylase Inhibitors	22
8	Additional Investigational Therapies	23
9	Therapy, Conclusions	24
10	Perspectives	24
	References	25

Abstract Mouse models of acute promyelocytic leukemia have been generated through transgenic, knock-in, retroviral, and xenograft strategies. These models have been used to elucidate mechanisms underlying leukemogenesis. Among the areas investigated are the role of reciprocal fusions; effects of target cells, expression levels, and mouse strains; cooperating events; and restrictive and permissive factors. These models have also been used to gain insight into the effects of the immune system on leukemic cells and the mechanism of response to retinoic acid. Furthermore, preclinical studies utilizing these mice have advanced therapy for myeloid leukemia.

Animal models of disease can be powerful tools for understanding pathogenesis and investigating therapies. Nevertheless, in 1997, when transgenic models of acute promyelocytic leukemia (APL) were first developed, it was initially unclear what impact such models could have on the field. APL seemed to be well understood. A recurrent t(15;17) chromosomal translocation resulted in a fusion of the promyelocytic leukemia gene (*PML*) to the gene encoding retinoic acid receptor α (*RARA*). The resulting PML-RARα fusion impaired the normal function of RARα in neutrophil differentiation. In addition, PML-RARα disrupted the nuclear bodies of which PML is a part and thereby abrogated the growth suppressive effects of PML. Furthermore, it had already been found that the event-free survival of patients with APL could be increased from approximately 20% with chemotherapy alone to approximately 70% with a combination of all-*trans* retinoic acid (ATRA) and chemotherapy (Degos et al. 1995). The models at first seemed simply to be interesting examples of replicating a human condition in mice.

In time, mouse models of APL have proved of greater value than anticipated (Fig. 1). They have helped us to understand the mechanisms by which PML-RARα and other X-RARα fusions contribute to leukemia. They have led to insights into the principles underlying cooperative leukemogenesis. The models have identified normal factors that permit or restrict leukemic transformation. APL has been identified as a disease in which the host immune system has the potential to exert an antileukemic effect. Perhaps most significantly, preclinical studies utilizing the models have both informed progress in treating human APL and have illuminated important principles in cancer therapy [see Pandolfi (2001), Pollock et al. (2001), and Lallemand-Breitenbach et al. (2005) for selected reviews of mouse APL models].

1
Models

Four approaches have been utilized to successfully generate mouse models of APL: transgenic, knock-in, bone marrow transduction, and xenograft (Table 1). Transgenic animals expressing *PML-RARA* under the control of the cathepsin G or migration inhibitory factor-related protein 8 (MRP8) promot-

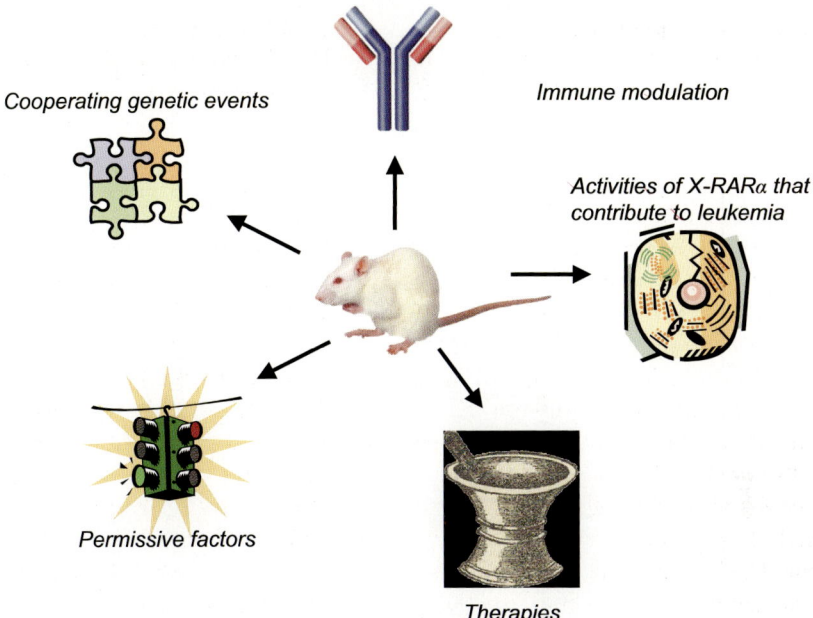

Fig. 1 Transgenic, knock-in, retroviral transduction, and xenograft mouse models have contributed in multiple ways to our understanding of the pathogenesis and therapy of acute promyelocytic leukemia

ers developed acute myeloid leukemias (Brown et al. 1997; Grisolano et al. 1997; He et al. 1997). Interestingly, expression of PML-RARα did not block neutrophilic differentiation by itself. Rather, PML-RARα expression resulted in a modest shift in the balance of myelopoiesis toward less mature elements. Only after significant latency (generally >6 months) and with incomplete penetrance (initially reported as 10%–30%) did AML develop. Importantly, many leukemic cells of *PML-RARA* mice were immature and contained numerous primary granules. This finding paralleled the abundance of primary granule-filled promyelocytes seen in human APL. Subsequently, in an effort to increase the penetrance of disease, *PML-RARA* was expressed under the control of cathepsin G regulatory elements by knock-in rather than by transgenesis (Westervelt et al. 2003). Although these knock-in mice expressed PML-RARα at a level only 3% of the cathepsin G *PML-RARA* transgenics, the penetrance of leukemia was increased to more than 90% in this model. A number of groups attempted to generate APL models by transducing murine bone marrow with retroviral vectors harboring the *PML-RARA* fusion gene. Eventually,

Table 1 Mouse models of acute promyelocytic leukemia (selected). Diagnoses are of most advanced disease stage

Model	Diagnosis	Incidence	Latency	Reference(s)
Transgenic				
Cathepsin G (C57BL/6)				
PML-RARA/Pml$^{+/+}$	Myl Leuk w/matur	13% at 1 year	~26 months (median)	He et al. 1997; Rego et al. 2001
PML-RARA/Pml$^{+/-}$	Myl Leuk w/matur	31% at 1 year	~16 months (median)	Rego et al. 2001
PML-RARA/Pml$^{-/-}$	Myl Leuk w/matur	53% at 1 year	~13 months (median)	Rego et al. 2001
PLZF-RARA	MPD-like Myl Leuk	Complete	6–18 months	He et al. 1998; Cheng et al. 1999
PLZF-RARA/RARA-PLZF	Myl Leuk w/matur	Complete	6–18 months	He et al. 2000
NPM-RARA	Myl Leuk wo/ or w/matur or MPD-like Myl Leuk	3 of 7	12–14 months	Cheng et al. 1999
NuMA-RARA	Myl Leuk w/matur[a]	Complete	10–14 months	Sukhai et al. 2004
Cathepsin G (C57BL/6:C3H/He Mix)				
PML-RARA	Myl Leuk w/matur	7%–32%[b] at ~2 years	~7–12 months (mean)	Grisolano et al. 1997; Pollock et al. 1999; Walter et al. 2004, 2005
PML-RARA/RARA-PML	Myl Leuk w/matur	57% at 2 years	~10 months (mean)	Pollock et al. 1999
PML-RARA+3 Gy XRT	Myl Leuk w/matur	67% at ~2 years	~7 months (median)	Walter et al. 2004
PML-RARA/FLT3 v	Myl Leuk w/matur	Complete	80 days (median)	Kelly et al. 2002
PML-RARA/PU.1$^{+/-}$	Myl Leuk w/matur	84% at ~2 years	~11 months (median)	Walter et al. 2005
MRP8 (FVB/N)				
PML-RARA	Myl Leuk wo/matur	67% at 1 year	~8 months (median)	Brown et al. 1997; Kogan et al. 2001

Table 1 (continued)

Model	Diagnosis	Incidence	Latency	Reference(s)
PML-RARA/BCL2	Myl Leuk wo/matur	Complete	~4 months (median)	Kogan et al. 2001
PML-RARAm4	Myl Leuk wo/matur	7 of 9	~7 months (median)	Kogan et al. 2000
PML-RARA/FLT3 v	Myl Leuk wo/ or w/matur	Complete	105 days (median)	Sohal et al. 2003
MRP8 (C57BL/6:DBA Mix)				
PML-RARA	Myl Leuk wo/matur	N/A	8–27 months	Zhu et al. 2005
PML-RARAK160R	MPD	Moderate to High	5–30 months	Zhu et al. 2005
Knock-In (Cathepsin G)				
PML-RARA (C57BL/6:129 Sv/J)	Myl Leuk w/matur	Complete	~10 months (median)	Westervelt et al. 2003
PML-RARA/NE$^{+/+}$ [c]	Myl Leuk w/matur	Complete	~7 months (median)	Lane and Ley et al. 2003
PML-RARA/NE$^{-/-}$ [c]	Myl Leuk w/matur	45% at ~1 year	6–10 months	Lane and Ley et al. 2003
Retroviral Transduction (129SvEv)				
PML-RARA	Myl Leuk wo/ or w/matur	81%	173 days (median)	Minucci et al. 2002
Xenograft (SCID or NOD-SCID)				
NB4 cells	Human APL	Complete	~1 month	Zhang et al. 1996

FLT3, activated allele of FLT3; MPD, myeloproliferative disease; MPD-like Myl Leuk, MPD-like myeloid leukemia; Myl Leuk w/matur, myeloid leukemia with maturation; Myl Leuk wo/matur, myeloid leukemia without maturation; N/A, not available; NE, gene encoding neutrophil elastase; Pml, gene encoding PML protein; PU.1, Sfpi1 locus; v, indicates that retroviral bone marrow transduction was used to add the allele to transgenic bone marrow; XRT, X-ray therapy, 3 Gy at 8–10 weeks of age

[a] These animals develop an unusual nonfatal leukemia

[b] Variation among the studies. Pertinent PML-RARA (alone) comparison groups were 15% vs PML-RARA/RARA-PML; 32% vs PML-RARA+XRT; 7% vs PML-RARA/PU.1$^{+/-}$

[c] Strain C57BL/6:129 Sv/J:129SvEv

it was found that retroviral transduction of immature (lineage-depleted) bone marrow cells of 129SvEv mice with transplantation into lethally irradiated recipients could lead to AMLs in 80% of recipient mice with a median latency of 6 months (Minucci et al. 2002). An alternative approach to animal models of human leukemia is to engraft human cells into immunocompromised mice. NB4 cells, which are a cell line derived from a human APL patient, can engraft in severe combined immunodeficiency (SCID) mice when injected into the peritoneal cavity, subcutaneously or intravenously (Kosugi et al. 2001; Zhang et al. 1996).

1.1
X-RARα Fusions

In addition to the *PML-RARA* fusion generated by the common t(15;17) of APL, alternative fusions are rarely observed in the human disease including *PLZF-RARA, NPM-RARA, NuMA-RARA* and *STAT5b-RARA*. These *RARA* chimeras are collectively referred to as *X-RARA* fusions. A number of limitations are evident in considering mouse models of APL as a means of understanding pathogenesis caused by these molecules. The models described above do not express the fusion genes from the endogenous promoters; hence the patterns of expression are different from those generated by the regulatory regions governing transcription of *PML* and other fusion partner genes. None of these models replicates the reciprocal translocations of the human disease that generate not only *X-RARA* fusions, but also *RARA-X* fusions accompanied by reduction of *RARA* and *X* loci to haploinsufficiency. In addition, mouse strain background, the impact of using human fusion genes rather than mouse genes, and differences in rodent and human biology all have the potential to influence and confound the results. Despite these limitations, the animal models have led to remarkable insights into APL biology.

The cathepsin G promoter has been used to generate not only *PML-RARA* transgenic mice, but also transgenic mice expressing *PLZF-RARA* (Cheng et al. 1999; He et al. 1998), *NPM-RARA* (Cheng et al. 1999), and *NuMA-RARA* (Sukhai et al. 2004). Work with the *PLZF-RARA* mice demonstrated that after 3–18 months, *PLZF-RARA* efficiently initiated myeloid leukemias that were well-differentiated. *NPM-RARA* could also lead to leukemias, with longer latency (12–15 months); these leukemias ranged from well-differentiated to predominantly immature. *NuMA-RARA* generated myeloid neoplasms with a progressive increase in promyelocytes (immature forms), but the myeloid leukemias with maturation that eventually manifested were nonfatal, in contrast to the diseases that arose in cathepsin G *PML-RARA, PLZF-RARA*, and *NPM-RARA* transgenic animals. The X-RARα fusions are all able to initiate myeloid neoplasia but differ in their efficiency of generating disease, the clinical course of the disease, and the likelihood that the disease will be characterized by a block in myeloid maturation.

1.2 Mechanisms of Leukemogenesis

Mouse models can be used to perform structure–function analyses of oncoproteins. This type of structure–function analysis has been pursued to an extent in mice transgenic for *PML-RARA*. In contrast to the ability of *PML-RARA* to initiate an APL-like disease and in contrast to the ability of all of the *X-RARA* fusions to cause myeloid neoplasia in mice, expression of a dominant-negative form of *RARA* under the MRP8 promoter resulted in only slight abnormalities of myelopoiesis and no disease (Kogan et al. 2000). This result indicated that although all of the X-RARα fusions can repress transcription from retinoic acid response elements (RAREs), repression at these sites is not sufficient for initiating leukemogenesis. Since they homodimerize (and can oligomerize), the X-RARα fusions bind a much broader array of DNA sequences than normal RXR/RAR heterodimers (Jansen et al. 1995; Kamashev et al. 2004; Lin and Evans 2000). This expanded binding site specificity may be an important reason that *RARA* fusions are a constant feature of human APL, rather than dominant-negative point mutations within *RARA*.

Transgenic mice have also been generated with a *PML-RARA* fusion that has a point mutation changing the lysine at position 160 of PML to arginine (Zhu et al. 2005). Lysine 160 is the location of a posttranslational modification of PML by addition of a ubiquitin-like peptide, SUMO (small ubiquitin-like modifier). Hence, the MRP8 *PML-RARA^{K160R}* transgenic animals provide a means to assess the importance of this site for leukemic transformation. Interestingly, *PML-RARA^{K160R}* mice can develop a well-differentiated myeloid neoplasm with some features in common with the disease observed in cathepsin G transgenics that express *PLZF-RARA*, *NPM-RARA*, or *NuMA-RARA*, but do not develop an APL-like disease with blocked differentiation. Therefore, K160 is an important structure for the ability of PML-RARα to initiate an AML with a block in maturation; sumoylation at this site is implicated to be key.

Structure–function studies performed in animals are vital to an accurate understanding of leukemogenesis. This assertion reflects our understanding that in vitro characteristics of transformation, including immortalization, do not always correlate with the ability of oncoproteins to initiate disease or block differentiation in vivo. The availability of retroviral-induced models of APL should speed additional in vivo studies of *X-RARA* fusions and derivatives.

1.3
Role of Reciprocal Fusions

In the majority of APL with t(15;17), the reciprocal *RARA-PML* fusion is expressed and *RARA-PLZF* is generally expressed in the rare cases of APL with t(11;17). Coexpression of *RARA-PML* as a cathepsin G-driven transgene with cathepsin G-driven *PML-RARA* increased the penetrance of leukemia from 15% to 57% without altering latency (Pollock et al. 1999). The disease that arose in the doubly transgenic mice was less differentiated and more rapidly fatal than that observed with *PML-RARA* alone. Strikingly, concordant findings were observed when a cathepsin G *RARA-PLZF* transgene was combined with cathepsin G *PLZF-RARA*. Without altering latency, the addition of the reciprocal fusion resulted in an acute leukemia with features of APL, rather than the well-differentiated leukemias observed in *PLZF-RARA* single transgenics (He et al. 2000). Both of these *RARA-X* fusions increased the likelihood that an aggressive AML would arise without decreasing the time to develop disease. These observations demonstrated that the reciprocal fusions (1) make important contributions to the morphologic phenotype that defines APL and (2) facilitate transformation without accelerating the rate-limiting steps required in these leukemia models.

1.4
Targeting, Expression Level, Strain Effects

Comparisons among the APL models of genetically engineered mice (GEM) demonstrate some of the complexities inherent in such systems. The degree of differentiation block appeared to be more pronounced in mice expressing *PML-RARA* under the control of the MRP8 promoter than in mice expressing *PML-RARA* under the control of the cathepsin G promoter; the penetrance of disease appeared to be somewhat higher in the MRP8 transgenics (Brown et al. 1997; Grisolano et al. 1997; He et al. 1997). Different MRP8 *PML-RARA* founders gave rise to different levels of transgene expression, and the line with the highest level of expression had the greatest incidence of leukemia. Yet, expression of *PML-RARA* as a knock-in allele under the control of cathepsin G resulted in very low-level expression but high leukemia penetrance (Westervelt et al. 2003). Although the effects of the different mouse strains used may have contributed to these differences, the findings suggest that the compartment in which an oncoprotein is expressed as well as the specific level of expression are important determinants of malignant transformation. It is of some interest that the 129 strain background was permissive for initiating leukemia by retroviral transduction of bone marrow (Minucci et al. 2002). Of note, 129 has been the most common source of murine embryonic stem cells, and although not directly assessed for *PML-RARA*, this strain might more readily yield myeloid leukemias after marrow transduction than other commonly used strains, including FVB/N and C57BL/6.

2
Cooperating Events

Mouse models in which a genetic event has been used to initiate a neoplasm are powerful tools for assessing the ability of chosen additional events to cooperate in transformation as well as for identifying spontaneous events that can complement an initiating lesion. Ideas regarding cooperative leukemogenesis have been tested in mouse APL models; these models have also yielded results that have served as a source of new hypotheses.

2.1
Hypothesis Testing

BCL-2 (B-cell CLL/lymphoma 2), a protein that inhibits apoptosis, is expressed in most APLs (Bensi et al. 1995; DiGiuseppe et al. 1996; Molica et al. 1996; Porwit-MacDonald et al. 1995; Wuchter et al. 1999). In addition, PML-RARα had been described as being able to induce apoptosis in many cell types (Ferrucci et al. 1997), and such cell death induction might limit the oncogenic effect of the fusion. For these reasons, it was hypothesized that BCL-2 might cooperate with PML-RARα to generate leukemias. The addition of MRP8 *BCL2* to mice expressing an MRP8 *PML-RARA* transgene resulted in decreased median latency to leukemia (in this study, 127 days for doubly transgenic mice vs 257 days in *PML-RARA* single transgenics) (Kogan et al. 2001). Furthermore, the penetrance was increased as all doubly transgenic mice developed leukemia before 7 months of age. An unanticipated finding in *BCL2/PML-RARA* transgenic animals was that the combination was initially associated with accumulation of immature myeloid cells (immature forms/blasts) in the bone marrow that did not behave in a leukemic manner (i.e., the peripheral red blood cell and platelet counts were maintained, and the immature forms/blasts did not disseminate beyond the marrow and spleen). This observation suggested that, as with malignancies of epithelial tissues, normal myeloid cells are dependent upon microenvironmental cues and that this dependence must be overcome during AML development.

Activation of the receptor tyrosine kinase FLT3 (fms-related tyrosine kinase 3) is observed in approximately 25% of human AML and approximately

33% of APL (Kiyoi et al. 1997; Kottaridis et al. 2001; Schnittger et al. 2002; Yamamoto et al. 2001; Yokota et al. 1997). The microgranular variant of APL shows an especially high rate of FLT3 mutations (~65%). FLT3 can be activated by internal tandem duplication (ITD) of a negative regulatory juxtamembrane region or by point mutation of the kinase domain. To assess the hypothesis that activated FLT3 would cooperate with PML-RARα to generate leukemia, bone marrow retroviral transduction was used to introduce activated FLT3 (an ITD mutant) into bone marrow of cathepsin G or MRP8 *PML-RARA* transgenic mice (Kelly et al. 2002; Sohal et al. 2003). Activated FLT3 accelerated the development of disease and increased penetrance in both of these transgenic models. Although potent, the activated FLT3+PMLRARα combination may not have immediately caused AML. Median latency was still 3 months (with a range of 2–10 months), and the leukemias appeared to be oligo- to monoclonal. This limited clonality raises the possibility that additional events were still required for leukemogenesis.

2.2
Non-engineered Cooperating Events

Leukemias arising in *PML-RARA* transgenic mice were examined for the presence of clonal abnormalities. Cytogenetic changes were also sought in *PML-RARA* mice in which additional changes had been engineered. Karyotypic alterations were observed by comparative genomic hybridization or spectral karyotyping in 23 of 27 (85%) MRP8 *PMLRARA* leukemias (Kogan et al. 2001; Le Beau et al. 2002). The most common changes were gain of mouse chromosome 15 or loss of a sex chromosome. Another frequent change was gain of chromosome 8. Loss of chromosome 2 in whole or in part was uncommon in this model (2 of 27, 7%). Spectral karyotyping of cathepsin G *PML-RARA* leukemias showed less frequent changes than in the MRP8 *PML-RARA* model: only 1 of 5 leukemias showed a predominant clonal population (Zimonjic et al. 2000). In the MRP8 *PML-RARA* model, the addition of *BCL2* resulted in complex karyotypic changes in almost all leukemias (15 of 17, 88%), rather than 15 of 27 (56%) complex karyotypes with *PML-RARA* alone. *RARA-PML* expression in the cathepsin G *PML-RARA* model was also associated with increased chromosomal changes; the frequency of clonal karyotypic abnormalities in these leukemias was 85% (Zimonjic et al. 2000). Interstitial deletion of chromosome 2 was seen in all 11 of 13 karyotypically abnormal *PML-RARA/RARA-PML* leukemias; these deletions were accompanied by gain of chromosome 15, tetraploidy, loss of a sex chromosome, or loss of chromosome 11, in some tumors. In contrast to the increased karyotypic alterations with *BCL2* or *RARA-*

PML, activation of growth factor signaling pathways with FLT3, an activated β_c chain of the granulocyte-macrophage colony-stimulating factor (GM-CSF)/interleukin (IL)-3/IL-5 receptor (a mutation not seen in human AML), or overexpressed IL-3 itself, resulted in a decreased frequency of karyotypic changes (Le Beau et al. 2003). It is of interest that the frequency and spectrum of karyotypic changes varied with what additional events were engineered into the animals.

A number of ideas are supported by these results. First, the fact that karyotypic abnormalities vary with the system studied indicates that there is more than one pathway to completing transformation initiated by *PML-RARA*. The presence of multiple paths of progression from initiation to leukemia is further supported by comparative gene expression profiles of leukemias of three models: *PML-RARA*, *PML-RARA+RARA-PML*, and *PML-RARA* mice treated with X-ray irradiation (XRT) (Walter et al. 2004). Patterns of messenger RNA (mRNA) transcript expression were significantly different among the three leukemia models, including between *PML-RARA+RARA-PML* and *PML-RARA+XRT* models that share a common interstitial deletion on chromosome 2. Second, the fact that certain models show increased chromosomal changes whereas others exhibit fewer karyotypic alterations implies that some cooperating events provide critical steps toward the malignant phenotype, whereas other changes can work indirectly by predisposing to the acquisition of further events. Activation of FLT3 is an example of the former and *RARA-PML* an example of the latter. (Events that predispose to additional genetic changes may themselves contribute directly to progression; e.g., BCL-2 may tolerize cells to chromosomal aberrations and also directly contribute to disease by repressing apoptosis.) Third, the identification of recurrent chromosomal changes in mouse models can reveal previously uninvestigated cooperating events. In the case of mouse APL models, the observed interstitial deletion of chromosome 2 resulted in an investigation of the gene encoding the PU.1 transcription factor (Walter et al. 2005). By crossing the cathepsin G *PML-RARA* transgene into mice lacking one copy of the gene for PU.1 (*Sfpi1*), it was shown that haploinsufficiency for this gene increases the penetrance of disease from 7% to 84%. Hence, changes in the RARα and PU.1 myeloid transcription factors can together contribute to transformation. An emerging theme of these and other studies is that one pathway to transformation involves cooperation of transcription factor abnormalities and activation of signaling pathways, whereas another pathway is created by combinations of transcription factors abnormalities.

2.3
Restrictive and Permissive Factors

Considering the mechanisms of malignant transformation, much attention has been paid to genetic mutations that underlie this process. Less focus has been placed on normal endogenous proteins that may either limit the effects of genetic mutations or permit their impact. The mouse APL models have been used to look at some of these factors. Crossing the cathepsin G *PML-RARA* transgene with mice lacking either one or both copies of *Pml* showed that the presence of endogenous PML at wildtype levels restricts progression (Rego et al. 2001). In the absence of one or both copies of *Pml*, the penetrance of the leukemias was increased and the latency was substantially decreased. Whereas in *PML-RARA/Pml$^{+/+}$* animals the incidence of leukemia was 12.5% in the first year of life with mean leukemia free survival (LFS) of 686 days, *PML-RARA/Pml$^{+/-}$* animals had a 1-year leukemia incidence of 31% with mean LFS of 499 days, and in *PML-RARA/Pml$^{-/-}$* animals the incidence and mean LFS were 53% and 434 days. Normal PML restricted the development of APL in this model, and reduction to haploinsufficiency for *PML* as a result of the t(15;17) translocation almost certainly contributes to human APL.

Neutrophil elastase was identified as a permissive factor for APL in the course of studies investigating the significance of cleavage of PML-RARα in myeloid cells (Lane and Ley 2003). When *PML-RARA* was introduced into U937 cells (a human myeloid cell line), a neutral serine protease cleaved the fusion protein in several positions. This protease was identified as neutrophil elastase. This enzyme is present and active in PML-RARα-expressing leukemia cells from humans and mice. Hence, this protein was hypothesized to influence APL pathogenesis. Intriguingly, breeding the cathepsin G *PML-RARA* knock-in allele into mice that lack neutrophil elastase reduced the incidence of leukemia in this model (penetrance of 100% in neutrophil elastase wildtype mice and 45% in neutrophil elastase-deficient mice at 350 days of age). These results indicated that neutrophil elastase is permissive for the development of APL, highlighting a previously unsuspected role for proteolytic enzymes in APL pathogenesis.

3
Pathogenesis, Conclusions

1. PML-RARα and other X-RARα fusions are able to initiate myeloid leukemias. This finding supports the hypothesis that t(15;17) and alternative chromosomal aberrations are initiating events in human APL.

2. PML-RARα and other X-RARα fusions do not themselves block neutrophil differentiation. This observation supports the hypothesis that interactions among genetic mutations are needed to block myeloid maturation.

3. PML-RARα may initiate myeloid leukemia with a block in maturation more readily than other X-RARα fusions. This inference raises the possibility that t(15;17) is a more potent initiator of acute myeloid leukemia than alternative fusions and as a result is the most frequently seen translocation in human APL.

4. Variations in PML-RARα structure can change the frequency of disease initiation or alter disease phenotype. This result supports the hypothesis that multiple activities of PML-RARα contribute to APL pathogenesis.

5. Reciprocal fusions, RARα-PML and RARα-PLZF, increase penetrance of acute leukemia in mice expressing the corresponding X-RARα fusion. Loss of PML increases the development of acute leukemia in mice expressing PML-RARα. These studies provide evidence that the reciprocal translocations contribute to APL not only by creation of the *X-RARA* fusion gene but also through reciprocal fusions and creating haploinsufficiency.

6. Cooperative events are associated with AML in humans and in mouse models of APL. This observation validates the use of mouse models for assessing hypotheses about events that may collaborate to transform myeloid cells.

7. Targeting of X-RARα protein expression, level of fusion protein expression, and the presence of normal endogenous proteins (including proteases) modulate leukemogenesis. These findings confirm the utility of mouse models for revealing novel aspects of leukemia pathogenesis.

4
Immune Modulation of APL

A few studies have indicated that the immune system can contribute to control and eradication of APL in mice. Leukemias that arose in *PML-RARA* transgenic animals can be readily transplanted into immunodeficient or into histocompatible immunocompetent recipient animals. One indication that the immune system can block APL cell growth was the observation that 100-fold fewer cells were required to transfer disease into SCID mice than were required for transfer into histocompatible immunocompetent mice (Pollock et al. 2005). A concordant study showed that liposomal ATRA (see below) was effective at inducing long-term remission in histocompatible immunocompetent mice engrafted with cathepsin G *PML-RARA/RARA-PML* leukemias: 88% of such mice treated with liposomal ATRA were alive at 1 year. In contrast, only 40% of SCID recipients experienced extended remissions (Westervelt et al. 2002). Thus, the adaptive immune system (T cells, B cells, or both) can cooperate with a targeted therapy to eradicate malignant disease.

Further work showed that DNA vaccines could be effective in treatment of mouse models of APL. DNA vaccination is a process in which plasmids that express potential antigens are injected intramuscularly (Wolff et al. 1990). The injected plasmids are taken up by some of the cells and begin to express the encoded antigens. This process can lead to both cell-mediated and humoral immune responses to these antigens. In one study, DNA vaccines encoded either full-length PML-RARα or a fusion of 33 amino acids surrounding the junction of PML and RARα to an immunogenic fragment of tetanus toxin (Padua et al. 2003). Vaccination with either of these plasmids extended survival of mice that had been injected with leukemic cells from MRP8 *PML-RARA* transgenic mice. Interestingly, the survival benefit was present not only in mice treated with the vaccine alone, but also in mice treated with a combination of DNA vaccination and ATRA. In another study of DNA vaccination, vaccines encoded PML-RARα, RARα-PML, PML, RARα, or a version of PML-RARα in which only the final 9 amino acids of the PML portion were fused to RARα (Pollock et al. 2005). Both the full-length PML-RARα and PML vaccines enhanced the leukemia-free survival of recipient mice, whereas the other constructs did not. Analyses of the immune responses of vaccinated animals indicated that, depending upon the model utilized and the vaccination strategy employed, PML or RARα portions of the human PML-RARα fusion protein can be immunogenic in mice (Padua et al. 2003; Pollock et al. 2005). The significance of these findings for human APL is uncertain: does the immunogenicity of APL in the mouse model simply reflect the immunogenicity of the human proteins, or does the immune response play an important role in control of human APL?

5
Therapies

The mouse APL models have been useful in confirming hypotheses regarding the mechanisms underlying the response of APL to ATRA, and in assessing the potential value of novel therapeutic approaches.

5.1
Mechanism of ATRA Response

Work in cell lines indicated that the ability of ATRA to cause differentiation of APL cells was dependent upon pharmacologic doses of ATRA binding to the PML-RARα fusion protein with resulting release of co-repressor complexes. This effect reverses repression at genes targeted by PML-RARα; resulting changes in gene expression underlie subsequent differentiation of APL cells. Studies in mice have provided additional evidence in support of these hypotheses. Expression of a version of PML-RARα deficient in ligand binding due to a point mutation [PML-RARαm4 (Shao et al. 1997)] resulted in leukemias that could not differentiate in response to ATRA (Kogan et al. 2000). A comparison of ATRA response in leukemic mice expressing PML-RARα, with response of leukemic mice expressing PLZF-RARα was also valuable (He et al. 1998). PML-RARα is able to dissociate from co-repressors at pharmacologic doses of ATRA, whereas PLZF-RARα maintains association with co-repressors through the PLZF portion of the fusion. Leukemic PML-RARα mice went into remission when treated with ATRA, whereas PLZF-RARα mice did not. This result paralleled the poor ATRA response of t(11;17) PLZF-RARα APLs in humans. Altogether, the differential response of *PML-RARA* and *PLZF-RARA* leukemias in mice and in humans is consistent with a critical role for co-repressor release in ATRA response. Interestingly, in both the *PML-RARAm4* and *PLZF-RARA* mouse models, the diseases were not entirely ATRA resistant, but the responsiveness was much diminished as compared to *PML-RARA* leukemias. Thus, although the ATRA regimen used for APL is ineffective for treating non-APL leukemias in humans, ATRA might have a broader role in treatment of AML when combined with other agents that foster differentiation.

There remains some controversy as to whether the differentiation of APL cells in response to ATRA is due solely to de-repression of genes abnormally repressed by PML-RARα, or whether there may also be a role for activation of important target genes by PML-RARα. Retinoic acid (RA) causes degradation of both PML-RARα and PLZF-RARα fusion proteins in mouse APL models (Rego et al. 2000). If de-repression alone were sufficient for full ATRA responsiveness, then the response of *PML-RARA* and *PLZF-RARA* leukemias might be expected to be more similar than what is actually observed. Hence, these data appear consistent with the hypothesis that both de-repression and activation play a role in the uniquely vigorous differentiation observed in APL cells that express PML-RARα.

5.2
Preclinical Studies

Ideas for improving treatment of APL have been tested in the mouse APL models; Table 2 summarizes information from many of these studies. An examination of Table 2 reveals differences in the models used, the timing of the initiation of treatment, the length of treatment, the agents examined, the route for agent administration, and the doses used. Despite these differences, in aggregate the studies provide information (1) pertinent to treating APL and (2) relevant to the design of preclinical trials in mice to develop therapies of other AMLs.

6
Arsenic Trioxide

APL shows a unique responsiveness to arsenic trioxide as well as to ATRA. One study examined the possibility that these two agents might be useful in combination by treating immunocompetent histocompatible mice engrafted with murine leukemias expressing *PML-RARA* under the MRP8 promoter. Mice were treated with ATRA in the form of subcutaneously implanted sustained-release pellets, intraperitoneally injected arsenic trioxide, or both (Lallemand-Breitenbach et al. 1999). Whereas ATRA and arsenic individually prolonged survival two- to threefold, the combination of these two agents resulted in extended disease-free survival in all mice that received the dual regimen. The combination of ATRA and arsenic was also tested in cathepsin G *PML-RARA* and *PLZF-RARA* models (Rego et al. 2000). In these experiments, treatment was given to either primary leukemic animals or to nude immunodeficient mice engrafted with leukemic cells. PLZF-RARα leukemias were resistant to ATRA, arsenic, or the combination. Although in this model combination therapy did not appear to eradicate the PML-RARα leukemias, the enhanced survival of animals treated with both agents was significantly longer than mice treated with either of the single agents. An additional study demonstrated that changes in the way ATRA is administered can have striking impacts on survival (Westervelt et al. 2002). By examining plasma ATRA levels in mice treated with implanted ATRA pellets, it was observed that the drug levels were five- to tenfold lower than those observed in the plasma of human patients receiving oral ATRA therapy. An alternative ATRA formulation was sought. In humans, liposomal ATRA had been associated with increased plasma concentrations, and in some patients, treatment with liposomal ATRA as a single agent caused prolonged hematologic and molecular remissions (Estey et al. 1999). This observation indicated that liposomal ATRA can be a more effective

Table 2 Therapeutic studies in mouse models of APL (selected)

Trial A (Lallemand-Breitenbach et al. 1999)

Treatments: ATRA (10-mg 21-day-release pellet, s.c.), arsenic trioxide (5 mg/kg per day×28 days, i.p.), or both

Treated 12 days after transplant into unirradiated histocompatible mice (10,000,000 cells, i.v.)

MRP8 *PML-RARA* leukemia

ATRA	Survival extended 42 days (median)
Arsenic	Survival extended 38 days (median)
Both	100% survival at 9 months

Trial B (Rego et al. 2000)

Treatments: ATRA (1.5 mg/kg per day×21 days, i.p.), arsenic trioxide [2.5 mg/kg per day (primary leukemias) or 5 mg/kg per day (transplants to nude mice)×21 days, i.p.], or both

Treatment of primary leukemic mice at leukemia onset

Cathepsin G *PML-RARA* leukemia (C57BL/6)

ATRA	Survival extended 35 days (mean)
Arsenic	Survival extended 28 days (mean)
Both	Survival extended 63 days (mean)

Cathepsin G *PLZF-RARA* leukemia (C57BL/6)

ATRA	Survival extended 15 days (mean)
Arsenic	Survival extended 6 days (mean)
Both	Survival extended 15 days (mean)

Treated 25 days after transplant into nude mice (50,000,000 cells, i.p.)

Cathepsin G *PML-RARA* leukemia (C57BL/6)

ATRA	Survival extended 23 days (mean)
Arsenic	Survival extended 15 days (mean)
Both	Survival extended 44 days (mean)

Cathepsin G *PLZF-RARA* leukemia (C57BL/6)

ATRA	Survival extended 4 days (mean)
Arsenic	Survival extended 3 days (mean)
Both	Survival extended 7 days (mean)

Of note: morphologic differentiation and remission of *PML-RARA* but not *PLZF-RARA* leukemias

Table 2 (continued)

Trial C (Westervelt et al. 2002)

Treatments: Liposomal ATRA (10 mg/kg per day×21 days, i.p.), arsenic trioxide (10 mg/kg per day× 21 days, i.p.) or both
Treated 21 days after transplant into unirradiated histocompatible mice (300,000 cells, i.p.)

Cathepsin G *PML-RARA/RARA-PML* leukemia

Lipo ATRA	88% survival at 1 year
Arsenic	14% survival at 1 year
Both	Equivalent to Lipo ATRA alone

Treated 21 days after transplant into SCID mice (300,000 cells, i.p.)

Cathepsin G *PML-RARA/RARA-PML* leukemia

Lipo ATRA	40% survival at 1 year
Arsenic	~7% survival at 1 year
Both	56% survival at 1 year

Trial D (He et al. 2001)

Treatments: ATRA (1.5 mg/kg per day×42 days, p.o.), ATRA (1.5 mg/kg per day×14 days, p.o.) followed by SAHA (a HDACI, 50 mg/kg per day× 28 days, i.p), or ATRA for 42 days with SAHA for 28 days (SAHA begun on day 15)
Treatment of primary leukemic mice at leukemia onset

Cathepsin G *PLZF-RARA/RARA-PLZF* leukemia

ATRA	(Control)
ATRA then SAHA	Survival extended 7 days beyond ATRA alone
ATRA plus SAHA	Survival extended 26 days beyond ATRA alone, remission

Trial E (Kosugi et al. 2001)

Treatments: ATRA (10 mg/kg per day×35 days, i.p.), FK228 (a HDACI, 0.5 mg/kg per day, 3×/week×35 days, i.p.), or both

Treatment of NB4 xenograft begun 1 day after transplant into NOD-SCID mice (10,000,000 cells, i.v.)

ATRA	No increase in survival
FK228	No increase in survival
Both	Survival extended 45 day

Trial F (Sohal et al. 2003)

Treatments: ATRA (10-mg 21-day-release pellet, s.c.), SU11657 (20 mg/kg per day×4 days, p.o.), or both
Treated at leukemia onset after transplant into sublethally irradiated histocompatible mice (1,000,000 cells, i.v.)

Table 2 (continued)

MRP8 *PML-RARA*/FLT3 v leukemia
    ATRA   Reduced leukemia in spleen, differentiation
    SU11657   Modest growth suppression
    Both   Remission

        ATRA response of various leukemias (Zhang et al. 1996; Kogan et al. 2000;
                    Kelly et al. 2002; Minucci et al. 2002)

MRP8 *PML-RARAm4* leukemia
Treatment: ATRA (5-mg 21-day-release pellet, s.c.)
Treated at leukemia onset after transplant into unirradiated histocompatible mice (5,000,000 cells, i.v.)
    ATRA   Survival extended >12 days, but without differentiation

Cathepsin G *PML-RARA*/FLT3 v leukemia
Treatment: ATRA (10-mg 60-day-release pellet, s.c.)
Treated at leukemia onset after transplant into sublethally irradiated histocompatible mice (1,000,000 cells, i.p.)
    ATRA   Decreased leukemia in spleen,
                              improved peripheral WBC differential

Retroviral *PML-RARA* leukemia
Treatment: ATRA (5-mg 21-day-release pellet, s.c.)
Treatment at leukemia onset after transplant into unirradiated histocompatible mice (10,000,000 cells, i.v.)
    ATRA   Survival extended 22 days

Treatment of NB4 xenograft begun 1 day after transplant into SCID mice (1,000,000 cells, i.p.)
Treatment: ATRA (10 mg/kg per day, 3×/week×4 weeks, i.p.)
    ATRA   Survival extended 8 days

        Other (Guillemin et al. 2002; Zhang et al. 1996; Insinga et al. 2005)
Treatments: 8-Cl-cAMP (240 µg/day×7 days, s.c.), both 8-Cl-cAMP and ATRA (10-mg 21-day-release pellet, s.c.), or aminophylline (2.5 mg/day×3 days, i.p.)
Treated at leukemia onset after transplant into unirradiated histocompatible mice (10,000,000 cells, i.v.)

MRP8 *PML-RARAm4* leukemia
    8-Cl-cAMP   Reduced leukemia in spleen, partial differentiation
    8-Cl-cAMP+ATRA Markedly reduced leukemia in spleen, differentiation

MRP8 *PML-RARA* leukemia
    Aminophylline   Reduced leukemia in spleen, partial differentiation

Table 2 (continued)

Treatment of NB4 xenograft begun 1 day after transplant into SCID mice (1,000,000 cells, i.p.)

Treatment: Doxorubicin (1 mg/kg per day, 3×/week×3 weeks)

    Doxorubicin   Survival extended 23 days

Retroviral *PML-RARA* leukemia

Treatment: valproic acid (400 mg/kg b.i.d.×21 days, i.p.)

Treatment at leukemia onset after transplant into unirradiated histocompatible mice (10,000,000 cells, i.v.)

    Valproic acid   Survival extended 25 days

8-Cl-cAMP, 8-chloro-adenosine 3′-5′ cyclic monophosphate; HDACI, histone deacetylase inhibitor; SAHA, suberoylanilide hydroxamic acid

---

treatment for APL than nonliposomal ATRA. (At present the liposomal formulation has seen only limited clinical application.) As noted in Sect. 4, when immunocompetent histocompatible mice engrafted with cathepsin G *PML-RARA/RARA-PML* leukemic cells were treated with liposomal ATRA, 88% were leukemia free at 1 year. In this setting, arsenic did not further enhance survival. However, the results in immunodeficient leukemic mice treated with liposomal ATRA plus arsenic were consistent with the other studies showing a benefit of ATRA+arsenic: there was a trend toward improved survival in dual-treated animals (Westervelt et al. 2002). In part based on the promising preclinical studies in mice, ATRA+arsenic in combination with chemotherapy was assessed in a human APL trial (Shen et al. 2004). This therapeutic approach to APL appeared to yield the best outcome observed to date for any human AML: Of the 21 patients who participated, all 20 who achieved morphologically complete remission experienced relapse-free survival with a follow up of 8–30 months (median 20 months).

7
Histone Deacetylase Inhibitors

Abnormal repression of transcription through enhanced recruitment and activity of histone deacetylases appears important for the pathogenesis of APL. Therefore, the efficacy of histone deacetylase inhibitors has been examined in an ATRA-resistant APL model (He et al. 2001). Primary cathepsin G *PLZF-RARA/RARA-PLZF* leukemic animals were treated with ATRA, the histone deacetylase inhibitor suberoylanilide hydroxamic acid (SAHA), or both. Although not curative in most animals, the combination therapy could induce remission and prolong survival to a greater extent than either agent alone. Another study of histone deacetylase inhibitors utilized the xenograft APL model (Kosugi et al. 2001). In this model, oral ATRA administration at the dose used had a moderate effect on subcutaneous growth of NB4 cells, and although NB4 cells are sensitive to ATRA, ATRA did not prolong survival of mice that received NB4 cells intravenously. The addition of the histone deacetylase inhibitor FK228 (also known as depsipeptide) to ATRA strongly suppressed subcutaneous growth. Further, when NB4 cells were injected intravenously, 3 of 7 dual-treated mice experienced long-term survival, in contrast to untreated or single-agent-treated animals. Thus, the mouse APL models support the idea that combining ATRA with a histone deacetylase inhibitor may be useful in treatment of some human leukemia patients.

8
Additional Investigational Therapies

Other agents and combinations have been tested in mouse APL models. Abnormal tyrosine kinases are an attractive target for therapy of leukemias, as evidenced by the effect of imatinib on human chronic myelogenous leukemia. SU11657 is a tyrosine kinase inhibitor that inhibits a class of receptor tyrosine kinases including FLT3, PDGFR, KIT, VEGFR1, and VEGFR2. The effect of SU11657 on leukemias that arose in cells expressing MRP8 *PML-RARA* plus an activated FLT3 was assessed (Sohal et al. 2003). Although SU11657 had limited effect as a single agent, the combination of SU11657 plus ATRA rapidly restored normal hematopoiesis in the bone marrow and resulted in a marked reduction in splenic involvement by the leukemic cells. A number of FLT3 inhibitors are under study in human clinical trials (Krause and Van Etten 2005). Cyclic adenosine monophosphate (cAMP) has growth suppressive and differentiative effects on myeloid leukemia cells. A RA-resistant leukemia that arose in an MRP8 *PML-RARAm4* transgenic mouse was examined in engrafted histocompatible recipients (Guillemin et al. 2002). Mice were treated with a low toxicity cAMP analog, [8-chloro-adenosine $3'$-$5'$ cyclic monophosphate (8-Cl-cAMP)], alone or in combination with ATRA or arsenic. Treatment with 8-Cl-cAMP had a moderate effect, whereas the combination of 8-Cl-cAMP with ATRA induced differentiation of the ATRA-resistant leukemic cells. Theophylline, an inhibitor of phosphodiesterase able to boost cAMP levels, has subsequently been used as an adjunct to therapy in some AML patients. Cotylenin A is a plant growth regulator that is able to induce differentiation of human myeloid leukemia cell lines and primary AML blasts. The xenograft mouse model of APL was used to show that cotylenin A can prolong survival in mice engrafted with the RA-sensitive NB4 cell line, or a RA-resistant version of NB4 (Honma et al. 2003). The possible utility of cotylenin A (or a derivative) as an antileukemic agent in humans is not yet clear. Another observation of uncertain clinical benefit is that hypoxia can facilitate differentiation of myeloid leukemic cells in vitro. A mouse APL model was recently used to show that the differentiative effects of hypoxia can potentially be used to extend survival in vivo (Liu et al. 2006).

9
Therapy, Conclusions

1. Animal models of leukemia can be used to assess the potential role of the immune system in controlling malignant cell growth, and to examine strategies to boost the immune response to AML. The use of mouse models in which the leukemic oncoproteins are themselves expressed from murine genes may enhance the relevance of such studies to future human clinical investigation.

2. APL models have been used in preclinical studies to assess the potential value of new AML therapies.

3. Many agents that enter human clinical trials are initially assessed as single agent therapies in phase I trials. In multiple preclinical trials in mouse APL models, agents that appear essentially ineffective as single agents can have very significant therapeutic effects when used in combination.

4. Preclinical studies in mice represent a valuable strategy for examining combination therapies that should be further investigated in human clinical trials. Such studies can be performed as a prelude to human trials, or mouse studies may be performed as adjuncts to matched human clinical trials. Adjunctive mouse trials can provide early endpoints and important additional data.

10
Perspectives

Animal models of APL are one part of the scientific landscape that contributes to our understanding of AML in general and APL in particular. These models are vital for examining how genetic events individually and in combination alter cellular behavior in the physiologic setting in which leukemia arises. Only in this in vivo context can hypotheses about pathogenesis be definitively proved or refuted. Furthermore, animal models of APL are equally important for assessing ideas regarding the value of novel therapies.

As we learn more about APL, added questions are raised. Among the areas that animal models will be used for in the coming years are:

1. Developing a better understanding of the cells from which relapses arise in APL and other AMLs. (These cells are sometimes referred to as leukemic stem cells.)

2. Identifying the critical transcriptional targets repressed by X-RARα proteins.

3. Elucidating effects on PML and its interaction partners that facilitate leukemic transformation.

4. Delineating how events cooperate at a molecular level to block differentiation and deregulate proliferation and survival.

5. Extending differentiation therapy to other leukemias.

Acknowledgements Thanks to Dr. Galit Rosen for Fig. 1 as well as Drs. Michael Bishop, Hugues de Thé, Jeffrey Lawrence, Frank McCormick, and Kevin Shannon for their continuing interest and support. Scott Kogan is a Scholar of the Leukemia and Lymphoma Society.

References

Bensi L, Longo R, Vecchi A, Messora C, Garagnani L, Bernardi S, Tamassia MG, Sacchi S (1995) Bcl-2 oncoprotein expression in acute myeloid leukemia. Haematologica 80:98–102

Brown D, Kogan S, Lagasse E, Weissman I, Alcalay M, Pelicci PG, Atwater S, Bishop JM (1997) a PMLRAR alpha transgene initiates murine acute promyelocytic leukemia. Proc Natl Acad Sci U S A 94:2551–2556

Cheng GX, Zhu XH, Men XQ, Wang L, Huang QH, Jin XL, Xiong SM, Zhu J, Guo WM, Chen JQ, Xu SF, So E, Chan LC, Waxman S, Zelent A, Chen GQ, Dong S, Liu JX, Chen SJ (1999) Distinct leukemia phenotypes in transgenic mice and different corepressor interactions generated by promyelocytic leukemia variant fusion genes PLZF-RARalpha and NPM-RARalpha. Proc Natl Acad Sci U S A 96:6318–6323

Degos L, Dombret H, Chomienne C, Daniel MT, Miclea JM, Chastang C, Castaigne S, Fenaux P (1995) All-trans-retinoic acid as a differentiating agent in the treatment of acute promyelocytic leukemia. Blood 85:2643–2653

DiGiuseppe JA, LeBeau P, Augenbraun J, Borowitz MJ (1996) Multiparameter flow-cytometric analysis of bcl-2 and Fas expression in normal and neoplastic hematopoiesis. Am J Clin Pathol 106:345–351

Estey EH, Giles FJ, Kantarjian H, O'Brien S, Cortes J, Freireich EJ, Lopez-Berestein G, Keating M (1999) Molecular remissions induced by liposomal-encapsulated all-trans retinoic acid in newly diagnosed acute promyelocytic leukemia. Blood 94:2230–2235

Ferrucci PF, Grignani F, Pearson M, Fagioli M, Nicoletti I, Pelicci PG (1997) Cell death induction by the acute promyelocytic leukemia-specific PML/RARalpha fusion protein. Proc Natl Acad Sci USA 94:10901–10906

Grisolano JL, Wesselschmidt RL, Pelicci PG, Ley TJ (1997) Altered myeloid development and acute leukemia in transgenic mice expressing PML-RAR alpha under control of cathepsin G regulatory sequences. Blood 89:376–387

Guillemin MC, Raffoux E, Vitoux D, Kogan S, Soilihi H, Lallemand-Breitenbach V, Zhu J, Janin A, Daniel MT, Gourmel B, Degos L, Dombret H, Lanotte M, De The H (2002) In vivo activation of cAMP signaling induces growth arrest and differentiation in acute promyelocytic leukemia. J Exp Med 196:1373–1380

He LZ, Tribioli C, Rivi R, Peruzzi D, Pelicci PG, Soares V, Cattoretti G, Pandolfi PP (1997) Acute leukemia with promyelocytic features in PML/RARalpha transgenic mice. Proc Natl Acad Sci USA 94:5302–5307

He LZ, Guidez F, Tribioli C, Peruzzi D, Ruthardt M, Zelent A, Pandolfi PP (1998) Distinct interactions of PML-RARalpha and PLZF-RARalpha with co-repressors determine differential responses to RA in APL. Nat Genet 18:126–135

He LZ, Bhaumik M, Tribioli C, Rego EM, Ivins S, Zelent A, Pandolfi PP (2000) Two critical hits for promyelocytic leukemia. Mol Cell 6:1131–1141

He LZ, Tolentino T, Grayson P, Zhong S, Warrell RP Jr, Rifkind RA, Marks PA, Richon VM, Pandolfi PP (2001) Histone deacetylase inhibitors induce remission in transgenic models of therapy-resistant acute promyelocytic leukemia. J Clin Invest 108:1321–1330

Honma Y, Ishii Y, Sassa T, Asahi K (2003) Treatment of human promyelocytic leukemia in the SCID mouse model with cotylenin A, an inducer of myelomonocytic differentiation of leukemia cells. Leuk Res 27:1019–1025

Insinga A, Monestiroli S, Ronzoni S, Gelmetti V, Marchesi F, Viale A, Altucci L, Nervi C, Minucci S, Pelicci PG (2005) Inhibitors of histone deacetylases induce tumor-selective apoptosis through activation of the death receptor pathway. Nat Med 11:71–76

Jansen JH, Mahfoudi A, Rambaud S, Lavau C, Wahli W, Dejean A (1995) Multimeric complexes of the PML-retinoic acid receptor alpha fusion protein in acute promyelocytic leukemia cells and interference with retinoid and peroxisome-proliferator signaling pathways. Proc Natl Acad Sci U S A 92:7401–7405

Kamashev D, Vitoux D, De The H (2004) PML-RARA-RXR oligomers mediate retinoid and rexinoid/cAMP cross-talk in acute promyelocytic leukemia cell differentiation. J Exp Med 199:1163–1174

Kelly LM, Kutok JL, Williams IR, Boulton CL, Amaral SM, Curley DP, Ley TJ, Gilliland DG (2002) PML/RARalpha and FLT3-ITD induce an APL-like disease in a mouse model. Proc Natl Acad Sci U S A 99:8283–8288

Kiyoi H, Naoe T, Yokota S, Nakao M, Minami S, Kuriyama K, Takeshita A, Saito K, Hasegawa S, Shimodaira S, Tamura J, Shimazaki C, Matsue K, Kobayashi H, Arima N, Suzuki R, Morishita H, Saito H, Ueda R, Ohno R (1997) Internal tandem duplication of FLT3 associated with leukocytosis in acute promyelocytic leukemia. Leukemia 11:1447–1452

Kogan SC, Hong SH, Shultz DB, Privalsky ML, Bishop JM (2000) Leukemia initiated by PMLRARalpha: the PML domain plays a critical role while retinoic acid-mediated transactivation is dispensable. Blood 95:1541–1550

Kogan SC, Brown DE, Shultz DB, Truong BTH, Lallemand-Breitenbach V, Guillemin MC, Lagasse E, Weissman IL, Bishop JM (2001) BCL-2 cooperates with promyelocytic leukemia retinoic acid receptor alpha chimeric protein (PMLRAR alpha) to block neutrophil differentiation and initiate acute leukemia. J Exp Med 193:531–543

Kosugi H, Ito M, Yamamoto Y, Towatari M, Ueda R, Saito H, Naoe T (2001) In vivo effects of a histone deacetylase inhibitor, FK228, on human acute promyelocytic leukemia in NOD / Shi-scid/scid mice. Jpn J Cancer Res 92:529–536

Kottaridis PD, Gale RE, Frew ME, Harrison G, Langabeer SE, Belton AA, Walker H, Wheatley K, Bowen DT, Burnett AK, Goldstone AH, Linch DC (2001) The presence of a FLT3 internal tandem duplication in patients with acute myeloid leukemia (AML) adds important prognostic information to cytogenetic risk group and response to the first cycle of chemotherapy: analysis of 854 patients from the United Kingdom Medical Research Council AML 10 and 12 trials. Blood 98:1752–1759

Krause DS, Van Etten RA (2005) Tyrosine kinases as targets for cancer therapy. N Engl J Med 353:172–187

Lallemand-Breitenbach V, Guillemin MC, Janin A, Daniel MT, Degos L, Kogan SC, Bishop JM, de The H (1999) Retinoic acid and arsenic synergize to eradicate leukemic cells in a mouse model of acute promyelocytic leukemia. J Exp Med 189:1043–1052

Lallemand-Breitenbach V, Zhu J, Kogan S, Chen Z, de The H (2005) Opinion: how patients have benefited from mouse models of acute promyelocytic leukaemia. Nat Rev Cancer 5:821–827

Lane AA, Ley TJ (2003) Neutrophil elastase cleaves PML-RARalpha and is important for the development of acute promyelocytic leukemia in mice. Cell 115:305–318

Le Beau MM, Bitts S, Davis EM, Kogan SC (2002) Recurring chromosomal abnormalities in leukemia in PML-RARA transgenic mice parallel human acute promyelocytic leukemia. Blood 99:2985–2991

Le Beau MM, Davis EM, Patel B, Phan VT, Sohal J, Kogan SC (2003) Recurring chromosomal abnormalities in leukemia in PML-RARA transgenic mice identify cooperating events and genetic pathways to acute promyelocytic leukemia. Blood 102:1072–1074

Lin RJ, Evans RM (2000) Acquisition of oncogenic potential by RAR chimeras in acute promyelocytic leukemia through formation of homodimers. Mol Cell 5:821–830

Liu W, Guo M, Xu YB, Dao L, Zhou ZN, Wu YL, Chen Z, Kogan SC, Chen GQ (2006) Induction of tumor arrest and differentiation with prolonged survival by intermittent hypoxia in a mouse model of acute myeloid leukemia. Blood 107:698–707

Minucci S, Monestiroli S, Giavara S, Ronzoni S, Marchesi F, Insinga A, Diverio D, Gasparini P, Capillo M, Colombo E, Matteucci C, Contegno F, Lo-Coco F, Scanziani E, Gobbi A, Pelicci PG (2002) PML-RAR induces promyelocytic leukemias with high efficiency following retroviral gene transfer into purified murine hematopoietic progenitors. Blood 100:2989–2995

Molica S, Mannella A, Dattilo A, Levato D, Iuliano F, Peta A, Consarino C, Magro S (1996) Differential expression of BCL-2 oncoprotein and Fas antigen on normal peripheral blood and leukemic bone marrow cells. A flow cytometric analysis. Haematologica 81:302–309

Padua RA, Larghero J, Robin M, le Pogam C, Schlageter MH, Muszlak S, Fric J, West R, Rousselot P, Phan TH, Mudde L, Teisserenc H, Carpentier AF, Kogan S, Degos L, Pla M, Bishop JM, Stevenson F, Charron D, Chomienne C (2003) PML-RARA-targeted DNA vaccine induces protective immunity in a mouse model of leukemia. Nat Med 9:1413–1417

Pandolfi PP (2001) In vivo analysis of the molecular genetics of acute promyelocytic leukemia. Oncogene 20:5726–5735

Pollock JL, Westervelt P, Kurichety AK, Pelicci PG, Grisolano JL, Ley TJ (1999) A bcr-3 isoform of RARalpha-PML potentiates the development of PML-RARalpha-driven acute promyelocytic leukemia. Proc Natl Acad Sci USA 96:15103–15108

Pollock JL, Westervelt P, Walter MJ, Lane AA, Ley TJ (2001) Mouse models of acute promyelocytic leukemia. Curr Opin Hematol 8:206–211

Pollock JL, Lane AA, Schrimpf K, Ley TJ (2005) Murine acute promyelocytic leukemia cells can be recognized and cleared in vivo by adaptive immune mechanisms. Haematologica 90:1042–1049

Porwit-MacDonald A, Ivory K, Wilkinson S, Wheatley K, Wong L, Janossy G (1995) Bcl-2 protein expression in normal human bone marrow precursors and in acute myelogenous leukemia. Leukemia 9:1191–1198

Rego EM, He LZ, Warrell RP Jr, Wang ZG, Pandolfi PP (2000) Retinoic acid (RA) and As2O3 treatment in transgenic models of acute promyelocytic leukemia (APL) unravel the distinct nature of the leukemogenic process induced by the PML-RARalpha and PLZF-RARalpha oncoproteins. Proc Natl Acad Sci U S A 97:10173–10178

Rego EM, Wang ZG, Peruzzi D, He LZ, Cordon-Cardo C, Pandolfi PP (2001) Role of promyelocytic leukemia (PML) protein in tumor suppression. J Exp Med 193:521–529

Schnittger S, Schoch C, Dugas M, Kern W, Staib P, Wuchter C, Loffler H, Sauerland CM, Serve H, Buchner T, Haferlach T, Hiddemann W (2002) Analysis of FLT3 length mutations in 1003 patients with acute myeloid leukemia: correlation to cytogenetics, FAB subtype, and prognosis in the AMLCG study and usefulness as a marker for the detection of minimal residual disease. Blood 100:59–66

Shao W, Benedetti L, Lamph WW, Nervi C, Miller WH Jr (1997) A retinoid-resistant acute promyelocytic leukemia subclone expresses a dominant negative PML-RAR alpha mutation. Blood 89:4282–4289

Shen ZX, Shi ZZ, Fang J, Gu BW, Li JM, Zhu YM, Shi JY, Zheng PZ, Yan H, Liu YF, Chen Y, Shen Y, Wu W, Tang W, Waxman S, De The H, Wang ZY, Chen SJ, Chen Z (2004) All-trans retinoic acid/As2O3 combination yields a high quality remission and survival in newly diagnosed acute promyelocytic leukemia. Proc Natl Acad Sci U S A 101:5328–5335

Sohal J, Phan VT, Chan PV, Davis EM, Patel B, Kelly LM, Abrams TJ, O'Farrell AM, Gilliland DG, Le Beau MM, Kogan SC (2003) A model of APL with FLT3 mutation is responsive to retinoic acid and a receptor tyrosine kinase inhibitor, SU11657. Blood 101:3188–3197

Sukhai MA, Wu X, Xuan Y, Zhang T, Reis PP, Dube K, Rego EM, Bhaumik M, Bailey DJ, Wells RA, Kamel-Reid S, Pandolfi PP (2004) Myeloid leukemia with promyelocytic features in transgenic mice expressing hCG-NuMA-RARalpha. Oncogene 23:665–678

Walter MJ, Park JS, Lau SK, Li X, Lane AA, Nagarajan R, Shannon WD, Ley TJ (2004) Expression profiling of murine acute promyelocytic leukemia cells reveals multiple model-dependent progression signatures. Mol Cell Biol 24:10882–10893

Walter MJ, Park JS, Ries RE, Lau SK, McLellan M, Jaeger S, Wilson RK, Mardis ER, Ley TJ (2005) Reduced PU.1 expression causes myeloid progenitor expansion and increased leukemia penetrance in mice expressing PML-RARalpha. Proc Natl Acad Sci U S A 102:12513–12518

Westervelt P, Pollock JL, Oldfather KM, Walter MJ, Ma MK, Williams A, DiPersio JF, Ley TJ (2002) Adaptive immunity cooperates with liposomal all-trans-retinoic acid (ATRA) to facilitate long-term molecular remissions in mice with acute promyelocytic leukemia. Proc Natl Acad Sci U S A 99:9468–9473

Westervelt P, Lane AA, Pollock JL, Oldfather K, Holt MS, Zimonjic DB, Popescu NC, DiPersio JF, Ley TJ (2003) High-penetrance mouse model of acute promyelocytic leukemia with very low levels of PML-RARalpha expression. Blood 102:1857–1865

Wolff JA, Malone RW, Williams P, Chong W, Acsadi G, Jani A, Felgner PL (1990) Direct gene transfer into mouse muscle in vivo. Science 247:1465–1468

Wuchter C, Karawajew L, Ruppert V, Büchner T, Schoch C, Haferlach T, Ratei R, Dörken B, Ludwig WD (1999) Clinical significance of CD95, Bcl-2 and Bax expression and CD95 function in adult de novo acute myeloid leukemia in context of P-glycoprotein function, maturation stage, and cytogenetics. Leukemia 13:1943–1953

Yamamoto Y, Kiyoi H, Nakano Y, Suzuki R, Kodera Y, Miyawaki S, Asou N, Kuriyama K, Yagasaki F, Shimazaki C, Akiyama H, Saito K, Nishimura M, Motoji T, Shinagawa K, Takeshita A, Saito H, Ueda R, Ohno R, Naoe T (2001) Activating mutation of D835 within the activation loop of FLT3 in human hematologic malignancies. Blood 97:2434–2439

Yokota S, Kiyoi H, Nakao M, Iwai T, Misawa S, Okuda T, Sonoda Y, Abe T, Kahsima K, Matsuo Y, Naoe T (1997) Internal tandem duplication of the FLT3 gene is preferentially seen in acute myeloid leukemia and myelodysplastic syndrome among various hematological malignancies. A study on a large series of patients and cell lines. Leukemia 11:1605–1609

Zhang SY, Zhu J, Chen GQ, Du XX, Lu LJ, Zhang Z, Zhong HJ, Chen HR, Wang ZY, Berger R, Lanotte M, Waxman S, Chen Z, Chen SJ (1996) Establishment of a human acute promyelocytic leukemia-ascites model in SCID mice. Blood 87:3404–3409

Zhu J, Zhou J, Peres L, Riaucoux F, Honore N, Kogan S, de The H (2005) A sumoylation site in PML/RARA is essential for leukemic transformation. Cancer Cell 7:143–153

Zimonjic DB, Pollock JL, Westervelt P, Popescu NC, Ley TJ (2000) Acquired, nonrandom chromosomal abnormalities associated with the development of acute promyelocytic leukemia in transgenic mice. Proc Natl Acad Sci USA 97:13306–13311

The PLZF Gene of t(11;17)-Associated APL

M. J. McConnell · J. D. Licht (✉)

Division of Hematology/Oncology, Northwestern University,
Feinberg School of Medicine, 303 E Superior St, Chicago, IL 60611, USA
j-licht@northwestern.edu

Abstract The PLZF gene is one of five partners fused to the retinoic acid receptor α in acute promyelocytic leukemia. PLZF encodes a DNA-binding transcriptional repressor and the PLZF-RARα fusion protein like other RARα fusions can inhibit the genetic program mediated by the wild tpe retinoic acid receptor. However an increasing body of literature indicates an important role for the PLZF gene in growth control and development. This information suggests that loss of PLZF function might also contribute to leukemogenesis.

Most cases of acute promyelocytic leukemia (APL) are caused by a chromosomal translocation that fuses the retinoic acid receptor α (*RARα*) gene on chromosome 11 with the *PML* gene on chromosome 15. An unusual case was identified with a t(11;17)(q23;q21) translocation, which resulted in fusion of RARα with a novel gene. This gene was cloned and named the *promyelocytic leukemia zinc finger* (*PLZF*) gene [7, 8], also known as *ZNF145* and more recently as *ZBTB16*. Since then, 17 cases of APL with a fusion between the *PLZF* and *RARα* genes have been described [11, 21, 22, 38, 45] representing less than 1% of cases of APL. Initial data suggested that unlike typical APL with the PML-RARα rearrangement, these patients had a poor prognosis, were resistant to treatment with all-*trans* retinoic acid (ATRA) and generally did not respond to chemotherapy [45]. However, subsequent data suggested that t(11;17)(q23;q21) disease can be chemotherapy-sensitive.

The promyelocytic blasts from t[11;17] APL patients show a regular nucleus and abundant cytoplasm with either coarse granules or many fine granules. A few cases also had Auer rods. Like the usual cases of APL, the promyelocytes were $CD34^-/CD13^+/CD33^+$ but were sometimes positive for the CD56 natural killer (NK) cell antigen. It was proposed that due to their characteristic regular nuclei and unusual immunophenotype, cases of APL with t(11;17)(q23;q21) should be given the subclassification M3r [69].

The *PLZF* gene is located on chromosome 11q23, about 1 Mb centromeric to the *MLL* (*mixed lineage leukemia*) gene. The *PLZF* locus was completely sequenced and the gene found to be contained in six exons spread over 201 kb of DNA. Several potential splice sites exist, with alternative transcripts detected in multiple tissues. The full-length transcript is 8 kb long, and has a 6-kb 5'-untranslated region of unknown function [81]. The most common alternative isoform, AS-I, is found in a large number of tissues, and is spliced in the 5'-untranslated region (UTR), which does not alter the PLZF coding sequence. The less common splice variants AS-II, AS-III, and AS-IV have a restricted pattern of tissue-specific expression. These variants maintain the open reading frame, but encode an N-terminally truncated PLZF protein [81].

The PLZF protein is a DNA-binding zinc finger transcription factor of 673 amino acids that generally acts as a transcriptional repressor [8]. The N-terminal 118 amino acids constitute the PLZF BTB (*broad-complex, tramtrack, bric a brac*) domain, also known as a POZ (*pox virus and zinc finger*) domain, which is essential for transcriptional repression [56]. Downstream of the BTB domain there is a second region also necessary for transcriptional repression, RD2, [44, 58], and at the C-terminus there are nine Kruppel-like C_2H_2 zinc fingers that contain the DNA-binding motif. DNA-binding activity is specified by the last three zinc fingers of PLZF, which direct binding to the PLZF consensus sequence $GTAC^T/_AGTAC$ [1].

The t(11;17)(q23;q21) translocation fuses the *PLZF* gene with the *RAR*α gene. In this rearrangement, the breakpoint in the *PLZF* locus falls between the regions coding for zinc fingers two and three, except in one case where the breakpoint was between zinc fingers three and four. In almost all cases, the chromosomal rearrangement is reciprocal, leading to expression of two fusion gene products, PLZF-RARα and RARα-PLZF. PLZF-RARα is made up of the transcriptional effector domains of PLZF linked to the DNA-binding and ligand-binding domains of RARα. This acts as a dominant-negative RARα, repressing the expression of genes normally activated by RARα. There is an important difference between PML-RARα, present in more than 98% of cases of APL, and PLZF-RARα. While PML-RARα will release co-repressors in response to ATRA and switch, at least transiently, to a transcriptional activator before undergoing ATRA-mediated degradation, PLZF-RARα, due to the presence of the inherent repression domains of PLZF, remains bound to co-repressors even in the presence of ATRA [20, 24, 29, 31, 47]. This aberrant transcriptional repression is associated with resistance of this form of APL to conventional ATRA treatment. The reciprocal fusion RARα-PLZF links the ligand-independent transcriptional activation domain of RARα to the last seven of the nine zinc fingers of PLZF, including the DNA-binding region. This fusion protein binds the same DNA sequences as PLZF, but does not have the PLZF repression domains. RARα-PLZF is an oncogenic version of PLZF, likely activating transcription of genes that are normally repressed by PLZF, due to the replacement of the PLZF repression domains with the activation domains of RARα.

Regulation and control of PLZF expression is incompletely understood. The gene is expressed in distinct temporal and spatial patterns in multiple tissues, both during embryogenesis and in the adult, but the factors that control these patterns have not been identified. The region immediately upstream of the transcription start site contains a TATA box and TFIID site, and several putative transcription factor binding sites, including AP-1 sites, multiple ETS-binding sites and an Evi-1 binding site [72, 81]. A 1.2-kb stretch of sequence 5′ to the transcription start site conferred relative specificity in hematopoietic cells, directing reporter activity only in cells that expressed PLZF, suggesting that this region contains at least the myeloid-specific elements. One critical element may be the EVI-1 site, since mutation of this site resulted in loss of PLZF promoter activity even in myeloid lines, but an exact role of EVI-1 in regulating PLZF expression has not been established [72]. Several recent reports indicate that PLZF transcripts can be upregulated by steroid hormone nuclear receptors, particularly in nonhematopoietic systems. Glucocorticoids, progesterone, and androgen have all been reported to rapidly upregulate PLZF expression in a variety of cell lines [17, 35, 77]. This effect may not be direct, since the glucocorticoid and progesterone receptors did not increase transcription from the PLZF promoter in a reporter assay [17].

In the hematopoietic system, PLZF is expressed in the $CD34^+$ human progenitor cell in approximately 50 small nuclear speckles, reminiscent of the PML nuclear bodies [46]. When $CD34^+$ cells were placed into culture and allowed to differentiate along myeloid and erythroid lineages, PLZF levels declined with terminal differentiation [12]. This is consistent with the expression of PLZF in myeloid cell lines—expression declines during differentiation of NB4 cells, and level of expression can be correlated to the stage of differentiation in erythroleukemic, promyelocytic and monocytic cell lines [8, 46, 67]. Together this suggests that PLZF may be important for the maintenance or survival of hematopoietic stem cells, early progenitors, or both. Interestingly, expression has also been observed in peripheral blood mononuclear cells [46]. PLZF seems to be re-expressed in monocytes, where it plays a role in regulating monocytic differentiation through direct interaction with the vitamin D3 receptor [78]. Additionally, PLZF expression increases throughout megakaryocytic development. Overexpression of PLZF in an erythro-megakaryocytic cell line induced megakaryocyte markers and expression of the thrombopoietin receptor, suggesting a role for PLZF in megakaryocyte development [43]. This appeared to be mediated through interaction between PLZF and the GATA-1 transcription factor.

PLZF-null mice do not exhibit an obvious hematopoietic phenotype, nor do they develop leukemia or other tumors. However, this does not rule out a role for PLZF in hematopoiesis. A second PLZF-like gene exists, which is expressed in a similar pattern during differentiation of hematopoietic progenitor cells. This gene, which has been variously called *PLZF2*, *FAZF* (for *Fanconi anemia zinc finger*) [30], *repressor of GATA* (*ROG*) [49, 59], and *testis-specific zinc finger protein* (*TZFP*) [49], is extremely close (1.4 kb) to the *MLL-2* gene at 19q13.1, suggesting that it arose by duplication of the *PLZF-MLL* locus at 11q23. The FAZF protein also has a BTB domain, and three Kruppel-like C_2H_2 zinc fingers highly homologous to the final three DNA-binding zinc fingers of PLZF. It can heterodimerize with PLZF, and can bind the same DNA sequences as PLZF in vitro [30]. FAZF is found in a pattern of nuclear foci similar to the PLZF speckles, and forced expression in a U937 cell had the same suppression of growth and induction of apoptosis as PLZF [12]. The phenotype of the *FAZF* knockout mouse demonstrates that while FAZF has a distinct role in other tissues, its expression and function overlap with PLZF in the $CD34^+$ progenitor cell [65]. This all suggests that FAZF might compensate for the lack of PLZF during hematopoietic development.

PLZF is expressed in a number of tissues outside the hematopoietic system. During development of the central nervous system PLZF is expressed in a segmental pattern in hindbrain [9], indicating possible regulation of transcription of the *Hoxb2* gene. A PLZF-binding site was found in the *Hoxb2* 5′ flanking region and PLZF could repress the *Hoxb2* promoter in cotransfection assays [36, 37]. PLZF expression is also notable in the limb buds where *Hox* genes have an essential role. Mice lacking PLZF display limb defects including the presence of extra as well as transformed digits [3]. Decreased expression of the *bone morphogenic protein 7* (*Bmp7*) gene, which controls cell proliferation and programmed cell death in the developing limb, was also noted. Homeotic changes were noted in the spine and were associated with a more posterior expression boundary for the *Hoxc6* and *Hoxc8* genes. The limb buds of *PLZF*-null mice also showed increased proliferation and decreased apoptosis consistent with data demonstrating PLZF to be a growth suppressor. This phenotype was associated with a more anterior pattern of expression of *Hoxd* genes in the developing hind limb, suggesting that PLZF might globally inhibit the expression of this class of Hox genes. Direct regulation of the *Hoxd* gene cluster by PLZF was demonstrated, reinforcing the role of PLZF in regulation of homeobox genes [4]. This may also reflect a similar role for PLZF in hematopoiesis, since *Hoxb2* among others, is also expressed in $CD34^+$ progenitor cells. These data also indicate, however, that as suspected and found for many other leukemia-associated proteins [51], such as MLL [80], *Hox* genes may be major targets of PLZF and its fusion protein with RARα.

PLZF is expressed in both prostate and uterine tissues, where as discussed above, expression was upregulated in response to steroid hormones. Glucocorticoid and progesterone treatment of endometrial stromal and myometrial cells led to increased PLZF levels [17]. PLZF may in part mediate growth suppression by these agents. PLZF was detected in the uterus in the mid and late secretory phase of the menstrual cycle but not in the proliferative phase, consistent with the general negative effect of PLZF on cell growth. Also consistent with an antiproliferative effect, PLZF overexpression in a prostate cancer cell line inhibited cell proliferation. In addition, PLZF was identified as a gene upregulated in prostate tissue by androgen treatment [39], and in breast cancer cells in response to glucocorticoids and progestins [77].

It was recently noted that PLZF, while expressed in normal melanocytes, is absent in melanoma, both in primary cells and in melanoma cell lines [18]. Overexpression of PLZF in melanoma lines caused a decrease in proliferation, blocked invasion and foci formation in semi-solid media, and enhanced melanocytic differentiation. Additionally, melanoma cells expressing PLZF had reduced growth in nude mice compared to parental cells, implying PLZF has tumor suppressor activity that was lost in this malignancy [18].

PLZF has traditionally been thought of as a nuclear protein, as befits a transcription factor, and in fact it is localized to the nucleus [46, 67] in the distinct nuclear speckled pattern described earlier. The speckled distribution is dependent on the presence of the BTB domain [16]. The identity and function of the PLZF speckle is as yet unclear, with some data suggesting that PLZF at least partially colocalizes with PML in PML nuclear bodies [42], while other data suggest that the two proteins are in adjacent but different structures in the nucleus [68]. In typical t(15;17) APL, PLZF is delocalized into a micro-speckled nuclear pattern similar to PML-RARα, suggesting that PLZF may normally be associated with PML.

As discussed, full-length PLZF has been best characterized as a repressor of gene expression. Two different portions of PLZF can act as repression domains when tethered to the GAL4 DNA-binding domain. The first is the BTB domain, which interacts with nuclear receptor co-repressors N-CoR, SMRT, and Sin3A as well as histone deacetylases (HDAC) 1 and 4 [6, 13, 20, 24, 31, 32, 47]. The BTB domain must dimerize to mediate repression [56]. Dimerization creates a highly conserved charged pocket, and mutations in the pocket impact repression activity. In the isolated BTB domain tethered to GAL4, mutation of critical residues in the pocket changed the domain from a repressor to an activator, and when the same mutations were made in full-length PLZF, the protein was inactive for transcriptional repression and subsequent growth suppression. A second repression domain in the center of the protein bears no similarity to other transcriptional effector domains and binds to a protein called ETO (the *e*ight-*t*wenty-*o*ne oncoprotein, also known as RUNX1T1). ETO, the fusion partner of AML1 in t(8;21)-associated M2 leukemia, acts a co-repressor for PLZF, and itself binds to mSin3A, N-CoR, and SMRT co-repressors [58]. PLZF repression is blocked by the AML1/ETO fusion protein, in part by inhibition of PLZF DNA binding and by removal of PLZF from the nuclear matrix [57]. This finding suggested that PLZF function might be disrupted in other forms of leukemia. Deletion of either the BTB domain or the second repression domain of PLZF severely impaired the ability of PLZF to repress transcription and to cooperate with ETO or other co-repressors [58]. It is believed that PLZF dimerizes and forms a multi-protein complex that includes co-repressors and histone deacetylases. In accordance with this model, specific histone deacetylase inhibitors such as trichostatin A can reverse repression by PLZF [14]. PLZF can dimerize with other ZF-BTB-containing proteins in vitro, notably BCL6 [15] and FAZF (Fanconi anemia zinc finger/ZBTB32) [30] but the consequence of this for PLZF activity remains to be clarified.

It should be noted that in addition to HDAC recruitment, other mechanisms of transcriptional repression by PLZF could be at play. Several other proteins have been found in complexes with PLZF. PLZF has a predicted molecular weight of 70 kDa, but binds to DNA as a high molecular weight complex of nearly 600 kDa [1]. Deletion of the BTB domain of PLZF reduced this DNA–protein complex to about 150 kDa, approximately one quarter of the size associated with the full-length protein. This suggests that the presence of BTB domain may allow two dimers of PLZF to form on a DNA-binding site. In accordance with these studies, atomic force microscopy analysis of PLZF binding to the *Hoxd11* promoter concluded that PLZF bound to DNA as a dimer, forming loops of naked DNA [4]. DNA looping through the formation of PLZF dimers or multimers might allow repression by PLZF to be propagated at distant sites. The identity of the other proteins in the 600-kDa complex is uncertain. One protein identified is the kinase protein cdc2, which may play a role in the phosphorylation of PLZF. Phosphorylation of PLZF is thought be critical for its function, as treatment of PLZF with a phosphatase leads to loss of DNA-binding activity [1]. In addition, a tyrosine phosphorylation was identified at the extreme C-terminus of the PLZF protein [70]. Cdc2 was previously implicated in transcriptional repression by phosphorylation of basal transcription factors [50], another possible mechanism by which PLZF might influence repression. In contrast, the RARα-PLZF protein, which is devoid of both the BTB and the RD2 domains of PLZF, forms a 40-kDa complex with DNA exactly as predicted from its molecular weight. It does not bind to cdc2 and is unaffected by phosphatase treatment [1]. These data suggest that RARα-PLZF is not subjected to the same regulation as wildtype

PLZF and is consistent with the notion that this leukemia-associated protein is a potent dominant-negative inhibitor of PLZF.

Several other proteins were also found to interact with PLZF and enhance its repressive action. VDUP1, also known as TRX2 (thioredoxin binding protein 2) is a nuclear and cytoplasmic protein mutated in hyperlipidemia syndromes. PLZF was identified in a two-hybrid screen as a VDUP1 partner [26], and although overexpressed PLZF and VDUP1 can interact, it is not yet certain if this is a significant interaction in vivo. Nevertheless, VDUP1 can augment repression by PLZF in reporter gene assays. Since VDUP1 binds thioredoxin, it is intriguing to speculate that thioredoxin could affect the redox state of PLZF, or link PLZF function to the cellular redox state. PLZF can also interact with the LIM (Lin11, Isl-1, and Mec-3) domain protein DRAL/FHL2, an interaction that requires both the BTB domain and the second repression domain of PLZF [55]. Co-expression of DRAL augmented transcriptional repression by PLZF. DRAL was localized in both the nucleus and cytoplasm, and serum stimulation of cells increased nuclear accumulation of DRAL, further increasing PLZF repression.

Additionally, PLZF interacts with Bmi-1, a member of the Polycomb protein family implicated in chromatin remodeling [4]. Work is ongoing in our laboratory and others to define a precise role for PLZF in repression-associated changes in chromatin structure.

Interestingly, there is a stretch of acidic residues C-terminal to the BTB domain of PLZF that, when tethered to GAL4, acts as a transcriptional activator [44]. Activation is not observed with full-length PLZF protein in the majority of biological systems. However, the presence of this domain raises the possibility that in some context, PLZF might activate gene expression. In this respect, it is worth noting that forced PLZF expression in the erythro-megakaryocytic TF-1 cell line leads to weak activation of a thrombopoietin (TpoR) reporter, correlated with the presence of a PLZF-binding site in the TpoR promoter and induction of TpoR expression after PLZF induction [43]. Similarly, it was demonstrated that PLZF can bind a consensus sequence from the *p85α (phosphoinositide 3-kinase) PI3K* promoter. Promoter activity is reduced when the PLZF site is lost, and PLZF is necessary for increasing p85α PI3K levels [70]. Transcriptional upregulation of *CBFA1* [*RUNX2*] was demonstrated by forced PLZF expression in C2C12 cells [35]. Although these systems do not provide a mechanism, or even evidence, of direct activation of gene expression by PLZF, the possibility that PLZF acts as a bifunctional transcription factor is intriguing. Work underway in our laboratory to purify interaction partners for PLZF may help address the possible mechanism of PLZF-mediated transcriptional activation.

There is a growing body of evidence that, in addition to the nucleus, PLZF can be found in the cytoplasm. In a process called "ectodomain shedding," a membrane-anchored ligand for the epidermal growth factor receptor (EGFR) HB-EGF (heparin-binding EGF-like growth factor) is cleaved, generating a small, roughly 7-kDa fragment of HB-EGF in the cytoplasm of the cell. This translocates to the nucleus where it binds PLZF through the first three (N-terminal) zinc fingers of PLZF [60, 61]. This causes export of PLZF from the nucleus in late S-phase of the cell cycle, resulting in the loss of PLZF-mediated transcriptional repression and consequent growth suppression [74]. This phenomenon can be stimulated by addition of the phorbol ester (TPA) to primary keratinocytes, a cell where PLZF is naturally expressed. This results in hyperplasia of the keratinocytes, consistent with the loss of PLZF-mediated growth suppression.

In addition, PLZF has been shown to interact with the cytoplasmic protein epsin1, a protein similar in structure to β-catenin, resulting in the relocalization of epsin1 and PLZF to the nucleus [34]. In a cardiac myocyte model, stimulation of cells with angiotensin II led to phosphorylation of cytoplasmic PLZF, association with epsin, and translocation of both PLZF and epsin to the nucleus, followed by upregulation of expression of the p85α subunit of PI3K [70]. Translocation was dependent on PLZF phosphorylation, since both inhibition of tyrosine kinase activity, and a nonphosphorylatable mutant of PLZF, prevented relocalization. Whether PLZF has some nontranscriptional role in the cytoplasm or whether removal to the cytoplasm is simply a way of negatively regulating its transcriptional activity has not been determined. Further, this cytoplasmic shuttling has not been documented in a hematopoietic cell, leaving its relevance to the progenitor cell and the development of APL unclear.

Modulation of PLZF action occurs via several mechanisms. As discussed above, changing the cellular localization of the protein is an effective way of reducing transcriptional activity. In addition, PLZF activity can be modulated by posttranslational modifications. PLZF is a phosphoprotein, and phosphorylation was shown to be essential for both nuclear localization and DNA binding [1]. Regulation of phosphorylation would presumably regulate PLZF activity, although this has not been demonstrated to date in vivo, nor are the kinases or phosphatases known.

Like other transcription factors, PLZF can be acetylated. The acetyltransferase p300 acetylates specific lysine residues in zinc fingers 6 and 9. The p300 is generally associated with activation of transcription; however, acetylation of PLZF by p300 increased its DNA-binding activity, which enhanced transcriptional repression and consequent growth suppression by PLZF [23]. Deacetylation of PLZF could potentially be carried out by any one of the HDAC proteins that have been shown to interact with PLZF [6, 47]. In addition, the class III HDAC SIRT1 has been shown to deacetylate PLZF [54]. The physiological stimuli that induce PLZF acetylation and deacetylation have not been identified.

In a recent paper, one group found that PLZF could be modified in vitro by the small ubiquitin-like molecule SUMO. The modification occurred at a lysine in RD2, the second repression domain of PLZF [40]. Sumoylation increased DNA binding, and mutation of this lysine residue (K242) resulted in decreased DNA binding and transcriptional repression, suggesting that sumoylation augments transcriptional repression by PLZF. Whether PLZF sumoylation occurs in vivo has not been determined, although PLZF is found in PML bodies, where a number of proteins are known to be sumoylated. Further, sumoylation is associated with transcriptional repression and repressive chromatin, again reminiscent of the action of PLZF [27].

Growth factor-mediated signaling may also modulate PLZF-mediated gene repression. We found that transcriptional repression by PLZF was inhibited by co-expression of a mutant, constitutively active form of the tyrosine kinase receptor Flt3. Flt3 is the most common mutation identified in human leukemia and mediates signaling through the ras-mitogen-activated protein (MAP) kinase pathway as well as through the Janus kinase/signal transducer and activator of transcription (JAK-STAT) pathway [19]. Co-expression of constitutively activated ras or stress kinases also blocks transcriptional repression by PLZF [32, 82]. Signaling by active Flt3 decreases the PLZF-SMRT interaction, and PLZF repression accordingly. There is an increase in the interaction between SMRT and the p65 subunit of nuclear factor (NF)-κB, resulting in the NF-κB-dependent relocalization of SMRT to the cytoplasm [73]. This may represent a general way in which signaling influences multiple transcriptional repressors that utilize the SMRT cofactor.

A more specific mechanism may be via the direct phosphorylation of PLZF. PLZF, expressed at high levels in the heart [67], is tyrosine phosphorylated and translocated to the nucleus in response to the cardiac hormone angiotensin II [70]. This phosphorylation was reported to be necessary for receptor signaling, upregulation of PI3K expression and subsequent p70 S6 kinase activation, an event associated with increasing protein synthesis. Activation of PI3K is a common event in myeloid leukemia [19], and is essential for leukemogenesis mediated by the Abl oncogene [41]. Whether PLZF can upregulate the PI3K pathway in hematopoietic cells has not been yet established, but is an interesting possibility. It will be important to determine whether the RARα-PLZF protein generated in APL will have a more striking effect on p85α expression. Activation of the PI3K pathways by RARα-PLZF might explain in part its ability to induce myeloproliferation [28].

PLZF has been shown to interact with other factors important in hematopoiesis. The nuclear receptor RARα binds the first three zinc fingers of PLZF, which results in a block in ATRA-induced RARα activation [52], a process central to differentiation of hematopoietic cells. The transcription factor GATA2, which is important for hematopoietic progenitor cell commitment [62], also interacts with PLZF, leading to a block in GATA2-mediated transactivation [75]. The effect of these interactions on PLZF repression activity has not been described, but downregulation of the action of other factors is a significant way in which PLZF could modulate hematopoietic development. Interestingly, both a physical interaction and functional crosstalk between RARα and GATA2 has been described in myeloid differentiation [76], suggesting that regulation of this process by PLZF would have a significant role in normal and malignant hematopoiesis.

The consequence of PLZF expression varies between cell type. In myeloid cells, PLZF expression results in inhibition of cell growth associated with cell cycle arrest, and a block in differentiation. Prolonged PLZF expression in the APL cell line NB4 causes an accumulation of cells in S-phase, pointing to a delay in S-phase progression [79]. 32Dcl3(G/GM) cells overexpressing the PLZF protein were highly growth inhibited, accumulated in G1, traversed S phase slowly, and had an increased rate of apoptosis [71]. Acute infection of these 32D cells with a PLZF-containing retrovirus was associated with arrest of cells in the S-phase of the cell cycle, implicating cyclin A as a potential target. PLZF can bind and repress the cyclin A2 promoter, and growth suppression mediated by PLZF was overcome by enforced expression of cyclin A2 [79]. Similar effects on cyclin A2 expression and cell cycle progression were observed in NIH3T3 cells expressing PLZF. Induction of PLZF in the monocytic U937 cell line led to growth suppression accompanied by G1 arrest [78]. Additionally, we found that c-myc expression is dramatically inhibited in this system, which correlates with occupancy of a PLZF-binding site in the c-myc promoter as shown by chromatin immunoprecipitation [53]. Hence PLZF may inhibit proliferation by repressing the expression of multiple cell cycle regulators.

PLZF expression inhibited myeloid differentiation induced by granulocyte colony-stimulating factor (G-CSF) or granulocyte-macrophage (GM)-CSF and led to the upregulation of the early hematopoietic marker Sca1 [71]. PLZF expression in the U937 cell line inhibited the ability of vitamin D3 (VD3) to stimulate monocyte differentiation of these cells, while leaving granulocyte differentiation in response to retinoic acid intact [78]. Similarly, forced PLZF expression inhibited VD3-mediated differentiation in HL60 cells [66]. PLZF-mediated inhibition of the action of VD3 was associated with the ability of the BTB domain of PLZF to bind to the vitamin D3 receptor (VDR) and inhibit transcriptional activation by VDR. PLZF did not block differentiation in response to ATRA in U937 cells.

In contrast to neutrophils where PLZF is downregulated relative to the progenitor $CD34^+$ cell, in circulating lymphocytes PLZF expression remains high, comparable to the level in $CD34^+$ cells [64]. Treatment of resting B lymphocytes with phorbol myristate acetate, an agent that induces proliferation and differentiation, decreased PLZF expression while upregulating expression of the PLZF target cyclin A [63].

The data concerning PLZF and apoptosis are inconsistent and suggest that the effect of PLZF on cell death may be cell type- and context-dependent. PLZF protected the interleukin (IL)-3 dependent 32D cell from apoptosis caused by growth factor withdrawal, although the basal apoptosis rate for 32D-PLZF cells in the presence of IL-3 was higher than the parental cell [71]. The U937T:PLZF inducible cell model shows an increase in apoptosis upon PLZF induction, but only after several days of continued expression [53], implying that induction of apoptosis is not a direct effect. Expression of the pro-apoptotic protein BID is repressed by PLZF in Jurkat cells, again suggesting an anti-apoptotic function for PLZF [64].

Together these data lead us to hypothesize that PLZF plays an essential role in the quiescence and resistance to apoptosis exhibited by hematopoietic stem cells. Expression of PLZF in the stem cell may be important for maintaining a pool of undifferentiated, self-renewing stem cells. This is highlighted by the knockout mouse, where the balance between quiescence and cycling of $CD34^+$ cells is reportedly disrupted, a feature shared by the FAZF-null mouse [65]. The importance of PLZF for maintenance of the hematopoietic stem cell is reflected in other stem cell systems. An essential role for PLZF has been demonstrated in the male germline stem cell. Both the $Plzf^{-/-}$ mouse and the luxoid mutant mouse (which has a *Plzf* mutation) have an age-dependent loss in self-renewal potential of the spermatogonia [5, 10]. This strongly supports the hypothesis that loss of PLZF leads to unrestricted exit from quiescence, diminishing the stem cell pool and causing premature progenitor loss due to the limited proliferative potential of committed progenitor cells. This effect of PLZF might be relevant to APL. Loss of one allele of PLZF might lead to deregulation of the stem cell; a decision in favor of proliferation may be made rather than quiescence. In this regard we note that while PLZF is a growth suppressor, the RARα-PLZF oncoprotein, which can bind to many of the same DNA-binding sites of wildtype PLZF, activates genes that PLZF represses and induces a myeloproliferative disease in mice.

Summary

The study of the t(11;17)-associated forms of APL and the PLZF protein has served as a paradigm for the role that aberrant transcriptional repression plays in hematological malignancy. The resistant phenotype of t(11;17) APL can be explained in part by a gain-of-function mutation of RARα in which the protein becomes a constitutive repressor of key genes required for normal myeloid maturation. However, closer study of PLZF has revealed additional layers of complexity in the development of APL. PLZF is clearly a growth suppressor that inhibits cell cycle progression in a number of processes including hematopoiesis, potentially by inhibiting expression of cyclins and c-myc. In APL, loss of PLZF expression and consequent growth suppression, combined with gain of the RARα-PLZF oncogene, plays an essential role in the aberrant gene expression associated with leukemia. PLZF expression is itself under temporal and spatial control, and the transcriptional function of the protein can be regulated by multiple posttranslational modifications and by relocalization within the cell. These findings also imply that PLZF and the related FAZF gene may be important for the proper control of growth and homeostasis of multiple tissues. Unresolved questions in regard to PLZF include its exact mode of repression, and key transcriptional targets and physiological stimuli that lead to its posttranslational modification and subsequent regulation of transcriptional function.

References

1. Ball HJ, Melnick A, Shaknovich R, Kohanski RA, Licht JD (1999) The promyelocytic leukemia zinc finger (PLZF) protein binds DNA in a high molecular weight complex associated with cdc2 kinase. Nucleic Acids Res 27:4106–4113
2. Reference deleted in proof
3. Barna M, Hawe N, Niswander L, Pandolfi PP (2000) Plzf regulates limb and axial skeletal patterning. Nat Genet 25:166–172
4. Barna M, Merghoub T, Costoya JA, Ruggero D, Branford M, Bergia A, Samori B, Pandolfi PP (2002) Plzf mediates transcriptional repression of HoxD gene expression through chromatin remodeling. Dev Cell 3:499–510
5. Buaas FW, Kirsh AL, Sharma M, McLean DJ, Morris JL, Griswold MD, de Rooij DG, Braun RE (2004) Plzf is required in adult male germ cells for stem cell self-renewal. Nat Genet 36:647–652
6. Chauchereau A, Mathieu M, de Saintignon J, Ferreira R, Pritchard LL, Mishal Z, Dejean A, Harel-Bellan A (2004) HDAC4 mediates transcriptional repression by the acute promyelocytic leukaemia-associated protein PLZF. Oncogene 23:8777–8784

7. Chen SJ, Zelent A, Tong JH, Yu HQ, Wang ZY, Derre J, Berger R, Waxman S, Chen Z (1993) Rearrangements of the retinoic acid receptor alpha and promyelocytic leukemia zinc finger genes resulting from t(11;17)(q23;q21) in a patient with acute promyelocytic leukemia. J Clin Invest 91:2260–2267
8. Chen Z, Brand NJ, Chen A, Chen SJ, Tong JH, Wang ZY, Waxman S, Zelent A (1993) Fusion between a novel Kruppel-like zinc finger gene and the retinoic acid receptor-alpha locus due to a variant t(11;17) translocation associated with acute promyelocytic leukaemia. EMBO J 12:1161–1167
9. Cook M, Gould A, Brand N, Davies J, Strutt P, Shaknovich R, Licht J, Waxman S, Chen Z, Gluecksohn-Waelsch S, et al (1995) Expression of the zinc-finger gene PLZF at rhombomere boundaries in the vertebrate hindbrain. Proc Natl Acad Sci U S A 92:2249–2253
10. Costoya JA, Hobbs RM, Barna M, Cattoretti G, Manova K, Sukhwani M, Orwig KE, Wolgemuth DJ, Pandolfi PP (2004) Essential role of Plzf in maintenance of spermatogonial stem cells. Nat Genet 36:653–659
11. Culligan DJ, Stevenson D, Chee YL, Grimwade D (1998) Acute promyelocytic leukaemia with t(11;17)(q23;q12-21) and a good initial response to prolonged ATRA and combination chemotherapy. Br J Haematol 100:328–330
12. Dai MS, Chevallier N, Stone S, Heinrich MC, McConnell M, Reuter T, Broxmeyer HE, Licht JD, Lu L, Hoatlin ME (2002) The effects of the Fanconi anemia zinc finger (FAZF) on cell cycle, apoptosis, and proliferation are differentiation stage-specific. J Biol Chem 277:26327–26334
13. David G, Alland L, Hong SH, Wong CW, DePinho RA, Dejean A (1998) Histone deacetylase associated with mSin3A mediates repression by the acute promyelocytic leukemia-associated PLZF protein. Oncogene 16:2549–2556
14. Deltour S, Guerardel C, Leprince D (1999) Recruitment of SMRT/N-CoR-mSin3A-HDAC-repressing complexes is not a general mechanism for BTB/POZ transcriptional repressors: the case of HIC-1 and gammaFBP-B. Proc Natl Acad Sci U S A 96:14831–14836
15. Dhordain P, Albagli O, Honore N, Guidez F, Lantoine D, Schmid M, de Thé HD, Zelent A, Koken MH (2000) Colocalization and heteromerization between the two human oncogene POZ/zinc finger proteins, LAZ3 (BCL6) and PLZF. Oncogene 19:6240–6250
16. Dong S, Zhu J, Reid A, Strutt P, Guidez F, Zhong HJ, Wang ZY, Licht J, Waxman S, Chomienne C, et al (1996) Amino-terminal protein-protein interaction motif (POZ-domain) is responsible for activities of the promyelocytic leukemia zinc finger-retinoic acid receptor-alpha fusion protein. Proc Natl Acad Sci U S A 93:3624–3629
17. Fahnenstich J, Nandy A, Milde-Langosch K, Schneider-Merck T, Walther N, Gellersen B (2003) Promyelocytic leukaemia zinc finger protein (PLZF) is a glucocorticoid- and progesterone-induced transcription factor in human endometrial stromal cells and myometrial smooth muscle cells. Mol Hum Reprod 9:611–623
18. Felicetti F, Bottero L, Felli N, Mattia G, Labbaye C, Alvino E, Peschle C, Colombo MP, Care A (2004) Role of PLZF in melanoma progression. Oncogene 23:4567–4576
19. Gilliland DG, Griffin JD (2002) Role of FLT3 in leukemia. Curr Opin Hematol 9:274–281

20. Grignani F, De Matteis S, Nervi C, Tomassoni L, Gelmetti V, Cioce M, Fanelli M, Ruthardt M, Ferrara FF, Zamir I, Seiser C, Lazar MA, Minucci S, Pelicci PG (1998) Fusion proteins of the retinoic acid receptor-alpha recruit histone deacetylase in promyelocytic leukaemia. Nature 391:815–818
21. Grimwade D, Biondi A, Mozziconacci MJ, Hagemeijer A, Berger R, Neat M, Howe K, Dastugue N, Jansen J, Radford-Weiss I, Lo Coco F, Lessard M, Hernandez JM, Delabesse E, Head D, Liso V, Sainty D, Flandrin G, Solomon E, Birg F, Lafage-Pochitaloff M (2000) Characterization of acute promyelocytic leukemia cases lacking the classic t(15;17): results of the European Working Party. Groupe Francais de Cytogenetique Hematologique, Groupe de Francais d'Hematologie Cellulaire, UK Cancer Cytogenetics Group and BIOMED 1 European Community-Concerted Action "Molecular Cytogenetic Diagnosis in Haematological Malignancies". Blood 96:1297–1308
22. Grimwade D, Gorman P, Duprez E, Howe K, Langabeer S, Oliver F, Walker H, Culligan D, Waters J, Pomfret M, Goldstone A, Burnett A, Freemont P, Sheer D, Solomon E (1997) Characterization of cryptic rearrangements and variant translocations in acute promyelocytic leukemia. Blood 90:4876–4885
23. Guidez F, Howell L, Isalan M, Cebrat M, Alani RM, Ivins S, Hormaeche I, McConnell MJ, Pierce S, Cole PA, Licht J, Zelent A (2005) Histone acetyltransferase activity of p300 is required for transcriptional repression by the promyelocytic leukemia zinc finger protein. Mol Cell Biol 25:5552–5566
24. Guidez F, Ivins S, Zhu J, Soderstrom M, Waxman S, Zelent A (1998) Reduced retinoic acid-sensitivities of nuclear receptor corepressor binding to PML- and PLZF-RARalpha underlie molecular pathogenesis and treatment of acute promyelocytic leukemia. Blood 91:2634–2642
25. Reference deleted in proof
26. Han SH, Jeon JH, Ju HR, Jung U, Kim KY, Yoo HS, Lee YH, Song KS, Hwang HM, Na YS, Yang Y, Lee KN, Choi I (2003) VDUP1 upregulated by TGF-beta1 and 1,25-dihydorxyvitamin D3 inhibits tumor cell growth by blocking cell-cycle progression. Oncogene 22:4035–4046
27. Hay RT (2005) SUMO: a history of modification. Mol Cell 18:1–12
28. He L, Bhaumik M, Tribioli C, Rego EM, Ivins S, Zelent A, Pandolfi PP (2000) Two critical hits for promyelocytic leukemia. Mol Cell 6:1131–1141
29. He LZ, Guidez F, Tribioli C, Peruzzi D, Ruthardt M, Zelent A, Pandolfi PP (1998) Distinct interactions of PML-RARalpha and PLZF-RARalpha with co-repressors determine differential responses to RA in APL. Nat Genet 18:126–135
30. Hoatlin ME, Zhi Y, Ball H, Silvey K, Melnick A, Stone S, Arai S, Hawe N, Owen G, Zelent A, Licht JD (1999) A novel BTB/POZ transcriptional repressor protein interacts with the Fanconi anemia group C protein and PLZF. Blood 94:3737–3747
31. Hong SH, David G, Wong CW, Dejean A, Privalsky ML (1997) SMRT corepressor interacts with PLZF and with the PML-retinoic acid receptor alpha (RARalpha) and PLZF-RARalpha oncoproteins associated with acute promyelocytic leukemia. Proc Natl Acad Sci U S A 94:9028–9033

32. Hong SH, Wong CW, Privalsky ML (1998) Signaling by tyrosine kinases negatively regulates the interaction between transcription factors and SMRT (silencing mediator of retinoic acid and thyroid hormone receptor) corepressor. Mol Endocrinol 12:1161–1171
33. Reference deleted in proof
34. Hyman J, Chen H, Di Fiore PP, De Camilli P, Brunger AT (2000) Epsin 1 undergoes nucleocytosolic shuttling and its eps15 interactor NH(2)-terminal homology (ENTH) domain, structurally similar to Armadillo and HEAT repeats, interacts with the transcription factor promyelocytic leukemia Zn(2)+ finger protein (PLZF). J Cell Biol 149:537–546
35. Ikeda R, Yoshida K, Tsukahara S, Sakamoto Y, Tanaka H, Furukawa K, Inoue I (2005) The promyelotic leukemia zinc finger promotes osteoblastic differentiation of human mesenchymal stem cells as an upstream regulator of CBFA1. J Biol Chem 280:8523–8530
36. Ivins S, Pemberton K, Guidez F, Howell L, Krumlauf R, Zelent A (2003) Regulation of Hoxb2 by APL-associated PLZF protein. Oncogene 22:3685–3697
37. Ivins S, Zelent A (1998) Promyelocytic leukaemia translocation gene, PLZF, encodes a transcriptional repressor targeting HOXB2 expression. Blood 92(Suppl 1):308a
38. Jansen JH, de Ridder MC, Geertsma WM, Erpelinck CA, van Lom K, Smit EM, Slater R, vd Reijden BA, de Greef GE, Sonneveld P, Lowenberg B (1999) Complete remission of t(11;17) positive acute promyelocytic leukemia induced by all-trans retinoic acid and granulocyte colony-stimulating factor. Blood 94:39–45
39. Jiang F, Wang Z (2004) Identification and characterization of PLZF as a prostatic androgen-responsive gene. Prostate 59:426–435
40. Kang SI, Chang WJ, Cho SG, Kim IY (2003) Modification of promyelocytic leukemia zinc finger protein (PLZF) by SUMO-1 conjugation regulates its transcriptional repressor activity. J Biol Chem 278:51479–51483
41. Kharas MG, Fruman DA (2005) ABL oncogenes and phosphoinositide 3-kinase: mechanism of activation and downstream effectors. Cancer Res 65:2047–2053
42. Koken MH, Reid A, Quignon F, Chelbi-Alix MK, Davies JM, Kabarowski JH, Zhu J, Dong S, Chen S, Chen Z, Tan CC, Licht J, Waxman S, de The H, Zelent A (1997) Leukemia-associated retinoic acid receptor alpha fusion partners, PML and PLZF, heterodimerize and colocalize to nuclear bodies. Proc Natl Acad Sci U S A 94:10255–10260
43. Labbaye C, Quaranta MT, Pagliuca A, Militi S, Licht JD, Testa U, Peschle C (2002) PLZF induces megakaryocytic development, activates Tpo receptor expression and interacts with GATA1 protein. Oncogene 21:6669–6679
44. Li JY, English MA, Ball HJ, Yeyati PL, Waxman S, Licht JD (1997) Sequence-specific DNA binding and transcriptional regulation by the promyelocytic leukemia zinc finger protein. J Biol Chem 272:22447–22455
45. Licht JD, Chomienne C, Goy A, Chen A, Scott AA, Head DR, Michaux JL, Wu Y, DeBlasio A, Miller WH Jr, Zelenetz AD, Wilman CL, Chen Z, J Chen S, Zelent A, Macintyre E, Veil A, Cortes J, Kantarjian H, Waxman S (1995) Clinical and molecular characterization of a rare syndrome of acute promyelocytic leukemia associated with translocation (11;17). Blood 85:1083–1094

46. Licht JD, Shaknovich R, English MA, Melnick A, Li JY, Reddy JC, Dong S, Chen SJ, Zelent A, Waxman S (1996) Reduced and altered DNA-binding and transcriptional properties of the PLZF-retinoic acid receptor-alpha chimera generated in t(11;17)-associated acute promyelocytic leukemia. Oncogene 12:323–336
47. Lin RJ, Nagy L, Inoue S, Shao W, Miller WH Jr, Evans RM (1998) Role of the histone deacetylase complex in acute promyelocytic leukaemia. Nature 391:811–814
48. Reference deleted in proof
49. Lin W, Lai CH, Tang CJ, Huang CJ, Tang TK (1999) Identification and gene structure of a novel human PLZF-related transcription factor gene, TZFP. Biochem Biophys Res Commun 264:789–795
50. Long JJ, Leresche A, Kriwacki RW, Gottesfeld JM (1998) Repression of TFIIH transcriptional activity and TFIIH-associated cdk7 kinase activity at mitosis. Mol Cell Biol 18:1467–1476
51. Look AT (1997) Oncogenic transcription factors in the human acute leukemias. Science 278:1059–1064
52. Martin PJ, Delmotte MH, Formstecher P, Lefebvre P (2003) PLZF is a negative regulator of retinoic acid receptor transcriptional activity. Nucl Recept 1:6
53. McConnell MJ, Chevallier N, Berkofsky-Fessler W, Giltnane JM, Malani RB, Staudt LM, Licht JD (2003) Growth suppression by acute promyelocytic leukemia-associated protein PLZF is mediated by repression of c-myc expression. Mol Cell Biol 23:9375–9388
54. McConnell MJ, Langley E, Martinez Martinez M, Kouzarides T, Licht JD (2004) ASH Annual Meeting Abstracts, 104:360
55. McLoughlin P, Ehler E, Carlile G, Licht JD, Schafer BW (2002) The LIM-only protein DRAL/FHL2 interacts with and is a corepressor for the promyelocytic leukemia zinc finger protein. J Biol Chem 277:37045–37053
56. Melnick A, Ahmad KF, Arai S, Polinger A, Ball H, Borden KL, Carlile GW, Prive GG, Licht JD (2000) In-depth mutational analysis of the promyelocytic leukemia zinc finger BTB/POZ domain reveals motifs and residues required for biological and transcriptional functions. Mol Cell Biol 20:6550–6567
57. Melnick A, Carlile GW, McConnell MJ, Polinger A, Hiebert SW, Licht JD (2000) AML-1/ETO fusion protein is a dominant negative inhibitor of transcriptional repression by the promyelocytic leukemia zinc finger protein. Blood 96:3939–3947
58. Melnick A, Westendorf JJ, Polinger A, Carlile GW, Arai S, Ball HJ, Lutterbach B, Licht JD, Hiebert SW (2000) The ETO protein disrupted in t(8;21)-associated acute myeloid leukemia is a co-repressor for the promyelocytic leukemia zinc finger protein. Mol Cell Biol 20:2075–2086
59. Miaw SC, Choi A, Yu E, Kishikawa H, Ho IC (2000) ROG, repressor of GATA, regulates the expression of cytokine genes. Immunity 12:323–333
60. Nanba D, Mammoto A, Hashimoto K, Higashiyama S (2003) Proteolytic release of the carboxy-terminal fragment of proHB-EGF causes nuclear export of PLZF. J Cell Biol 163:489–502
61. Nanba D, Toki F, Higashiyama S (2004) Roles of charged amino acid residues in the cytoplasmic domain of proHB-EGF. Biochem Biophys Res Commun 320:376–382

62. Ohneda K, Yamamoto M (2002) Roles of hematopoietic transcription factors GATA-1 and GATA-2 in the development of red blood cell lineage. Acta Haematol 108:237–245
63. Parrado A, Noguera ME, Delmer A, McKenna S, Davies J, Le Gall I, Bentley P, Whittaker JA, Sigaux F, Chomienne C, Padua RA (2000) Deregulated expression of promyelocytic leukemia zinc finger protein in B-cell chronic lymphocytic leukemias does not affect cyclin A expression. Hematol J 1:15–27
64. Parrado A, Robledo M, Moya-Quiles MR, Marin LA, Chomienne C, Padua RA, Alvarez-Lopez MR (2004) The promyelocytic leukemia zinc finger protein down-regulates apoptosis and expression of the proapoptotic BID protein in lymphocytes. Proc Natl Acad Sci U S A 101:1898–1903
65. Piazza F, Costoya JA, Merghoub T, Hobbs RM, Pandolfi PP (2004) Disruption of PLZP in mice leads to increased T-lymphocyte proliferation, cytokine production, and altered hematopoietic stem cell homeostasis. Mol Cell Biol 24:10456–10469
66. Puccetti E, Obradovic D, Beissert T, Bianchini A, Washburn B, Chiaradonna F, Boehrer S, Hoelzer D, Ottmann OG, Pelicci PG, Nervi C, Ruthardt M (2002) AML-associated translocation products block vitamin D(3)-induced differentiation by sequestering the vitamin D(3) receptor. Cancer Res 62:7050–7058
67. Reid A, Gould A, Brand N, Cook M, Strutt P, Li J, Licht J, Waxman S, Krumlauf R, Zelent A (1995) Leukemia translocation gene, PLZF, is expressed with a speckled nuclear pattern in early hematopoietic progenitors. Blood 86:4544–4552
68. Ruthardt M, Orleth A, Tomassoni L, Puccetti E, Riganelli D, Alcalay M, Mannucci R, Nicoletti I, Grignani F, Fagioli M, Pelicci PG (1998) The acute promyelocytic leukaemia specific PML and PLZF proteins localize to adjacent and functionally distinct nuclear bodies. Oncogene 16:1945–1953
69. Sainty D, Liso V, Cantu-Rajnoldi A, Head D, Mozziconacci MJ, Arnoulet C, Benattar L, Fenu S, Mancini M, Duchayne E, Mahon FX, Gutierrez N, Birg F, Biondi A, Grimwade D, Lafage-Pochitaloff M, Hagemeijer A, Flandrin G (2000) A new morphologic classification system for acute promyelocytic leukemia distinguishes cases with underlying PLZF/RARA gene rearrangements. Group Francais de Cytogenetique Hematologique, UK Cancer Cytogenetics Group and BIOMED 1 European Community-Concerted Action "Molecular Cytogenetic Diagnosis in Haematological Malignancies". Blood 96:1287–1296
70. Senbonmatsu T, Saito T, Landon EJ, Watanabe O, Price E Jr, Roberts RL, Imboden H, Fitzgerald TG, Gaffney FA, Inagami T (2003) A novel angiotensin II type 2 receptor signaling pathway: possible role in cardiac hypertrophy. EMBO J 22:6471–6482
71. Shaknovich R, Yeyati PL, Ivins S, Melnick A, Lempert C, Waxman S, Zelent A, Licht JD (1998) The promyelocytic leukemia zinc finger protein affects myeloid cell growth, differentiation, and apoptosis. Mol Cell Biol 18:5533–5545
72. Takahashi S, Licht JD (2002) The human promyelocytic leukemia zinc finger gene is regulated by the Evi-1 oncoprotein and a novel guanine-rich site binding protein. Leukemia 16:1755–1762
73. Takahashi S, McConnell MJ, Harigae H, Kaku M, Sasaki T, Melnick AM, Licht JD (2004) The Flt3 internal tandem duplication mutant inhibits the function of transcriptional repressors by blocking interactions with SMRT. Blood 103:4650–4658

74. Toki F, Nanba D, Matsuura N, Higashiyama S (2005) Ectodomain shedding of membrane-anchored heparin-binding EGF like growth factor and subcellular localization of the C-terminal fragment in the cell cycle. J Cell Physiol 202:839–848
75. Tsuzuki S, Enver T (2002) Interactions of GATA-2 with the promyelocytic leukemia zinc finger (PLZF) protein, its homologue FAZF, and the t(11;17)-generated PLZF-retinoic acid receptor alpha oncoprotein. Blood 99:3404–3410
76. Tsuzuki S, Kitajima K, Nakano T, Glasow A, Zelent A, Enver T (2004) Cross talk between retinoic acid signaling and transcription factor GATA-2. Mol Cell Biol 24:6824–6836
77. Wan Y, Nordeen SK (2002) Overlapping but distinct gene regulation profiles by glucocorticoids and progestins in human breast cancer cells. Mol Endocrinol 16:1204–1214
78. Ward JO, McConnell MJ, Carlile GW, Pandolfi PP, Licht JD, Freedman LP (2001) The acute promyelocytic leukemia-associated protein, promyelocytic leukemia zinc finger, regulates 1,25-dihydroxyvitamin D(3)-induced monocytic differentiation of U937 cells through a physical interaction with vitamin D(3) receptor. Blood 98:3290–3300
79. Yeyati PL, Shaknovich R, Boterashvili S, Li J, Ball HJ, Waxman S, Nason-Burchenal K, Dmitrovsky E, Zelent A, Licht JD (1999) Leukemia translocation protein PLZF inhibits cell growth and expression of cyclin A. Oncogene 18:925–934
80. Yu BD, Hess JL, Horning SE, Brown GA, Korsmeyer SJ (1995) Altered Hox expression and segmental identity in Mll-mutant mice. Nature 378:505–508
81. Zhang T, Xiong H, Kan LX, Zhang CK, Jiao XF, Fu G, Zhang QH, Lu L, Tong JH, Gu BW, Yu M, Liu JX, Licht J, Waxman S, Zelent A, Chen E, Chen SJ (1999) Genomic sequence, structural organization, molecular evolution, and aberrant rearrangement of promyelocytic leukemia zinc finger gene. Proc Natl Acad Sci U S A 96:11422–11427
82. Zhou Y, Gross W, Hong SH, Privalsky ML (2001) The SMRT corepressor is a target of phosphorylation by protein kinase CK2 (casein kinase II). Mol Cell Biochem 220:1–13

SUMO, the Three Rs and Cancer

J.-S. Seeler (✉) · O. Bischof · K. Nacerddine · A. Dejean

Nuclear Organisation and Oncogenesis Unit, INSERM U.579, Institut Pasteur,
28 rue du Dr. Roux, 75724 Paris Cedex 15, France
seeler@pasteur.fr

1	Introduction	49
2	At the Chromosomal Level	51
2.1	Chromosome Cohesion and Condensation	51
2.2	Specialized Chromatin, Centromeres and Telomeres	56
3	DNA Replication and Repair	57
4	SUMO and Cancer: Caretakers and Gatekeepers	59
5	Conclusion	63
	References	64

Abstract SUMO modification (sumoylation) plays important roles in nucleo-cytoplasmic transport, maintenance of sub-nuclear architecture, the regulation of gene expression and in DNA replication, repair and recombination. Here we review recent evidence for SUMO's role in protecting genomic integrity at both the chromosomal and the DNA level. Furthermore, the involvement of sumoylation and of specific SUMO targets in cancer is discussed.

1
Introduction

Protein modification by SUMO (small ubiquitin-like modifier, sumoylation) is conserved in all eukaryote cells and is essential for all dividing cells. Sumoylation involves the sequential action of SUMO activating (E1), conjugating (E2) and ligase (E3) activities to produce a covalent conjugate of one or more SUMO moieties with a target protein via an isopeptide linkage between the carboxy-terminal glycine of SUMO to a specific lysine residue of the target. Sumoylation is a highly dynamic process since the steady-state level of SUMO-conjugated proteins is maintained by the sum of SUMO conjugating (E1, E2, E3) and de-conjugating activities (the SUMO proteases, or SENPs/Ulps). Unlike ubiquitylation, which relies on a similar but distinct modification pathway, sumoylation does not tag proteins for proteasomal degradation, but rather, like all post-translational modifications, alters the target protein's interacting properties.

A simple, unifying function of sumoylation has remained elusive, and it appears that the spectrum of functions for this modification is as wide as that of its targets. To date, some 100 SUMO substrates have been reported, but despite this wealth of information, mechanistic insight into SUMO function is accumulating only slowly. One reason for this is surely technical: detailed analysis is hampered by cellular de-sumoylating activities that generally permit only a small fraction of a given protein to remain in the modified state and further, because specific probes that distinguish modified from non-modified proteins do not as yet exist. Nevertheless, it can be said that sumoylation, like all other ubiquitin-like modifications, is intimately tied to the basic activities and challenges faced by eukaryotic cells. First, the 'nuclear' condition requires regulating nucleo-cytoplasmic transport. Hence, sumoylation regulates nuclear import and export, and conversely, nuclear transport regulates sumoylation [90]. Second, the large and complex eukaryotic genome must be carefully managed, first to ensure its faithful transmission to the next generation, and second for the regulation of gene expression programmes essential for cell proliferation and differentiation. SUMO has thus been shown to play critical roles in the maintenance of genomic integrity and in transcriptional regulation, two processes that involve DNA transactions at the higher-order chromatin level.

Sumoylation of most targets has been shown to require a specific consensus sequence, the ψKxE/D motif, where ψ is a large hydrophobic residue (Leu, Ile, Val) and K is the target Lysine, often separated by one amino acid (x) from an acidic residue (Glu or Asp) [92]. Given that the SUMO pathway relies on only one type of E1 (the Aos1/Uba2 heterodimer) and E2 (Ubc9) activity, the demonstration of a third class of factors, the E3 ligase enzymes, has provided an additional level of control for sumoylation substrate specificity besides the above-mentioned consensus sequence. Three classes of E3 enzymes have been described to date: (1) the SIZ/PIAS (protein inhibitor of activated Stat) [51, 112, 100] and related SP-RING domain proteins [2, 128], (2) RanBP1 [89] and (3) Pc2 [54]. All possess specific subcellular localization properties, suggesting that sumoylation is subject, in part, to strict spatial control within the cell. The further study of these E3 ligases as well as their associated proteins will undoubtedly provide much needed information on the regulation of SUMO modification in vivo.

Neoplastic transformation is both the consequence and the cause of genomic instability. Therefore, understanding how a large and complex genome is faithfully transmitted, and how transmission errors are either prevented or sensed and corrected, is key to understanding carcinogenesis and the development of rational therapeutic strategies. Given the context of the present volume, we will focus this review on the roles played by SUMO and the sumoylation machinery in the regulation of DNA replication, repair and recombination. For the involvement of SUMO in transcriptional regulation [119, 33], nucleo-cytoplasmic trafficking and protein targeting [90] and recent structural insight into the sumoylation reaction [71], the reader is referred to detailed previous reviews. Starting with perhaps the most visible role of sumoylation, the maintenance of proper chromosome structure and function, we will then discuss some of the possible mechanisms responsible at the DNA level. Finally, we will attempt to relate some of these findings to the involvement of SUMO and its substrates in oncogenic or tumour-suppressive mechanisms.

2
At the Chromosomal Level

Defects in DNA replication and repair often manifest themselves at the time of cell division when sister chromatids separate and cells undergo cytokinesis. Reverse genetic approaches using model organisms have thus provided the primary, phenomenological evidence that sumoylation is intimately involved in chromosome structure and function. Mitotic defects, such as anaphase bridges and cohesion defects that lead to chromosome loss or fragmentation, have been associated with mutations in essentially all genes that encode SUMO pathway components (see Table 1 and below). Moreover, cells hypomorphic for, or lacking SUMO, E1, E2 or E3, or Ulp functions, display hypersensitivities to DNA-damaging agents (ionizing radiation, UV or genotoxic chemicals) that either activate cell cycle checkpoints or are the cause of aberrant mitosis (or both). There has been significant progress in our understanding of the underlying molecular mechanisms, and we will first discuss some key findings that link sumoylation with chromosome cohesion, condensation and separation as well as centromere and telomere function.

2.1
Chromosome Cohesion and Condensation

The packaging and replication of higher eukaryotic chromosomes requires a carefully orchestrated series of events mediated by the highly conserved structural maintenance of chromosomes (SMC) proteins and their co-factors [66]. These proteins, divided into three subgroups, ensure

Table 1 Phenotypes of SUMO pathway mutations

Gene/mutation	Phenotypes	References
Saccharomyces cerevisiae		
SMT3 (sumo)	Essential; large budded cells, sister chromatid separation defects	[9]
AOS1 (E1)	Essential; enlarged cells, that are ultimately lysed	[52]
UBA2 (E1)	Essential; G2/M growth arrest with large bud	[23]
UBC9 (E2)	Essential; G2/M phase arrest, large budded cells with a single nucleus, a short spindle and replicated DNA	[99]
SIZ1 (E3) SIZ2/NFI1 (E3)	Single mutants viable; double mutant viable, slower, temperature-sensitive growth, sporulation defect; growth defects rescued by deletion of yeast 2-µm plasmid	[51, 112, 18]
MMS21 (E3)	Essential; mutants DNA damage sensitive (MMS, UV, and bleomycin)	[128]
ULP1 (Ulp)	Essential; ulp1-ts cells arrest in G2/M, single nucleus near bud neck; short spindle	[61]
ULP2/SMT4	Temperature-sensitive growth; severe sporulation defect; abnormal cell and mitotic spindle morphology; plasmid/mini-chromosome loss; hypersensitivity to DNA-damaging agents; impaired Smc4 condensin targeting to rDNA	[62, 97, 109]
Schizosaccharomyces pombe		
pmt3 (SUMO)	Severe growth defects; aberrant cellular and nuclear morphology; chromosome missegregation; centromere/kinetochore defects; increased telomere length	[113]
rad31 (E1)	Viable; growth defects; minichromosome loss; cell and nuclear abnormal morphologies; infrared and UV sensitive	[101]
hus5 (E2)	hus5Δ growth impaired; mitotic abnormalities and misshapen elongated cells; hus5-ts sensitive to HU and infrared	[1]
nse2 (E3)	Essential; Nse2SA mutant cells sensitive to HU and DNA damaging agents	[2, 72]

Table 1 (continued)

Gene/mutation	Phenotypes	References
pli1 (E3)	Viable, no obvious mitotic growth defects; sensitive to TBZ; enhanced minichromosome loss; telomere length increase	[126]
ulp1 (Ulp)	Ulp1Δ show slow growth, severe cell and nuclear abnormalities; sensitivity to UV	[114]
Caenorhabditis elegans		
smo-1 (SUMO)	Essential; maternally rescued mutant develop into sterile adults with abnormal somatic gonad, germ line; lack vulval–uterine connection; protruding vulva	[15, 30, 53]
uba2 (E1)	Embryonic lethality, secondary phenotype: everted vulva	[53]
ubc9 (E2)	Embryonic lethality after gastrulation; maternally rescued mutant with pleiotropic defects in larval development and adult morphology	[53]
gei-17 (CePIAS, E3)	Embryonic lethality; protruding vulva; body morphology defect	[30]
Drosophila melanogaster		
Semushi, *Lesswright* (dUbc9 E2)	Essential; meiotic defects; anterior segmentation defects; melanotic tumours in the haemolymphe at the third instar stage; impairment of bicoid nuclear import; activation of Rel-related proteins	[26, 3, 47]
Su(var)2–10 (dPIAS E3)	Essential; late larval/early pupal lethality; melanotic tumours; chromosome condensation/segregation defects; telomere clustering defects	[40]
Arabidopsis thaliana		
AtSCE1 (E2)	Reduced expression accentuates ABA-mediated growth inhibition	[65]
AtSIZ1 (E3)	Exaggerated prototypical Pi starvation responses, including cessation of primary root growth	[77]
ESD4 (Ulp)	Extreme early flowering and alterations in shoot development	[81]

Table 1 (continued)

Gene/mutation	Phenotypes	References
Chicken		
Ubc9 (E2)	DT-40 cells: cytokinesis defects, multiple nuclei; apoptosis	[42]
Mouse		
Ubc9 (E2)	Early embryonic lethality E5.5; chromosome condensation/segregation defects; nuclear envelope dysmorphy. Disassembly of nucleoli and PML nuclear bodies; perturbation of the RanGTPase nucleo-cytoplasmic gradient	[132]
PIASy (E3)	Viable, fertile; minor Wnt signalling defect	[94, 124]
PIASx (E3)	Viable, fertile; reduced testis weight	[95]
SENP1/SuPr-2 (Ulp)	Embryonic lethality E12.5/E14.5; placental abnormalities	[127]
Human		
SUMO1	Cleft lip and palate phenotype associated with balanced t(2, 8)(q33.1; q24.3) chromosomal translocation disrupting the *SUMO1* locus (*SUMO1* haploinsufficiency)	[133]
SUMO-4 M55V	Polymorphism associated with susceptibility to type 1 diabetes	[13, 82]
SENP1-MESDC2	Constitutional t(12;15)(q13;q25) translocation associated with infantile teratoma	[118]
SUSP1-TCBA1	Chimeric fusion protein of HT-1 T-cell lymphoblastic lymphoma cell line associated with 6q21–22 breakpoint region	[111]

ABA, abscisic acid; HU, hydroxyurea; PML, promyelocytic leukaemia protein; TBZ, thiabendazole the cohesion of sister chromatids (cohesins, SMC1, SMC3), their subsequent condensation in preparation for anaphase chromosome segregation (condensins, SMC2, SMC4) and play important roles in DNA repair (SMC 5–6 complex [72, 86]). The activity of these complexes, together with non-SMC proteins (NSEs), is intimately linked, since, for example, chromosome condensation must occur after the successful resolution of sister chromatids, which, in turn, depends on the proper loading and partial unloading (after DNA synthesis) of cohesin subunits. Hence, dysfunction of proteins involved in cohesion (e.g. Pds5 or Scc1/Mcd1) leads to condensation defects [41, 37]. Recent work (reviewed in [43]) has also underscored the importance of sister chromatid cohesion in the repair of DNA double-strand breaks.

A number of the proteins involved have been shown recently to be modified by SUMO or to participate in the sumoylation of specific targets (see below). Moreover, several earlier studies had already implicated SUMO and sumoylation in chromosome dynamics. For example, the budding yeast SUMO gene (*SMT3*) was first described as a high-copy suppressor of a mutation in the gene for the centromeric Mif2p (CENP-C homologue) protein [76]. A genetic screen for defects in chromosome cohesion similarly yielded *SMT3* [9] and disruption of *SMT4*, the gene for the Smt4p/Ulp2p de-sumoylase, led to impaired condensin targeting to the ribosomal DNA (rDNA) loci [109], a phenotype that could be partially rescued by synthetic over-expression of *SIZ1*, the gene later shown to encode one of the PIAS-type SUMO E3 ligases in budding yeast. In flies, mutation of the putative PIAS family SUMO E3 ligase Su(var)2–10 leads to chromosome segregation defects, enhanced minichromosome loss and abnormal telomere clustering [40], and flies carrying a mutant Ubc9 (E2) allele (*lwr, lesswright*) exhibit dominant suppression of a meiotic non-disjunction phenotype that is the result of a second-site mutation in the meiotic spindle apparatus [3].

A recent study [106] of the budding yeast Pds5 protein provided one possible SUMO target in chromosome cohesion. Pds5 is required for stabilizing the cohesin-chromatin interactions, and it was shown that over-expression of the SUMO protease gene *SMT4* partially rescues the mitotic cohesion defect of a temperature-sensitive *PDS5* mutation. Moreover, Pds5 was also shown to be sumoylated, with a peak of sumoylation at anaphase. This suggests that Pds5 de-sumoylation (promoted by Smt4p/Ulp2) is required for cohesion maintenance, and conversely, that Pds5 sumoylation promotes the dissolution of cohesion required for mitosis.

Another SUMO substrate involved in chromosome cohesion is topoisomerase II (Topo-II; budding yeast Top2), a key enzyme required for the decatenation of sister chromatids prior to chromosome condensation and segregation. The study of budding yeast cells arrested at the G2/M DNA damage checkpoint revealed that mutants for the *SMT4* SUMO protease gene displayed defects in centromeric cohesion, suggesting that over-expressing the (hypo-sumoylated-) SUMO substrate normally targeted by Smt4 might rescue this defect [7]. Indeed, a screen for high-copy suppressors yielded *TOP2*, and the authors showed that expression of a non-modifiable Top2 also partially compensated for the cohesion defect. These observations suggest that sumoylation is necessary both for the resolution of chromatid fibres after DNA synthesis and for the control of untimely separation of sister chromatids in centromeric regions. Consistent with these findings, mammalian centromeres had been shown previously to be enriched in SUMO and sumoylated proteins [27]. Studies using the *Xenopus* system demonstrated that inhibition of sumoylation (using a dominant-negative, catalytically inactive form of Ubc9) leads to chromosome dissociation defects, possibly also as a result of Topo-II hypo-sumoylation [5]. This work, seemingly at odds with that in yeast, also provided evidence that a sub-pool of Topo-II might work non-catalytically by establishing cohesion as a (non-decatenating) protein scaffold that requires sumoylation for dissolution.

2.2
Specialized Chromatin, Centromeres and Telomeres

The special chromatin structure of certain chromosomal regions such as the rDNA loci, the centromeres and telomeres, makes particular demands on the cellular DNA replication, repair and cohesion/condensation systems. One challenge, for example, is to avoid illegitimate homologous recombination between repeated sequences in *cis* or between sister chromatids (in G2), that could lead to loss of genetic material. As mentioned in the previous section, sumoylation is associated with the proper loading of condensins to rDNA [109], and the sumoylation of Ycs4, a budding yeast condensin subunit, has been shown to be involved in the proper condensation and segregation of rDNA [19]. Mutation of the newly described SUMO E3 ligase Mms21p in budding yeast (discussed further in the following section) leads to defects in both nucleolar and telomere structure [128]. Severe nucleolar disaggregation could also be observed in day 5 mouse embryos homozygously inactivated for Ubc9 [132].

Centromeric chromatin, which is the site of kinetochore assembly and microtubule attachment [12], seems particularly sensitive to disruptions of the sumoylation pathway. For example, loss of SUMO (Pmt3p) or of the PIAS-type E3 ligase Pli1p in fission yeast leads to aberrant mitoses, enhanced minichromosome loss, sensitivity to the microtubule poison thiabendazole (TBZ) and loss of transcriptional silencing [113, 126]. Strikingly, mutation of *Pli1*, which is correlated with severe reduction of global cellular sumoylation, also causes a significant increase in gene conversion (homologous recombination) events at the centromeric central core and inner repeat sequences [126]. Sumoylation thus appears to be directly involved in the control of homologous recombination (see the following section). Indeed, this pathway is not only required for the survival of *pli1* mutants but also in de-sumoylating enzyme *ulp1* mutants of budding yeast [105], possibly because it represents the 'last recourse' repair mechanism for replication damage incurred in the absence of sumoylation.

Telomeres consist of specialized heterochromatin that function to protect the ends of linear chromosomes from erosion (i.e. DNA synthesis-associated shortening, the 'end-replication' problem; reviewed in [104]) and the inappropriate activation of DNA damage checkpoints. While sumoylation appears not to affect telomere length in budding yeast [51, 128], SUMO or *pli1* mutants of fission yeast display rapid telomere elongation [113, 126]. Recent work further showed this to require telomerase (B. Xhemalce, E.M. Riising, P. Baumann, A. Dejean, B. Arcangioli and J. Seeler, manuscript submitted), but whether this enzyme or other telomere-associated proteins represent(s) the SUMO target(s) involved, remains an open question. Nonetheless, given the role of telomeres in the control of cell life span (senescence) and in tumour biology, it will be interesting to know whether higher eukaryotic cells possess similar sumoylation-dependent mechanisms for the regulation of telomere length.

3
DNA Replication and Repair

The DNA genome is under constant threat of damage from extrinsic and intrinsic factors, and thus cells have evolved complex systems for damage avoidance and repair. The choice of which system to use depends not only on the type of DNA lesion, but also on the cell cycle phase in which it occurs. Double-strand breaks (DSBs) occurring in G1, for instance, are usually repaired by non-homologous end-joining (NHEJ), whereas in G2, homologous recombination (HR) may make use of the sister chromatids to effect error-free repair. Moreover, it must be borne in mind that DNA repair pathways themselves render cells vulnerable to genomic instability if reaction intermediates [single-stranded DNA (ssDNA), nicks, gaps, double-strand breaks, cleavable complexes, Holliday junctions, etc.] are not properly resolved or at least protected. For example, in budding yeast, mutation of the DNA helicase SGS1 suppresses a mutation in the type 1 topoisomerase TOP3. Epistasis and biochemical analysis has further revealed that *SGS1* and *TOP3* operate in the same pathway and that the activity of Sgs1 creates recombinogenic intermediates that are toxic if not processed by Top3 [31, 28]. DNA replication also has a dual role, as replication fork passage can, on the one hand, provide a second chance to repair previously undetected single-stranded lesions, but, on the other hand, transform these same lesions into more dangerous ones (like DSBs or mutations). Moreover, stalling of replication forks in front of 'normal' sequence secondary structures (e.g. repeats), protein/DNA complexes or upon temporary nucleotide depletion can be harmful since, if left unprotected, such forks may collapse and expose stretches of recombinogenic ssDNA.

One mechanism to restart stalled replication forks uses enzymes encoded by the *RAD6* epistasis group, which form part of a ubiquitylation system required for post-replicative repair (reviewed in [116]). One branch of this system, considered error-prone, uses alternative DNA polymerases for DNA synthesis across the lesions by (so-called translesion synthesis, TLS), while another mechanism uses the information from the undamaged sister duplex to carry out error-free repair. A key study [45] revealed the DNA synthesis processivity clamp PCNA (proliferating cell nuclear antigen, or *pol30* in budding yeast) to be the critical ubiquitin target in this process. Poly-ubiquitin modification of PCNA (via the non-standard K63 linkage, and hence unaffected by proteasomal degradation) was shown to be required for error-free repair of induced DNA lesions. By contrast, mono-ubiquitylated PCNA (achieved by mutating the *UBC13, MMS2* or *RAD5* genes required for ubiquitin polymerization) preferentially channelled repair towards the TLS error-prone system [108, 55, 123]. Interestingly, the ubiquitylated lysine residue of PCNA (K164) was found also to be sumoylated, as was a (non-ubiquitylated) second site (K127). Analysis of the damage sensitivities of PCNA single (K164R) and double (K164/127R) lysine mutations further suggested that sumoylation of PCNA exerts an inhibitory effect on error-free repair, since the non-modifiable double mutant was less sensitive to damaging agents than the K164R single mutant. Consistent with this, mutation of the *SIZ1* gene encoding a SUMO E3 ligase alleviated the damage sensitivity of the PCNA K164R single mutant, and additional genetic experiments showed that this damage sensitivity suppression requires HR, i.e. does not occur in a *RAD52* mutant background. These and other results [38] thus suggested that PCNA sumoylation inhibits HR, and two recent studies [87, 84] provided a mechanism by which this occurs. Based on the finding that mutating the *SRS2* helicase gene (like mutating *SIZ1*) alleviated PCNA K164R damage sensitivity by activating repair by HR, these studies demonstrated that sumoylated PCNA interacts directly with Srs2. Previous work [58, 117] had shown that Srs2 mediates the disruption of Rad51-ssDNA filaments, thus inhibiting this early step in HR. These results thus support a model by which the modification state (mono-, poly-ubiquitin or SUMO) of PCNA regulates the cross-talk between error-prone (TLS) and error-free (HR) post-replicative repair pathways. It will be interesting to see whether this mechanism applies also to other eukaryotes. For example, PCNA is ubiquitylated in mammals [45], but there is as yet no evidence that it is also sumoylated. Nonetheless, several systems support the notion that sumoylation has an inhibitory effect on HR [64, 126]. Perhaps in these systems it is the sumoylation of Rad51, Rad52 or of the helicases (WRN, BLM, RecQl4, see also the next section), rather than that of PCNA, that has taken over this role [102, 64, 56, 44, 24].

The most direct effect of sumoylation on a DNA repair protein was found with thymine DNA glycosylase (TDG), a key enzyme in the base excision repair (BER) pathway. This enzyme recognizes mismatched base pairs (e.g. G:T or G:U) and cleaves the thymine or uracil glycosidic bond for their removal, leaving an abasic (G:_, apurinic, or AP) site. Sumoylation was shown to be required for the enzyme's controlled release from the AP site [39], since premature release would carry the risk of leaving an unprotected, potentially mutagenic gap in the DNA. Subsequent detailed structural studies [6, 107] further confirmed that SUMO attachment to TDG leads to a specific conformational change that reduces the affinity for DNA and thus paves the way for the orderly repair process.

Further evidence for the involvement of SUMO in DNA repair came by the demonstration that a novel SUMO E3 ligase, Mms21 in budding yeast [128] (Nse2 in fission yeast, [2]), forms part of the Smc5/6 complex mentioned previously. Mms21/Nse2 is essential for normal growth, but mutant alleles cause enhanced sensitivity to DNA damaging agents, consistent with previous results implicating the Smc5/6 complex components in mitotic and meiotic chromosome segregation, rDNA disjunction and DNA repair [72, 86, 115]. It was shown that budding yeast Mms21 catalyses sumoylation of Smc5 and yKu70, a bridging protein involved in NHEJ DSB repair, and the fission yeast Nse2 catalyses that of the Smc6 and Nse3 subunits of the Smc5/6 complex. While the functional consequences of these modifications remain unclear, it is interesting that the Smc5/6 complex also contains a RING finger-containing putative ubiquitin E3 ligase (Nse1), thus opening the possibility that this complex, like PCNA, may provide another example of the functional interplay between ubiquitin and SUMO modification.

4
SUMO and Cancer: Caretakers and Gatekeepers

As seen from the previous account, there has been significant progress in our understanding of the role of sumoylation in a variety of biological processes.

In this part of the review we attempt to relate some of these findings to oncogenic and tumour-suppressor mechanisms, at the heart of which lies genomic and organismal integrity [16].

Tumourigenesis is strictly limited to complex organisms with renewable tissues that contain dividing or proliferation competent cells. Cancer can be simplistically defined as a case of aberrant cell hyperproliferation that develops in post-natal tissues and causes organismal disorder that, in most cases, leads to the death of the organism. Complex organisms have evolved specific tumour-suppressor mechanisms to curb uncontrolled cell proliferation. The molecules involved in these mechanisms can be broadly divided into caretakers and gatekeepers [57].

Caretaker tumour suppressors act predominantly on the genome, in principle, by preventing, sensing and repairing DNA damage. Gatekeeper tumour suppressors, on the other hand, act on cells by regulating and implementing apoptosis or cellular senescence. Apoptosis kills and ultimately eliminates cancerous cells, while cellular senescence irreversibly arrests cell growth and thus immobilizes cancerous cells (for further details see, for example, recent reviews on apoptosis and cellular senescence as tumour-suppressor mechanisms [16, 20, 22, 67]). To date, several caretaker proteins have been validated as SUMO substrates, the RecQ-like DNA-dependent helicases Bloom (*BLM*) and Werner (*WRN*) [24, 56, 125], topoisomerases I (Topo-I) [69] and -II (Topo-II) [68], PARP, Ku80, TRAX and XRCC1 [34].

The Bloom gene is mutated in a rare hereditary disorder, Bloom syndrome (BS). BS cells are hypermutable, showing numerous chromatid gaps and breaks and many sister chromatid exchanges (SCEs) [25]. The BLM helicase is a nuclear protein that is differentially regulated during the cell cycle and is distributed throughout the nucleoplasm as well as concentrated in PML nuclear bodies [10, 32]. One of the salient feature of the BLM helicase is its colocalization with proteins involved in DNA damage repair after treatment of cells with DNA damaging agents [122]. Within minutes after DNA damage, BLM starts to appear in foci harbouring γH2AX, RAD50 complex, RAD51, FANCD2 and BRCA1 [21, 29, 88]. Elegant experiments by Eladad et al. [24] provided evidence that sumoylation of BLM plays an essential role for intra-nuclear trafficking and the authors established SUMO modification as a negative regulator of BLM's function in the maintenance of genomic stability. Moreover, cells lacking functional PML show an increased number of sister-chromatid exchanges, most likely due to mislocalization of the BLM protein [129] and it is therefore tempting to speculate that PML nuclear bodies (NBs) act as a storage and modification site for sumoylated BLM.

Defects in *WRN*, another SUMO substrate [56, 125], have also been linked to a hereditary disorder, Werner's syndrome (WS). WS shares several features with BS, most notably a high incidence of cancer. In addition, WS cells, like BS cells, are hypermutable. However, there are marked differences. WS individuals are asymptomatic before puberty, but thereafter develop a panoply of age-related disorders, including cardiovascular disease, cataracts, and osteoporosis. At the biochemical level *WRN* distinguishes itself from other RecQ-like helicases by possessing, apart from its helicase activity, also an N-terminal 3′-5′ exonuclease activity. Several studies have linked *WRN* function to various DNA metabolic processes as for example replication, restoration of stalled replication forks, rDNA transaction mechanisms, homologous recombination and telomere maintenance [8, 83]. WRN is a nuclear protein that is located predominantly in the nucleolus in interphase cells. Upon DNA damage, however, it delocalizes into discrete DNA damage induced foci in the nucleoplasm [36, 70]. Its redistribution appears to be at least in part driven by p14ARF induced sumoylation [125] supporting the notion that WRN plays a crucial role in the cellular response to DNA damage in that its activity is modulated by DNA damage-induced post-translational modifications and possibly WRN-interacting proteins. Moreover, these findings imply that there is an intimate relationship between rDNA metabolism and homeostasis of the cell, which is in part communicated by the modification status of WRN.

Topo-I and -II play essential roles during DNA replication, transcription, recombination and mitosis by relaxation of negatively and positively supercoiled DNA [121]. Topo-II exists in two isoforms α and β, the α isoform being the predominant in proliferating cells [110]. Whereas Topo-I transiently cleaves only a single strand of duplex DNA, Topo-II cleaves both DNA strands simultaneously. Topoisomerases are found in multi-protein complexes that include RP-A, BLM and the RAD51/DMC-I complex among others [79, 73]. Several studies have demonstrated an increased topoisomerase inhibitor sensitivity of cells defective in DNA damage repair proteins, replication checkpoints, or both. For this reason topoisomerases now constitute major cellular targets for numerous anti-cancer drugs, e.g. Topo-I for camptothecin (CPT) and its analogues or Topo-II for VP-16 [63]. Recent results have implicated sumoylation in the regulation of Topo-I [46, 49, 78] and -II activity [4, 5]. In the case of Topo-I, a simple model in which conjugation or de-conjugation of SUMO alters enzymatic activity cannot explain experimental outcomes. Rather, it appears that transient cycles of Topo-I sumoylation and de-sumoylation at different sites within the protein regulate the dynamic association with other protein complexes, thereby modulating the various Topo-dependent processes. Topo-II sumoylation has been shown to play critical roles in centromeric function and sister chromatid segregation during mitosis (mentioned in Sect. 2.1), as well as for the proteasome-dependent turnover of Topo-IIb [4, 5, 48].

For other proteins mentioned in the list above, no clear function has been established for their SUMO-modified forms. Given, however, the functional consequences of SUMO modification on other caretaker tumour suppressors, there is every reason to believe that, in these cases, SUMO will also play a critical role in altering their mode of action.

The ultimate tumour-suppressor gatekeepers in mammalian cells are p53 and the retinoblastoma protein pRB. Both proteins are instrumental in implementing an apoptosis and cellular senescence response as a result of aberrant proliferation, and their genes are found frequently mutated or inactivated in human cancer [103].

The p53 tumour suppressor—a transcription factor that establishes programmes for apoptosis, cellular senescence and repair in response to a variety of cellular insults—is subject to SUMO modification [74], particularly as a consequence of DNA damage [59]. Post-translational SUMO modification was shown to be regulated by MDM2 (murine double minute 2) and p14^{ARF}, two pivotal upstream regulators of p53 stability [17]. MDM2 and its sibling MDMX are themselves subject to sumoylation, but the functional importance of their modification remains unclear. One functional consequence of p53 sumoylation appears to be the modulation of p53 transcriptional activity, but this remains a matter of debate [35, 80, 93, 96]. It also remains an open question as to what extent and in what cellular context(s) sumoylation is important for proper p53 function. Several scenarios are possible. For example, a restricted local modification may alter a specific function of a p53 subset or the entire pool of p53 may undergo transient sumoylation, in both cases to control, for example, p53 residence time in specific protein/protein or protein/DNA complexes. Of further interest is under which physiological conditions (apart from DNA damage) p53 becomes sumoylated and whether sumoylated p53 accumulates during apoptosis or cellular senescence, as has been shown for other post-translational modifications [85, 120]. In this context, work from our laboratory [131] has recently shown that the SUMO E3 ligase PIASy induces premature senescence, and further, that sumoylated p53 plays a role in the execution of this senescence programme.

Identified as the first tumour-suppressor protein, pRB has since been shown to be a master regulator for cellular senescence [14]. Its functionality is predominantly controlled by way of post-translational modifications, in particular phosphorylation. Hypophosphorylated pRB corresponds here with its active state, whereas hyperphosphorylation renders pRB inactive. Recently, also sumoylation of pRB has found its way into spotlight. Ledl et al. [60] identified SUMO modification as a negative regulator of pRB activity. It remains to be seen, however, to what extent sumoylated pRB is found under physiological conditions and what role pRB-SUMO plays in these conditions.

An important mediator for p53 and pRB function is PML [11]. The PML gene was initially identified in patients with acute promyelocytic leukaemia (APL) in which it is fused to the retinoic acid receptor α (RARα) gene as a result of the t(15;17) chromosomal translocation [75]. One of the main features of PML is its concentration within discrete subnuclear structures, termed PML NBs, which are disrupted in a retinoic acid-reversible manner in APL cells [75]. PML was also found among the first proteins subject to sumoylation, and PML modification was shown to be required for proper formation of NBs, recruitment of NB-associated proteins [98] and the expression of the full-blown leukaemogenic potential of the PML-RARα fusion protein [130]. Moreover, PML was implicated in telomere maintenance of cancer cells exhibiting the ALT phenotype (alternative way of telomere lengthening via homologous recombination) [91], where it was found to colocalize with telomeres in so-called ALT-associated promyelocytic leukaemia bodies (APBs). Disruption of this interaction was recently demonstrated by over-expression of a permanent PML NB resident SP100 in ALT cells, leading to repression of ALT-mediated lengthening of telomeres in these cells [50]. Given that both PML and SP100 are important SUMO targets, it would be interesting to see whether sumoylation also plays a significant role in APB function.

5
Conclusion

The studies carried out to date clearly establish sumoylation as a critical regulatory mechanism in pathways protecting genomic integrity. In some cases, e.g. PCNA, this has led to the development of specific models for SUMO function, while in others, we have merely caught a glimpse of the possible roles of this modification. Model organisms and proteomic approaches will continue to provide important tools for the elucidation of the SUMO substrates involved and for the identification of the downstream targets of the modified proteins. The transposition of these findings to models of human disease such as cancer and neurodegenerative disorders should thus provide important insight into the involvement of this modification in both normal and pathological contexts.

Acknowledgements Our apologies to the many authors whose work could not be cited here. Our thanks to Blerta Xhemalce and Benoît Arcangioli for stimulating discussion and permission to cite unpublished work. Work in our laboratory is supported by grants from ARC, LNCC, AICR, the EEC and the Fondation de France. K.N. was supported by the French Ministry of Research and Technology.

References

1. al-Khodairy F, Enoch T, Hagan IM, Carr AM (1995) The Schizosaccharomyces pombe hus5 gene encodes a ubiquitin conjugating enzyme required for normal mitosis. J Cell Sci 108:475–486
2. Andrews EA, Palecek J, Sergeant J, Taylor E, Lehmann AR, Watts FZ (2005) Nse2, a component of the Smc5-6 complex, is a SUMO ligase required for the response to DNA damage. Mol Cell Biol 25:185–196
3. Apionishev S, Malhotra D, Raghavachari S, Tanda S, Rasooly RS (2001) The Drosophila UBC9 homologue lesswright mediates the disjunction of homologues in meiosis I. Genes Cells 6:215–224
4. Azuma Y, Arnaoutov A, Anan T, Dasso M (2005) PIASy mediates SUMO-2 conjugation of Topoisomerase-II on mitotic chromosomes. EMBO J 24:2172–2182
5. Azuma Y, Arnaoutov A, Dasso M (2003) SUMO-2/3 regulates topoisomerase II in mitosis. J Cell Biol 163:477–487
6. Baba D, Maita N, Jee JG, Uchimura Y, Saitoh H, Sugasawa K, Hanaoka F, Tochio H, Hiroaki H, Shirakawa M (2005) Crystal structure of thymine DNA glycosylase conjugated to SUMO-1. Nature 435:979–982
7. Bachant J, Alcasabas A, Blat Y, Kleckner N, Elledge SJ (2002) The SUMO-1 isopeptidase Smt4 is linked to centromeric cohesion through SUMO-1 modification of DNA topoisomerase II. Mol Cell 9:1169–1182
8. Bachrati CZ, Hickson ID (2003) RecQ helicases: suppressors of tumorigenesis and premature aging. Biochem J 374:577–606
9. Biggins S, Bhalla N, Chang A, Smith DL, Murray AW (2001) Genes involved in sister chromatid separation and segregation in the budding yeast *Saccharomyces cerevisiae*. Genetics 159:453–470
10. Bischof O, Kim SH, Irving J, Beresten S, Ellis NA, Campisi J (2001) Regulation and localization of the bloom syndrome protein in response to DNA damage. J Cell Biol 153:367–380
11. Bischof O, Nacerddine K, Dejean A (2005) Human papillomavirus oncoprotein E7 targets the promyelocytic leukemia protein and circumvents cellular senescence via the Rb and p53 tumor suppressor pathways. Mol Cell Biol 25:1013–1024
12. Bjerling P, Ekwall K (2002) Centromere domain organization and histone modifications. Braz J Med Biol Res 35:499–507
13. Bohren KM, Nadkarni V, Song JH, Gabbay KH, Owerbach D (2004) A M55 V polymorphism in a novel SUMO gene (SUMO-4) differentially activates heat shock transcription factors and is associated with susceptibility to type I diabetes mellitus. J Biol Chem 279:27233–27238
14. Bringold F, Serrano M (2000) Tumor suppressors and oncogenes in cellular senescence. Exp Gerontol 35:317–329
15. Broday L, Kolotuev I, Didier C, Bhoumik A, Gupta BP, Sternberg PW, Podbilewicz B, Ronai Z (2004) The small ubiquitin-like modifier (SUMO) is required for gonadal and uterine-vulval morphogenesis in Caenorhabditis elegans. Genes Dev 18:2380–2391
16. Campisi J (2005) Aging, tumor suppression and cancer: high wire-act! Mech Ageing Dev 126:51–58

17. Chen L, Chen J (2003) MDM 2-ARF complex regulates p53 sumoylation. Oncogene 22:5348–5357
18. Chen XL, Reindle A, Johnson ES (2005) Misregulation of 2 micron circle copy number in a SUMO pathway mutant. Mol Cell Biol 25:4311–4320
19. D'Amours D, Stegmeier F, Amon A (2004) Cdc14 and condensin control the dissolution of cohesin-independent chromosome linkages at repeated DNA. Cell 117:455–469
20. Danial NN, Korsmeyer SJ (2004) Cell death: critical control points. Cell 116:205–219
21. Davalos AR, Campisi J (2003) Bloom syndrome cells undergo p53-dependent apoptosis and delayed assembly of BRCA1 and NBS1 repair complexes at stalled replication forks. J Cell Biol 162:1197–1209
22. Dimri GP (2005) What has senescence got to do with cancer? Cancer Cell 7:505–512
23. Dohmen RJ, Stappen R, McGrath JP, Forrova H, Kolarov J, Goffeau A, Varshavsky A (1995) An essential yeast gene encoding a homolog of ubiquitin-activating enzyme. J Biol Chem 270:18099–18109
24. Eladad S, Ye TZ, Hu P, Leversha M, Beresten S, Matunis MJ, Ellis NA (2005) Intranuclear trafficking of the BLM helicase to DNA damage-induced foci is regulated by SUMO modification. Hum Mol Genet 14:1351–1365
25. Ellis NA, German J (1996) Molecular genetics of Bloom's syndrome. Hum Mol Genet 5 Spec No:1457–1463
26. Epps JL, Tanda S (1998) The Drosophila semushi mutation blocks nuclear import of bicoid during embryogenesis. Curr Biol 8:1277–1280
27. Everett RD, Earnshaw WC, Pluta AF, Sternsdorf T, Ainsztein AM, Carmena M, Ruchaud S, Hsu WL, Orr A (1999) A dynamic connection between centromeres and ND10 proteins. J Cell Sci 112:3443–3454
28. Fabre F, Chan A, Heyer WD, Gangloff S (2002) Alternate pathways involving Sgs1/Top3, Mus81/Mms4, and Srs2 prevent formation of toxic recombination intermediates from single-stranded gaps created by DNA replication. Proc Natl Acad Sci U S A 99:16887–16892
29. Franchitto A, Pichierri P (2002) Bloom's syndrome protein is required for correct relocalization of RAD50/MRE11/NBS1 complex after replication fork arrest. J Cell Biol 157:19–30
30. Fraser AG, Kamath RS, Zipperlen P, Martinez-Campos M, Sohrmann M, Ahringer J (2000) Functional genomic analysis of C. elegans chromosome I by systematic RNA interference. Nature 408:325–330
31. Gangloff S, McDonald JP, Bendixen C, Arthur L, Rothstein R (1994) The yeast type I topoisomerase Top3 interacts with Sgs1, a DNA helicase homolog: a potential eukaryotic reverse gyrase. Mol Cell Biol 14:8391–8398
32. Gharibyan V, Youssoufian H (1999) Localization of the Bloom syndrome helicase to punctate nuclear structures and the nuclear matrix and regulation during the cell cycle: comparison with the Werner's syndrome helicase. Mol Carcinog 26:261–273
33. Gill G (2003) Post-translational modification by the small ubiquitin-related modifier SUMO has big effects on transcription factor activity. Curr Opin Genet Dev 13:108–113

34. Gocke CB, Yu H, Kang J (2005) Systematic identification and analysis of mammalian small ubiquitin-like modifier substrates. J Biol Chem 280:5004–5012
35. Gostissa M, Hengstermann A, Fogal V, Sandy P, Schwarz SE, Scheffner M, Del Sal G (1999) Activation of p53 by conjugation to the ubiquitin-like protein SUMO-1. EMBO J 18:6462–6471
36. Gray MD, Wang L, Youssoufian H, Martin GM, Oshima J (1998) Werner helicase is localized to transcriptionally active nucleoli of cycling cells. Exp Cell Res 242:487–494
37. Guacci V, Koshland D, Strunnikov A (1997) A direct link between sister chromatid cohesion and chromosome condensation revealed through the analysis of MCD1 in S. cerevisiae. Cell 91:47–57
38. Haracska L, Torres-Ramos CA, Johnson RE, Prakash S, Prakash L (2004) Opposing effects of ubiquitin conjugation and SUMO modification of PCNA on replicational bypass of DNA lesions in Saccharomyces cerevisiae. Mol Cell Biol 24:4267–4274
39. Hardeland U, Steinacher R, Jiricny J, Schar P (2002) Modification of the human thymine-DNA glycosylase by ubiquitin-like proteins facilitates enzymatic turnover. EMBO J 21:1456–1464
40. Hari KL, Cook KR, Karpen GH (2001) The Drosophila Su(var)2–10 locus regulates chromosome structure and function and encodes a member of the PIAS protein family. Genes Dev 15:1334–1348
41. Hartman T, Stead K, Koshland D, Guacci V (2000) Pds5p is an essential chromosomal protein required for both sister chromatid cohesion and condensation in Saccharomyces cerevisiae. J Cell Biol 151:613–626
42. Hayashi T, Seki M, Maeda D, Wang W, Kawabe Y, Seki T, Saitoh H, Fukagawa T, Yagi H, Enomoto T (2002) Ubc9 is essential for viability of higher eukaryotic cells. Exp Cell Res 280:212–221
43. Hirano T (2005) Cell biology: holding sisters for repair. Nature 433:467–468
44. Ho JC, Warr NJ, Shimizu H, Watts FZ (2001) SUMO modification of Rad22, the Schizosaccharomyces pombe homologue of the recombination protein Rad52. Nucleic Acids Res 29:4179–4186
45. Hoege C, Pfander B, Moldovan GL, Pyrowolakis G, Jentsch S (2002) RAD6-dependent DNA repair is linked to modification of PCNA by ubiquitin and SUMO. Nature 419:135–141
46. Horie K, Tomida A, Sugimoto Y, Yasugi T, Yoshikawa H, Taketani Y, Tsuruo T (2002) SUMO-1 conjugation to intact DNA topoisomerase I amplifies cleavable complex formation induced by camptothecin. Oncogene 21:7913–7922
47. Huang L, Ohsako S, Tanda S (2005) The lesswright mutation activates Rel-related proteins, leading to overproduction of larval hemocytes in Drosophila melanogaster. Dev Biol 280:407–420
48. Isik S, Sano K, Tsutsui K, Seki M, Enomoto T, Saitoh H (2003) The SUMO pathway is required for selective degradation of DNA topoisomerase IIbeta induced by a catalytic inhibitor ICRF-193(1). FEBS Lett 546:374–378
49. Jacquiau HR, van Waardenburg RC, Reid RJ, Woo MH, Guo H, Johnson ES, Bjornsti MA (2005) Defects in SUMO (small ubiquitin-related modifier) conjugation and deconjugation alter cell sensitivity to DNA topoisomerase I-induced DNA damage. J Biol Chem 280:23566–23575

50. Jiang WQ, Zhong ZH, Henson JD, Neumann AA, Chang ACM, Reddel RR (2005) Suppression of alternative lengthening of telomeres by sp100-mediated sequestration of the MRE11/RAD50/NBS1 complex. Mol Cell Biol 25:2708–2721
51. Johnson ES, Gupta AA (2001) An E3-like factor that promotes SUMO conjugation to the yeast septins. Cell 106:735–744
52. Johnson ES, Schwienhorst I, Dohmen RJ, Blobel G (1997) The ubiquitin-like protein Smt3p is activated for conjugation to other proteins by an Aos1p/Uba2p heterodimer. EMBO J 16:5509–5519
53. Jones D, Crowe E, Stevens TA, Candido EP (2002) Functional and phylogenetic analysis of the ubiquitylation system in Caenorhabditis elegans: ubiquitin-conjugating enzymes, ubiquitin-activating enzymes, and ubiquitin-like proteins. Genome Biol 3:
54. Kagey MH, Melhuish TA, Wotton D (2003) The polycomb protein Pc2 is a SUMO E3. Cell 113:127–137
55. Kannouche PL, Wing J, Lehmann AR (2004) Interaction of human DNA polymerase eta with monoubiquitinated PCNA: a possible mechanism for the polymerase switch in response to DNA damage. Mol Cell 14:491–500
56. Kawabe Y, Seki M, Seki T, Wang WS, Imamura O, Furuichi Y, Saitoh H, Enomoto T (2000) Covalent modification of the Werner's syndrome gene product with the ubiquitin-related protein, SUMO-1. J Biol Chem 275:20963–20966
57. Kinzler KW, Vogelstein B (1997) Cancer-susceptibility genes. Gatekeepers and caretakers. Nature 386:761–763
58. Krejci L, Van Komen S, Li Y, Villemain J, Reddy MS, Klein H, Ellenberger T, Sung P (2003) DNA helicase Srs2 disrupts the Rad51 presynaptic filament. Nature 423:305–309
59. Kwek SS, Derry J, Tyner AL, Shen Z, Gudkov AV (2001) Functional analysis and intracellular localization of p53 modified by SUMO-1. Oncogene 20:2587–2599
60. Ledl A, Schmidt D, Muller S (2005) Viral oncoproteins E1A and E7 and cellular LxCxE proteins repress SUMO modification of the retinoblastoma tumor suppressor. Oncogene 24:3810–3818
61. Li SJ, Hochstrasser M (1999) A new protease required for cell-cycle progression in yeast. Nature 398:246–251
62. Li SJ, Hochstrasser M (2000) The yeast ULP2 (SMT4) gene encodes a novel protease specific for the ubiquitin-like Smt3 protein. Mol Cell Biol 20:2367–2377
63. Li TK, Liu LF (2001) Tumor cell death induced by topoisomerase-targeting drugs. Annu Rev Pharmacol Toxicol 41:53–77
64. Li W, Hesabi B, Babbo A, Pacione C, Liu J, Chen DJ, Nickoloff JA, Shen Z (2000) Regulation of double-strand break-induced mammalian homologous recombination by UBL1, a RAD51-interacting protein. Nucleic Acids Res 28:1145–1153
65. Lois LM, Lima CD, Chua NH (2003) Small ubiquitin-like modifier modulates abscisic acid signaling in Arabidopsis. Plant Cell 15:1347–1359
66. Losada A, Hirano T (2005) Dynamic molecular linkers of the genome: the first decade of SMC proteins. Genes Dev 19:1269–1287
67. Lowe SW, Cepero E, Evan G (2004) Intrinsic tumour suppression. Nature 432:307–315
68. Mao Y, Desai SD, Liu LF (2000) SUMO-1 conjugation to human DNA topoisomerase II isozymes. J Biol Chem 275:26066–26073

69. Mao Y, Sun M, Desai SD, Liu LF (2000) SUMO-1 conjugation to topoisomerase I: a possible repair response to topoisomerase-mediated DNA damage. Proc Natl Acad Sci U S A 97:4046–4051
70. Marciniak RA, Lombard DB, Johnson FB, Guarente L (1998) Nucleolar localization of the Werner syndrome protein in human cells. Proc Natl Acad Sci U S A 95:6887–6892
71. Matunis MJ, Pickart CM (2005) Beginning at the end with SUMO. Nat Struct Mol Biol 12:565–566
72. McDonald WH, Pavlova Y, Yates JR 3rd, Boddy MN (2003) Novel essential DNA repair proteins Nse1 and Nse2 are subunits of the fission yeast Smc5-Smc6 complex. J Biol Chem 278:45460–45467
73. Meetei AR, Sechi S, Wallisch M, Yang D, Young MK, Joenje H, Hoatlin ME, Wang W (2003) A multiprotein nuclear complex connects Fanconi anemia and Bloom syndrome. Mol Cell Biol 23:3417–3426
74. Melchior F, Hengst L (2002) SUMO-1 and p53. Cell Cycle 1:245–249
75. Melnick A, Licht JD (1999) Deconstructing a disease: RARalpha, its fusion partners, and their roles in the pathogenesis of acute promyelocytic leukemia. Blood 93:3167–3215
76. Meluh PB, Koshland D (1995) Evidence that the MIF2 gene of Saccharomyces cerevisiae encodes a centromere protein with homology to the mammalian centromere protein CENP-C. Mol Biol Cell 6:793–807
77. Miura K, Rus A, Sharkhuu A, Yokoi S, Karthikeyan AS, Raghothama KG, Baek D, Koo YD, Jin JB, Bressan RA, Yun DJ, Hasegawa PM (2005) The Arabidopsis SUMO E3 ligase SIZ1 controls phosphate deficiency responses. Proc Natl Acad Sci U S A 102:7760–7765
78. Mo YY, Yu Y, Shen Z, Beck WT (2002) Nucleolar delocalization of human topoisomerase I in response to topotecan correlates with sumoylation of the protein. J Biol Chem 277:2958–2964
79. Moens PB, Kolas NK, Tarsounas M, Marcon E, Cohen PE, Spyropoulos B (2002) The time course and chromosomal localization of recombination-related proteins at meiosis in the mouse are compatible with models that can resolve the early DNA-DNA interactions without reciprocal recombination. J Cell Sci 115:1611–1622
80. Müller S, Berger M, Lehembre F, Seeler JS, Haupt Y, Dejean A (2000) c-Jun and p53 activity is modulated by SUMO-1 modification. J Biol Chem 275:13321–13329
81. Murtas G, Reeves PH, Fu YF, Bancroft I, Dean C, Coupland G (2003) A nuclear protease required for flowering-time regulation in Arabidopsis reduces the abundance of small ubiquitin-related modifier conjugates. Plant Cell 15:2308–2319
82. Owerbach D, Pina L, Gabbay KH (2004) A 212-kb region on chromosome 6q25 containing the TAB2 gene is associated with susceptibility to type 1 diabetes. Diabetes 53:1890–1893
83. Ozgenc A, Loeb LA (2005) Current advances in unraveling the function of the Werner syndrome protein. Mutat Res 577:237–251
84. Papouli E, Chen S, Davies AA, Huttner D, Krejci L, Sung P, Ulrich HD (2005) Crosstalk between SUMO and ubiquitin on PCNA is mediated by recruitment of the helicase srs2p. Mol Cell 19:123–133

85. Pearson M, Carbone R, Sebastiani C, Cioce M, Fagioli M, Saito S, Higashimoto Y, Appella E, Minucci S, Pandolfi PP, Pelicci PG (2000) PML regulates p53 acetylation and premature senescence induced by oncogenic Ras. Nature 406:207–210
86. Pebernard S, McDonald WH, Pavlova Y, Yates JR 3rd, Boddy MN (2004) Nse1, Nse2, and a novel subunit of the Smc5-Smc6 complex, Nse3, play a crucial role in meiosis. Mol Biol Cell 15:4866–4876
87. Pfander B, Moldovan GL, Sacher M, Hoege C, Jentsch S (2005) SUMO-modified PCNA recruits Srs2 to prevent recombination during S phase. Nature 436:428–433
88. Pichierri P, Franchitto A, Rosselli F (2004) BLM and the FANC proteins collaborate in a common pathway in response to stalled replication forks. EMBO J 23:3154–3163
89. Pichler A, Gast A, Seeler JS, Dejean A, Melchior F (2002) The nucleoporin RanBP2 has SUMO1 E3 ligase activity. Cell 108:109–120
90. Pichler A, Melchior F (2002) Ubiquitin-related modifier SUMO1 and nucleocytoplasmic transport. Traffic 3:381–387
91. Reddel RR, Bryan TM (2003) Alternative lengthening of telomeres: dangerous road less travelled. Lancet 361:1840–1841
92. Rodriguez MS, Dargemont C, Hay RT (2001) SUMO-1 conjugation in vivo requires both a consensus modification motif and nuclear targeting. J Biol Chem 276:12654–12659
93. Rodriguez MS, Desterro JM, Lain S, Midgley CA, Lane DP, Hay RT (1999) SUMO-1 modification activates the transcriptional response of p53. EMBO J 18:6455–6461
94. Roth W, Sustmann C, Kieslinger M, Gilmozzi A, Irmer D, Kremmer E, Turck C, Grosschedl R (2004) PIASy-deficient mice display modest defects in IFN and Wnt signaling. J Immunol 173:6189–6199
95. Santti H, Mikkonen L, Hirvonen-Santti S, Toppari J, Janne OA, Palvimo JJ (2003) Identification of a short PIASx gene promoter that directs male germ cell-specific transcription in vivo. Biochem Biophys Res Commun 308:139–147
96. Schmidt D, Müller S (2002) Members of the PIAS family act as SUMO ligases for c-Jun and p53 and repress p53 activity. Proc Natl Acad Sci USA 99:2872–2877
97. Schwienhorst I, Johnson ES, Dohmen RJ (2000) SUMO conjugation and deconjugation. Mol Gen Genet 263:771–786
98. Seeler JS, Dejean A (2001) SUMO: of branched proteins and nuclear bodies. Oncogene 20:7243–7249
99. Seufert W, Futcher B, Jentsch S (1995) Role of a ubiquitin-conjugating enzyme in degradation of S- and M-phase cyclins. Nature 373:78–81
100. Sharma M, Li X, Wang Y, Zarnegar M, Huang CY, Palvimo JJ, Lim B, Sun Z (2003) hZimp10 is an androgen receptor co-activator and forms a complex with SUMO-1 at replication foci. EMBO J 22:6101–6114
101. Shayeghi M, Doe CL, Tavassoli M, Watts FZ (1997) Characterisation of Schizosaccharomyces pombe rad31, a UBA-related gene required for DNA damage tolerance. Nucleic Acids Res 25:1162–1169
102. Shen Z, Pardington-Purtymun PE, Comeaux JC, Moyzis RK, Chen DJ (1996) UBL1, a human ubiquitin-like protein associating with human RAD51/RAD52 proteins. Genomics 36:271–279
103. Sherr CJ (2004) Principles of tumor suppression. Cell 116:235–246

104. Smogorzewska A, de Lange T (2004) Regulation of telomerase by telomeric proteins. Annu Rev Biochem 73:177–208
105. Soustelle C, Vernis L, Freon K, Reynaud-Angelin A, Chanet R, Fabre F, Heude M (2004) A new Saccharomyces cerevisiae strain with a mutant Smt3-deconjugating Ulp1 protein is affected in DNA replication and requires Srs2 and homologous recombination for its viability. Mol Cell Biol 24:5130–5143
106. Stead K, Aguilar C, Hartman T, Drexel M, Meluh P, Guacci V (2003) Pds5p regulates the maintenance of sister chromatid cohesion and is sumoylated to promote the dissolution of cohesion. J Cell Biol 163:729–741
107. Steinacher R, Schar P (2005) Functionality of human thymine DNA glycosylase requires SUMO-regulated changes in protein conformation. Curr Biol 15:616–623
108. Stelter P, Ulrich HD (2003) Control of spontaneous and damage-induced mutagenesis by SUMO and ubiquitin conjugation. Nature 425:188–191
109. Strunnikov AV, Aravind L, Koonin EV (2001) Saccharomyces cerevisiae SMT4 encodes an evolutionarily conserved protease with a role in chromosome condensation regulation. Genetics 158:95–107
110. Taagepera S, Rao PN, Drake FH, Gorbsky GJ (1993) DNA topoisomerase II alpha is the major chromosome protein recognized by the mitotic phosphoprotein antibody MPM-2. Proc Natl Acad Sci U S A 90:8407–8411
111. Tagawa H, Miura I, Suzuki R, Suzuki H, Hosokawa Y, Seto M (2002) Molecular cytogenetic analysis of the breakpoint region at 6q21–22 in T-cell lymphoma/leukemia cell lines. Genes Chromosomes Cancer 34:175–185
112. Takahashi Y, Toh-e A, Kikuchi Y (2001) A novel factor required for the SUMO1/Smt3 conjugation of yeast septins. Gene 275:223–231
113. Tanaka K, Nishide J, Okazaki K, Kato H, Niwa O, Nakagawa T, Matsuda H, Kawamukai M, Murakami Y (1999) Characterization of a fission yeast SUMO-1 homologue, pmt3p, required for multiple nuclear events, including the control of telomere length and chromosome segregation. Mol Cell Biol 19:8660–8672
114. Taylor DL, Ho JC, Oliver A, Watts FZ (2002) Cell-cycle-dependent localisation of Ulp1, a Schizosaccharomyces pombe Pmt3 (SUMO)-specific protease. J Cell Sci 115:1113–1122
115. Torres-Rosell J, Machin F, Farmer S, Jarmuz A, Eydmann T, Dalgaard JZ, Aragon L (2005) SMC5 and SMC6 genes are required for the segregation of repetitive chromosome regions. Nat Cell Biol 7:412–419
116. Ulrich HD (2004) How to activate a damage-tolerant polymerase: consequences of PCNA modifications by ubiquitin and SUMO. Cell Cycle 3:15–18
117. Veaute X, Jeusset J, Soustelle C, Kowalczykowski SC, Le Cam E, Fabre F (2003) The Srs2 helicase prevents recombination by disrupting Rad51 nucleoprotein filaments. Nature 423:309–312
118. Veltman IM, Vreede LA, Cheng J, Looijenga LH, Janssen B, Schoenmakers EF, Yeh ET, van Kessel AG (2005) Fusion of the SUMO/Sentrin-specific protease 1 gene SENP1 and the embryonic polarity-related mesoderm development gene MESDC2 in a patient with an infantile teratoma and a constitutional t(12;15)(q13;q25). Hum Mol Genet 14:1955–1963
119. Verger A, Perdomo J, Crossley M (2003) Modification with SUMO. EMBO Rep 4:137–142

120. Vousden KH (2002) Activation of the p53 tumor suppressor protein. Biochim Biophys Acta 1602:47–59
121. Wang JC (2002) Cellular roles of DNA topoisomerases: a molecular perspective. Nat Rev Mol Cell Biol 3:430–440
122. Wang Y, Cortez D, Yazdi P, Neff N, Elledge SJ, Qin J (2000) BASC, a super complex of BRCA1-associated proteins involved in the recognition and repair of aberrant DNA structures. Genes Dev 14:927–939
123. Watanabe K, Tateishi S, Kawasuji M, Tsurimoto T, Inoue H, Yamaizumi M (2004) Rad18 guides poleta to replication stalling sites through physical interaction and PCNA monoubiquitination. EMBO J 23:3886–3896
124. Wong KA, Kim R, Christofk H, Gao J, Lawson G, Wu H (2004) Protein inhibitor of activated STAT Y (PIASy) and a splice variant lacking exon 6 enhance sumoylation but are not essential for embryogenesis and adult life. Mol Cell Biol 24:5577–5586
125. Woods YL, Xirodimas DP, Prescott AR, Sparks A, Lane DP, Saville MK (2004) p14 Arf promotes small ubiquitin-like modifier conjugation of Werners helicase. J Biol Chem 279:50157–50166
126. Xhemalce B, Seeler JS, Thon G, Dejean A, Arcangioli B (2004) Role of the fission yeast SUMO E3 ligase Pli1p in centromere and telomere maintenance. EMBO J 23:3844–3853
127. Yamaguchi T, Sharma P, Athanasiou M, Kumar A, Yamada S, Kuehn MR (2005) Mutation of SENP1/SuPr-2 reveals an essential role for desumoylation in mouse development. Mol Cell Biol 25:5171–5182
128. Zhao X, Blobel G (2005) A SUMO ligase is part of a nuclear multiprotein complex that affects DNA repair and chromosomal organization. Proc Natl Acad Sci USA 102:4777–4782
129. Zhong S, Hu P, Ye TZ, Stan R, Ellis NA, Pandolfi PP (1999) A role for PML and the nuclear body in genomic stability. Oncogene 18:7941–7947
130. Zhu J, Zhou J, Peres L, Riaucoux F, Honore N, Kogan S, de The H (2005) A sumoylation site in PML/RARA is essential for leukemic transformation. Cancer Cell 7:143–153
131. Bischof O, Schwamborn K, Martin N, Werner A, Sustmann C, Grosschedl R, Dejean A (2006) The E3 SUMO ligase PIASy is a regulator of cellular senescence and apoptosis. Mol Cell 22:783–794
132. Nacerddine K, Lehembre F, Bhaumik M, Artus J, Cohen-Tannoudji M, Babinet C, Pandolfi PP, Dejean A (2005) The SUMO pathway is essential for nuclear integrity and chromosome segregation in mice. Dev Cell 9:769–779
133. Alkuraya FS, Saadi I, Lund JJ, Turbe-Doan A, Morton CC, Maas RL (2006) *SUMO1* haploinsufficiency leads to cleft lip and palate. Science 313:1751

Emerging Role for MicroRNAs in Acute Promyelocytic Leukemia

C. Nervi[1] (✉) · F. Fazi[1] · A. Rosa[2] · A. Fatica[2] · I. Bozzoni[2]

[1]Department of Histology and Medical Embryology, University of Rome "La Sapienza" and San Raffaele Bio-medical Park Foundation, Via di Castel Romano 100, 00128 Rome, Italy
clara.nervi@uniroma1.it

[2]Institute Pasteur Cenci-Bolognetti, Department of Genetics and Molecular Biology and I.B.P.M., University of Rome "La Sapienza", P.le A. Moro 5, 00185 Rome, Italy

1	Introduction	74
2	microRNAs	75
3	microRNAs and Hematopoietic Lineage Specificity	77
4	Regulation of miR-223 Expression Levels in Acute Promyelocytic Leukemia	78
5	C/EBPα and NFI-A	79
6	miR-223 Upstream Region	81
7	Concluding Remarks	82
	References	83

Abstract Hematopoiesis is highly controlled by lineage-specific transcription factors that, by interacting with specific DNA sequences, directly activate or repress specific gene expression. These transcription factors have been found mutated or altered by chromosomal translocations associated with leukemias, indicating their role in the pathogenesis of these malignancies. The post-genomic era, however, has shown that transcription factors are not the only key regulators of gene expression. Epigenetic mechanisms such as DNA methylation, posttranslational modifications of histones, remodeling of nucleosomes, and expression of small regulatory RNAs all contribute to the regulation of gene expression and determination of cell and tissue specificity. Deregulation of these epigenetic mechanisms cooperates with genetic alterations to the establishment and progression of tumors. MicroRNAs (miRNAs) are negative regulators of the expression of genes involved in development, differentiation, proliferation, and apoptosis. Their expression appears to be tissue-specific and highly regulated according to the cell's developmental lineage and stage. Interestingly, miRNAs expressed in hematopoietic cells have been found mutated or altered by chromosomal translocations associated with leukemias. The expression levels of a specific miR-223 correlate with the differentiation fate of myeloid precursors. The activation of both pathways of transcriptional regulation by the myeloid lineage-specific transcription factor C/EBPα (CCAAT/enhancer-binding protein-α), and posttranscriptional regulation by miR-223 appears essential for granulocytic differentiation and clinical response of acute promyelocytic leukemia (APL) blasts to all-*trans* retinoic acid (ATRA). Together, this evidence underlies transcription factors, chromatin remodeling, and miRNAs as ultimate determinants for the correct organization of cell type-specific gene arrays and hematopoietic differentiation, therefore providing new targets for the diagnosis and treatment of leukemias.

1
Introduction

Recent progress in molecular biology has shown that control of gene expression at the RNA level, which includes alternative splicing, messenger RNA (mRNA) stability, translation, etc., by expanding protein diversity and abundance, plays a crucial role in cell metabolism and in the ability of the cell to rapidly respond to external stimuli. Many of these processes require the participation of small noncoding RNA molecules (sRNAs) that, in most cases, act as true regulators.

Recently, a new family of microscopic sRNAs [~22 nucleotides (nt) long] has been described that controls gene expression at the posttranscriptional level by cleaving or repressing mRNA in a sequence-specific manner (Sontheimer and Carthew 2005; Meister and Tuschl 2004). The sRNA-mediated pathways are triggered by the presence of double-stranded RNA (dsRNA) molecules that are processed into small interfering RNAs (siRNAs) or microRNAs (miRNAs), depending on the origin of the dsRNA. While siRNAs are produced in response to exogenous DNA (transgenes, viruses) or against transposons mobilization, miRNAs are synthesized by endogenous cellular genes and are involved in physiological processes (Bartell 2004; Sontheimer and Carthew 2005). miRNAs have been shown to regulate mRNA and protein abundance and to participate in many regulatory circuits controlling developmental timing, cell proliferation and differentiation, apoptosis, stress response, hematopoiesis, and patterning of the nervous system (Ambros 2004). The existence of numerous tissue- and developmental stage-specific miRNAs and the evolutionary conservation of many miRNAs argue for numerous additional, yet unidentified, functions of this class of transcripts. Notably, miRNA activity has also been correlated to the pathogenesis of cancer, since miRNAs with oncogenic and tumor-suppressor activity have been identified. Hence, a new molecular taxonomy of human cancers based on miRNA profiling has been proposed (Caldas and Brenton 2005; Calin et al. 2005).

2
microRNAs

Hundreds of miRNAs operating in different organisms have been identified through cloning, genetic, and bioinformatic methods. According to current predictions, 800 or more miRNAs operate in primates and each miRNA may target dozens of mRNAs. Hence, it is estimated that the expression of as many as 30% of human genes may be controlled by miRNAs (Lewis et al. 2005).

Coding regions for miRNA have very peculiar and heterogeneous genomic organizations. Many of them are found in intronic regions and may be transcribed as part of the host gene; however, the majority are located in intergenic regions or in annotated genes but in an antisense orientation, strongly suggesting that they form independent transcription units. miRNAs have been shown to be transcribed by RNA polymerase II (RNA pol II) from transcriptional units that differ from those of protein-coding genes in that they do not possess canonical TATA boxes and are intronless. Nowadays, very little is known about their transcriptional regulation, including the factors responsible for basal and tissue-specific expression (Lewis et al. 2005; Bartell 2004).

The first step in miRNA biogenesis is the nuclear cleavage of a long precursor molecule with partially double-stranded inverted repeat regions (pri-miRNA), which liberates a 60- to 70-nt stem-loop intermediate known as pre-miRNA. This maturation event is performed by a multiprotein complex containing the Drosha nuclear endonuclease and the double-stranded RNA binding domain protein (dsRBD) DGCR8 whose cleavage defines one end of the mature miRNA. This pre-miRNA is actively exported through the exportin-5 pathway and, once in the cytoplasm, is cleaved by the endoribonuclease Dicer to produce a dsRNA in the form of approximately 22-nt RNA duplexes with 2-nt overhanging 3′-ends (Meister and Tuschl 2004). The RNA strand that has the less stable 5′-end is recruited as a single-stranded molecule into the RNA-induced silencing (RISC) effector complex assembled through processes that are dependent on Dicer and other dsRNA-binding proteins, members of the Argonaute (AGO) family, and other factors (Filipowicz 2005; Okamura et al. 2004; Lee et al. 2004). The miRNA pathway is summarized in Fig. 1.

Nearly all animal miRNAs investigated to date regulate gene expression by imperfect base-pairing to the 3′-untranslated region (3′-UTR) of target

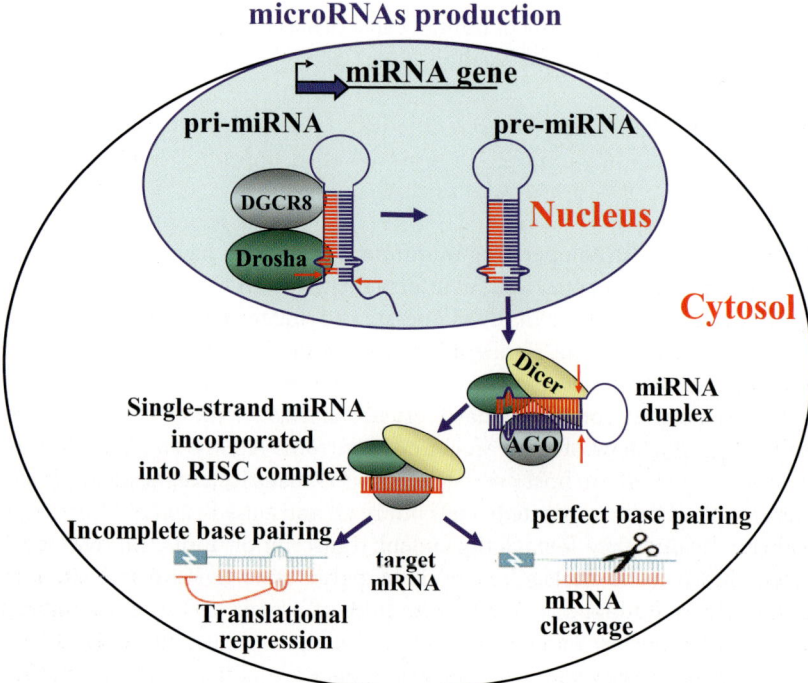

Fig. 1 miRNA production. The initial product of a miRNA gene is a long precursor molecule (*pri-miRNA*) transcribed in the nucleus. It forms a stem-loop structure that is recognized and processed by a protein complex containing the RNAse III Drosha and the dsRBD protein DGCR8 that specifically cleaves the hairpin-shaped RNAs at the basis of the stem loop (indicated by the *red arrows*), thus liberating a 60- to 70-nt precursor miRNA (*pre-miRNA*). Each mature miRNA resides in one of the two sites of the pre-miRNA (represented in *red*). Pre-miRNA is exported to the cytoplasm and cleaved by the RNAse III Dicer, generating a ~22-nt miRNA duplex. The RNA strand (in *red*) is recruited as a single-stranded molecule into the RNA-induced silencing (*RISC*) effector complex and assembled through processes that are dependent on Dicer and other dsRNA-binding proteins, members of the AGO family, and other factors. Perfect or incomplete base pairing between the miRNA and its target respectively directs RISC to either destroy the mRNA or impede its translation into protein

mRNAs and, as a consequence of this binding, they inhibit protein synthesis. On the other hand, perfect pairing to the target mRNA directs cleavage and degradation as in the case of miR-196a and of the majority of plant miRNAs (Ambros 2004).

3
microRNAs and Hematopoietic Lineage Specificity

Since the discovery of *lin-4* and *let-7* in *Caenorhabditis elegans*, the founding members of the miRNA family, and search for their role in the control timing of larval development, the control of development and cell fate has appeared as a common theme for the activity of this novel family of small noncoding RNAs (Bartell 2004). The number of miRNAs identified is continuously growing and their existence has now been proved in all eukaryotic cells. While some of these miRNAs shows ubiquitous expression, others are involved in post-embryonic developmental decisions or are present in specific tissues or cell types (Pasquinelli et al. 2005).

In 2004, Bartel and coworkers studied the expression of four miRNAs (miRs-16, -142, -223 and -181a) cloned from murine bone marrow (Chen et al. 2004). This study is informative for the hematopoietic lineage specific-expression pattern of three of the four miRNAs. In fact, while miR-16 is ubiquitously expressed in all hematopoietic cells and in a wide range of mouse tissues, miR-142 and miR-223 are almost undetectable in nonhematopoietic tissues, except for lung. miR-142 is indeed highly expressed in fetal liver, spleen, bone marrow, and thymus, and miR-223 expression is nearly exclusively associated with the bone marrow. miR-181 is highly expressed in the thymus (mostly containing T lymphocytes), in B lymphocytes from bone marrow, in the spleen but also in the brain and in the lung (Chen et al. 2004).

The analysis of the expression patterns of the miR-142-5, miR-181a, and miR-223 (the human counterparts of the murine miR-181, miR-142s, and miR-223), in hematopoietic cells from normal donors has shown a strong analogy with the murine model system. Indeed, miR-142-5 is found widely expressed in all human hematopoietic cells, miR-181a is present in hematopoietic stem/progenitors CD34$^+$ fraction isolated from bone marrow and human T lymphocytes, while miR-223 is absent in B and T cells but present in the bone marrow with the highest levels in the CD34$^-$ cell fraction, mostly representative of lineage-committed precursors and mature hematopoietic cells (Fazi et al. 2005). More recently, a study by Felli et al. indicates that miR-221 and miR-222 are abundant in hematopoietic stem/progenitors and that their expression levels relate to erythroid differentiation. Moreover, this study indicates the kit receptor mRNA as a functional target of miR-221 and miR-222 in normal erythropoiesis (Felli et al. 2005).

The demonstration that miRNAs are differentially expressed in hematopoietic cells in vivo suggests that miRNAs may play important roles in hematopoiesis and lineage differentiation. Several experimental evidences support this hypothesis: (1) ectopic expression of miR-181 in mouse hematopoietic/stem progenitors cells increases the fraction of B-lineage cells in vitro and in vivo (Chen et al 2004); (2) down-modulation of miR-221 and miR-222 expression levels promotes erythropoiesis of human CD34$^+$ progenitor cells (Felli et al. 2005); (3) up-regulation of miR-223 in human myeloid progenitors promotes granulocytic differentiation (Fazi et al. 2005).

4
Regulation of miR-223 Expression Levels in Acute Promyelocytic Leukemia

Myelopoiesis, which involves growth and maturation of granulocytic and monocytic lineages, is largely controlled by unique combinations of transcription factors such as acute myeloid leukemia (AML)1, PU-1, CCAAT/enhancer-binding protein-α (C/EBPα), core binding factor (CBF)β, retinoic acid (RA) receptor α (RARα), etc., that cooperatively regulate promoters or enhancers present on myeloid-specific genes (Tenen et al. 1997; Salomoni and Pandolfi 2000). Evidence linking miR-223 activation to the RA signaling pathway and C/EBPα in human granulopoiesis was mainly obtained in the acute promyelocytic leukemia (APL) model system (Fazi et al. 2005). APL results from the clonal expansion of hematopoietic progenitors that are blocked at the promyelocytic stage of differentiation. APL is characterized by chromosomal translocations, all involving the RARα gene, resulting in the formation of fusion products that abnormally recruit both histone deacetylase (HDAC) and DNA methyltransferase activities on RA-target promoters. Pharmacological doses of RA overcome this repression and induce terminal differentiation of PML/RARα-positive APL blasts, representing the majority of APLs (Melnick and Licht 1999; Di Croce et al. 2002). The remarkable clinical response to RA treatment, which occurs through the granulocytic differentiation of the leukemic clone, is indeed another important feature of APL (Melnick and Licht 1999; Sanz et al. 2005).

Recent evidence obtained in primary APL blasts undergoing granulocytic differentiation by RA treatment in vivo and in vitro indicates that RA specifically upregulates miR-223 without affecting the expression levels of miR-181a or miR-142. Of note is that:

1. miR-223 expression is strongly increased by RA treatment in RA-responsive myeloid cell lines such as NB4 and HL-60 cells. NB4 is a cell line derived from an APL patient containing the t(15;17) and expressing the promyelocytic leukemia (PML)/RARα fusion product. HL-60 is a myeloid cell line morphologically and biochemically very similar to the APL blasts lacking the t(15;17) but expressing a functional RARα.

2. miR-223 levels are not changed by RA treatment in Kasumi-1 or U937 cells, two myeloid cell lines unresponsive to the effect of RA on granulocytic differentiation (Ferrara et al. 2001).
3. miR-223 levels and granulocytic differentiation are not induced by RA treatment in NB4-MR4 and HL-60R, two RA-resistant subclones of NB4 and HL-60 cells, respectively. These resistant cell lines contain mutations abrogating RA-binding activities of PML/RARα and RARα, respectively (Shao et al. 1997; Tsai et al. 1992).
4. Vitamin D treatment, which induces differentiation of these myeloid cell lines toward the monocytic lineage, does not significantly change the levels of miR-223, thus suggesting a direct involvement of RA binding to either a functional PML-RARα or endogenous wildtype RARα in the upregulation of miR-223 expression during granulopoiesis.

Of note too is that the stable ectopic expression of miR-223 increases the granulocytic differentiation of NB4 cells, while miR-223 knockdown inhibits the response of NB4 cells to the differentiation effect of RA (Fazi et al. 2005). Altogether, these findings directly correlate the levels of miR-223 with the differentiation fate of myeloid precursors.

5
C/EBPα and NFI-A

Important questions in miRNA biology concern, on the one hand, the characterization of the factors controlling miRNAs' expression levels and, on the other, the identification of their target mRNAs. Study of miR-223 expression in APL cells identified two transcriptional factors responsible for the differential expression of this miRNA during granulopoiesis, C/EBPα and nuclear factor I-A (NFI-A) (Fig. 2). Interestingly, one of these activators turned out also to be a target for miR-223 translational repression, thus establishing a regulatory loop circuitry crucial in the control of differentiation.

C/EBPα is a member of the bZIP (basic leucine zipper) family of transcriptional regulators that includes C/EBPβ, ε, γ, and δ. All the members of this family play important roles in development, growth, and differentiation of many cell types. C/EBPα expression has a key role in granulopoiesis. C/EBPα is activated in early myeloid precursors and direct them to granulopoiesis with a concomitant block of monocytic differentiation (Tenen 2003; Radomska et al. 1998). Indeed, C/EBPα knockout mice lack neutrophils and eosinophils but retain monocytes (Zhang et al. 1997; Tenen 2003). Interestingly, C/EBPα is rapidly upregulated during RA-mediated granulocytic differentiation of

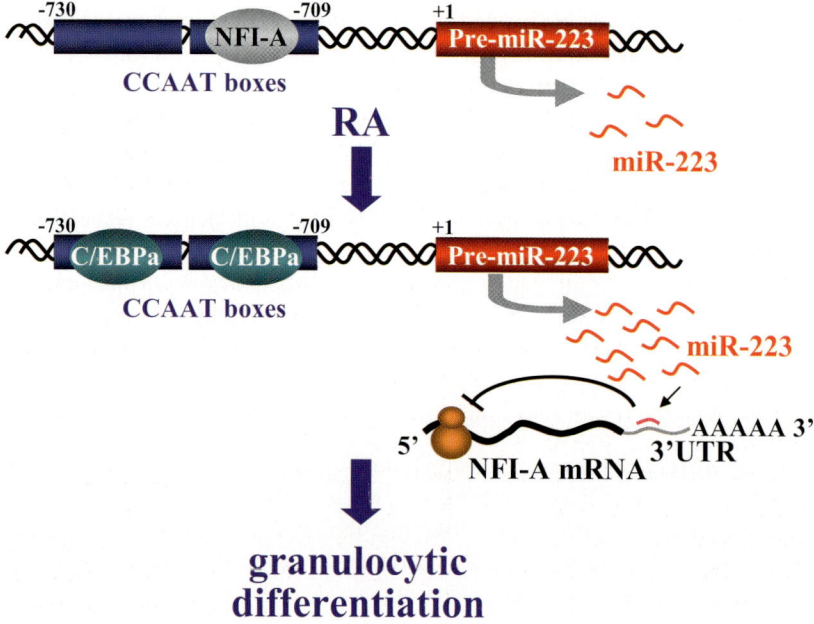

Fig. 2 Schematic representation of the regulatory circuitry involving microRNA-223 and transcription factors NFI-A and C/EBPα in RA-induced granulocytic differentiation of APL blast. The RA-induced activity of the miRNA-223 promoter is mediated by a region lying between bp −730 and −709 relative to the 5′-end of the pre-miR-223. This region contains two putative CCAAT binding sites (*CCAAT boxes*) for C/EBPα and NFI-A. In untreated APL cells, NFI-A constitutively interacts with its site on this sequence, while C/EBPα is not present. NFI-A binding is released upon RA treatment and substituted by that of C/EBPα. This displacement results in the upregulation of miR-223, translational repression of NFI-A mRNA, and granulocytic differentiation of APL blasts

APL blasts, and its constitutive expression in myeloid progenitors results in the induction of granulocytic development and inhibition of monocytic and erythroid development (Radomska et al. 1998). Moreover, overexpression of C/EBPα in transgenic APL mice mimics RA's effect on granulocytic differentiation of APL blasts (Truong et al. 2003). Functionally, C/EBPα binds as a homodimer or heterodimer with other C/EBP proteins or transcription factors at specific two half CCAAT sites on promoters also including differentiation-related genes such as granulocyte colony-stimulating factor (G-CSF) receptor, myeloperoxidase, and neutrophil elastase (Tenen 2003).

The other miR-223 regulator, NFI-A, belongs to the NFI family of proteins, which is composed by four independent genes (NFI-A, -B, -C, and X).

Members of this family are transcriptional factors involved in the replication of adenoviral DNA and in changes of cell growth, oncogenic processes, and disease state (Gronostajski 2000). NFI-A binds as dimers or heterodimers with other members of the NF-I family or other transcriptional factors, to the dyad symmetric consensus sequence TTGGC(N5)GCCAA on duplex DNA (Gronostajski 2000). However, NFI-A specifically binds individual half-sites (TTGGC or GCCAA) and competes with C/EBPs in binding to the CCAAT element (Garlatti et al. 1993). Binding sites for NFI proteins have been identified in genes expressed in virtually every tissue and organ system of vertebrates. An involvement of NFIs in the control of gene expression by a number of hormones and physiological modulators has been also proposed (Gronostajski 2000), but NFIs' role in hematopoiesis has never been demonstrated.

Notably, NFI-A was found among the hundreds of predicted regulatory targets of miR-223 (Lewis et al. 2005; Krek et al. 2005). The analysis of the levels of the NFI-A protein and mRNA before and after RA treatment of NB4 cells suggests that NFI-A is a miR-223 target. The amount of the NFI-A protein decreases with time after RA treatment, whereas the accumulation of its mRNA is unaffected: these are typical features for a miRNA-mediated translational repression of a predicted mRNA target. A reconstitution assay in which miR-223 was co-expressed with a reporter construct containing the 3'-UTR of the NFI-A mRNA fused to the luciferase coding region, allowed the validation of NFI-A as a miR-223 target.

6
miR-223 Upstream Region

The analysis of the sequence upstream of miR-223 revealed the presence of two putative CCAAT binding sites for C/EBPα. One of these two binding elements overlaps with a putative NFI-A binding site (Meisterernst et al. 1988; Garlatti et al. 1993; Gronostajski 2000). Notably, this region mediates the responsiveness to RA (Fazi et al. 2005). Furthermore, C/EBPα interacts with these sites in vivo, and its binding perfectly correlates in time with the start of miR-223 upregulation and granulopoiesis of NB4 cells induced by RA. NFI-A constitutively interacts with this sequence in vivo and its binding is competed by C/EBPα upon RA treatment. Notably, in RA-resistant cells, which are unable to undergo differentiation, the NFI-A factor remains on the miR-223 promoter and no C/EBPα binding is detected. In agreement, RNA interference (RNAi) experiments proved that NFI-A and C/EBPα do indeed act as miR-223 transactivators before and after RA-treatment, respectively. The knockdown of C/EBPα results in decreased levels of miR-223 after RA treatment, whereas the decrease of NFI-A results in reduced levels of miR-223 in the absence of RA. These findings support the hypothesis of a competition between the two transcriptional factors in the regulation of the miRNA expression, NFI-A producing low levels of miR-223 and C/EBPα being the differentiation-specific activator of its expression. In line with this, both RNAi against NFI-A and ectopic expression of miR-223 in APL cells enhance granulocytic differentiation, whereas miR-223 knockdown inhibits the differentiation response to RA. These findings indicate that miR-223 plays a crucial role during granulopoiesis and point to the NFI-A repression as an important molecular pathway mediating gene reprogramming in APL blasts.

7
Concluding Remarks

miRNAs are evolutionarily conserved gene regulatory molecules acting both spatially and temporally during development that also show restricted expression profiles in adult tissues. Since modification of the miRNA expression profiles have been found related to neoplastic transformation, miRNAs and their target genes are now regarded as a potential new class of tumor suppressors or oncogenes (Chen 2005; Caldas and Brenton 2005).

Interestingly, lineage-specific transcription factors regulating normal hematopoietic differentiation and miRNAs expressed in hematopoietic cells have been found mutated or consistently altered by chromosomal translocations associated with leukemias, indicating their role in the pathogenesis of these malignancies (Rabbitts 1994; Salomoni and Pandolfi 2000; Tenen 2003; Calin et al. 2005). Indeed, miR-142, miR-15, and miR-16 are present at sites of translocation breakpoints or deletions connected to human lymphocytic leukemias. Mutations of miR-15 and miR-16 have been also described in the same leukemia (Calin et al. 2005). In APL, the activation of both pathways of transcriptional regulation by the lineage-specific transcription factor C/EBPα, and posttranscriptional regulation by miR-223 appear essential for granulocytic differentiation and clinical response to RA (Tenen 2003; Fazi et al. 2005). Interestingly, different wide screening approaches performed to establish miRNA expression profiles show a unique miRNA signature relevant for the pathogenesis, diagnosis, and prognosis of myeloid and lymphoid leukemias (Lu et al. 2005; Calin et al. 2005). This underlies both transcription factors and miRNAs as ultimate determinants of the correct organization of cell type-specific gene arrays that control hematopoietic differentiation, therefore providing new targets for the diagnosis and treatment of leukemias.

References

Ambros V (2004) The function of animal miRNAs. Nature 431:350–355
Bartell DP (2004) MicroRNAs: genomics, biogenesis, mechanism and function. Cell 116:281–297
Caldas C, Brenton JD (2005) Sizing up miRNAs as cancer genes. Nat Med 11:712–714
Calin GA, Ferracin M, Cimmino A, Di Leva G, Shimizu M, Wojcik SE, Iorio MV, Visone R, Sever NI, Fabbri M, Iuliano R, Palumbo T, Pichiorri F, Roldo C, Garzon R, Sevignani C, Rassenti L, Alder H, Volinia S, Liu CG, Kipps TJ, Negrini M, Croce CM (2005) A MicroRNA signature associated with prognosis and progression in chronic lymphocytic leukemia. N Engl J Med 353:1793–1801
Chen CZ (2005) MicroRNAs as oncogenes and tumor suppressors. N Engl J Med 353:1768–1771
Chen CZ, Li L, Lodish HF, Bartell DP (2004) MicroRNAs modulate hematopoietic lineage differentiation. Science 303:83–86
Di Croce L, Raker VA, Corsaro M, Fazi F, Fanelli M, Faretta M, Fuks F, Lo Coco F, Kouzarides T, Nervi C, Minucci S, Pelicci PG (2002) Methyltransferase recruitment and DNA hypermethylation of target promoters by an oncogenic transcription factor. Science 295:1079–1082
Fazi F, Rosa A, Fatica A, Gelmetti V, De Marchis ML, Nervi C, Bozzoni I (2005) A minicircuitry comprising microRNA-223 and transcription factors NFI-A and C/EBPα regulates human granulopoiesis. Cell 123:819–831
Felli N, Fontana L, Pelosi E, Botta R, Bonci D, Facchiano F, Liuzzi F, Lulli V, Morsilli O, Santoro S, Valtieri M, Calin GA, Liu CG, Sorrentino A, Croce CM, Peschle C (2005) MicroRNAs 221 and 222 inhibit normal erythropoiesis and erythroleukemic cell growth via Kit receptor downmodulation. Proc Natl Acad Sci U S A 102:18081–18086
Ferrara FF, Fazi F, Bianchini A, Padula F, Gelmetti V, Minucci S, Mancini M, Pelicci PG, Lo Coco F, Nervi C (2001) Histone deacetylase targeted treatment restores retinoic acid signaling and differentiation in acute myeloid leukemia. Cancer Res 61:2–7
Filipowicz W (2005) RNAi: the nuts and bolts of the RISC machine. Cell 122:17–20
Garlatti M, Tchesnokov V, Daheshia M, Feilleux-Duche S, Hanoune J, Aggerbeck M, Barouki R (1993) CCAAT/enhancer-binding protein-related proteins bind to the unusual promoter of the aspartate aminotransferase housekeeping gene. J Biol Chem 268:6567–6574
Gronostajski RM (2000) Roles of the NFI/CTF gene family in transcription and development. Gene 249:31–45
Krek A, Grun D, Poy MN, Wolf R, Rosenberg L, Epstein EJ, MacMenamin P, da Piedade I, Gunsalus KC, Stoffel M, Rajewsky N (2005) Combinatorial microRNA target predictions. Nat Genet 37:495–500
Lee YS, Nakahara K, Pham JW, Kim K, He Z, Sontheimer EJ, Carthew RW (2004) Distinct roles for Drosophila Dicer-1 and Dicer-2 in the siRNA/miRNA silencing pathways. Cell 117:69–81
Lewis BP, Burge CB, Bartel DP (2005) Conserved seed pairing, often flanked by adenosines, indicates that thousands of human genes are microRNA targets. Cell 120:15–20

Lu J, Getz G, Miska EA, Alvarez-Saavedra E, Lamb J, Peck D, Sweet-Cordero A, Ebert BL, Mak RH, Ferrando AA, Downing JR, Jacks T, Horvitz HR, Golub TR (2005) MicroRNA expression profiles classify human cancers. Nature 435:834–838

Meister G, Tuschl T (2004) Mechanisms of gene silencing by double-stranded RNA. Nature 431:343–349

Meisterernst M, Gander I, Rogge L, Winnacker EL (1988) A quantitative analysis of nuclear factor I/DNA interactions. Nucleic Acids Res 16:4419–4435

Melnick A, Licht JD (1999) Deconstructing a disease: RARα, its fusion partners, and their roles in the pathogenesis of acute promyelocytic leukemia. Blood 93:3167–3215

Okamura K, Ishizuka A, Siomi H, Siomi MC (2004) Distinct roles for Argonaute proteins in small RNA-directed RNA cleavage pathways. Genes Dev 18:1655–1666

Pasquinelli AE, Hunter S, Bracht J (2005) MicroRNAs: a developing story. Curr Opin Genet Dev 15:200–205

Rabbitts TH (1994) Chromosomal translocations in human cancer. Nature 372:143–149

Radomska HS, Huettner CS, Zhang P, Cheng T, Scadden DT, Tenen DG (1998) CCAAT/enhancer binding protein alpha is a regulatory switch sufficient for induction of granulocytic development from bipotential myeloid progenitors. Mol Cell Biol 18:4301–4314

Salomoni P, Pandolfi PP (2000) Transcriptional regulation of cellular transformation. Nat Med 6:742–744

Sanz MA, Tallman MS, Lo-Coco F (2005) Tricks of the trade for the appropriate management of newly diagnosed acute promyelocytic leukemia. Blood 105:3019–3025

Shao W, Benedetti L, Lamph WW, Nervi C, Miller WHJ (1997) A retinoid-resistant acute promyelocytic leukemia subclone expresses a dominant negative PML-RARα mutation. Blood 89:4282–4289

Sontheimer EJ, Carthew RW (2005) Silence from within: endogenous siRNAs and miRNAs. Cell 122:9–12

Tenen DG (2003) Disruption of differentiation in human cancer: AML shows the way. Nat Rev Cancer 3:89–101

Tenen DG, Hromas R, Licht JD, Zhang DE (1997) Transcription factors, normal myeloid development, and leukemia. Blood 90:489–519

Truong BT, Lee YJ, Lodie TA, Park DJ, Perrotti D, Watanabe N, Koeffler HP, Nakajima H, Tenen DG, Kogan SC (2003) CCAAT/Enhancer binding proteins repress the leukemic phenotype of acute myeloid leukemia. Blood 101:1141–1148

Tsai S, Bartelmez S, Heyman RA, Damm K, Evans RM, Collins SJ (1992) A mutated retinoic acid receptor-α exhibiting dominant-negative activity alters the lineage development of a multipotent hematopoietic cell line. Genes Dev 6:2258–2269

Zhang DE, Zhang P, Wang ND, Hetherington CJ, Darlington GJ, Tenen DG (1997) Absence of granulocyte colony-stimulating factor signaling and neutrophil development in CCAAT enhancer binding protein alpha-deficient mice. Proc Natl Acad Sci U S A 94:569–574

The Theory of APL Revisited

P. P. Scaglioni · P. P. Pandolfi (✉)

Cancer Biology and Genetics Program, Memorial Sloan-Kettering Cancer Center, Sloan-Kettering Institute, 1275 York Avenue, 10021, NY New York, USA
p-pandolfi@ski.mskcc.org

1	Introduction	86
2	The Fusion Proteins of APL Are Oncogenes of the Early Myeloid Hematopoietic Compartment	87
3	X-RARα Proteins Are Necessary but Not Sufficient to Cause Leukemia and Represent Biologically Distinct RARα Mutants	88
4	RARα-X Proteins Do Play a Critical Role in APL Leukemogenesis, but Are Not Sufficient for Full-Blown Transformation	88
5	Multiple Genetic Hits in APL Pathogenesis	89
6	X Molecules Are Involved in the Control of the Cell Mitogenic and Survival Signals, and of Genomic Stability	90
7	The Crosstalk Between X and RAR/RXR Pathways	91
8	X Haploinsufficiency and Functional Interference of X-RARα and RARα-X with X-Regulated Pathways Is Critical for APL Leukemogenesis	92
9	The X Moiety Lends to the X-RARα Fusion Protein Distinct Gain-of-Function Proteins	93
10	Conclusions and Future Directions	93
10.1	Identification and Validation of Cooperative Events and X-RARα and RARα Target Genes	95
10.2	Beyond APL: A Role for the Genes of APL in Other Malignancies	95
References		96

Abstract Acute promyelocytic leukemia (APL) is associated with reciprocal and balanced chromosomal translocations always involving the retinoic acid receptor α (RARα) gene on chromosome 17 and variable partner genes (X genes) on distinct chromosomes. RARα fuses to the PML gene in the majority of APL cases, and in a few cases to the PLZF, NPM, NuMA and STAT5b genes. As a consequence, X-RARα and RARα-X fusion genes are generated encoding aberrant chimeric proteins that exert critical oncogenic functions. Here we will integrate some of the most recent findings in APL research in a unified model and discuss some of the outstanding questions that remain to be addressed.

1
Introduction

Acute promyelocytic leukemia (APL) is associated with a reciprocal and balanced translocation always involving the retinoic acid receptor α (RARα) gene on chromosome 17, which translocates to the PML gene (promyelocytic leukemia gene, originally named *myl*) on chromosome 15 (de The et al. 1991; Goddard et al. 1991; Kakizuka et al. 1991; Pandolfi et al. 1991). In a few variant cases, RARα fuses to the promyelocytic leukemia zinc finger (PLZF) gene, nucleophosmin (NPM) gene, nuclear mitotic apparatus (NuMA) gene, and signal transducer and activator of transcription 5b (STAT5b) gene, which are located on chromosomes 11, 5, 11, and 17 respectively (Chen et al. 1993; Redner et al. 1996; Wells et al. 1997; Arnould et al. 1999). In view of the reciprocity of these translocations, X-RARα and RARα-X fusion genes are generated and coexpressed in the APL blasts in the majority of cases. Although rare, these variant translocations have been tremendously informative, allowing a comparative analysis of molecular and biological similarities and differences among the various fusion proteins. Since the RARα gene always breaks within the same intron, the various fusion proteins are coherent in the RARα moiety but do not bear structural similarities in the X moiety, and yet the disease associated with these molecular lesions is APL.

The RARα portion of the X-RARα fusion protein can mediate heterodimerization with RXR, as well as DNA and ligand binding through the retinoic acid (RA) and DNA binding domains (Perez et al. 1993). Therefore, the X-RARα fusion products invariably retain the ability to potentially interfere with the RAR/RXR pathways. The various X-RARα proteins also display the capacity of heterodimerizing with the respective X proteins (e.g., PML-RARα with PML etc.). This is due to the fact that X proteins are normally capable of homodimerizing and that the region that mediates X protein homodimerization is invariably retained in the X moieties fused to RARα (Liu and Chan 1991; Perez et al. 1993; Bardwell and Treisman 1994; Redner et al. 1996; Wells et al. 1997; Arnould et al. 1999). Thus, X-RARα can potentially interfere with both X and RARα pathways. Since the identification of PML-RARα, it has been hypothesized that the X-RARα fusion protein would act as a double dominant-negative (DN) mutant on PML and RARα pathways. This hypothesis was put forward on the basis of the observation that PML-RARα, unlike RARα, acts as a transcriptional repressor at physiologic concentration of the ligand (RA), and that PML-RARα can also cause the disruption of the PML nuclear bodies (NBs) where PML normally accumulates. As we will discuss, this notion has to be reconciled with more recent findings that have defined that the PML-RARα aberrant transcriptional activity is also due to "gain of function" properties. Furthermore, progress has been made at defining the repressive mechanisms of PML-RARα.

The RARα-X fusion protein also shares important functional regions with the various X proteins fused to the A transactivation domain of RARα and can therefore play an active cooperative role in APL pathogenesis.

A number of firm conclusions and definitive answers have been obtained throughout the years concerning the cooperative events and mechanisms underlying APL pathogenesis. Analysis of knockout (KO) and transgenic animal models (TM) has been invaluable to this end. Here we will summarize these conclusions and integrate them on the basis of information accrued in the last few years. We will also discuss the outstanding questions and the possible directions of APL research in the years to come.

2
The Fusion Proteins of APL Are Oncogenes of the Early Myeloid Hematopoietic Compartment

The generation of mouse models that faithfully recapitulate APL pathogenesis led to important conclusions regarding the role of various X-RARα and RARα-X fusion proteins in APL pathogenesis. This analysis allowed us to conclude that expression of the fusion proteins must be directed and possibly restricted to the appropriate cellular compartment, namely the early myeloid progenitor pool, for them to exert their full oncogenic potential. Expression of the PML-RARα fusion protein in the myeloid promyelocytic compartment leads to APL-like disease in transgenic mice (Grisolano et al. 1997; He et al. 1997; Brown et al. 1997), while ubiquitous and unrestricted expression of the fusion gene results in embryonic lethality (He et al. 1997; P.P. Pandolfi, unpublished observation). Expression of PML-RARα in early pluripotent hematopoietic progenitors or in mature myeloid cells did not result in leukemia either (P. Greer, personal communication; Early et al. 1996). Most recently, it was also reported that retroviral transduction of PML-RARα in murine hematopoietic progenitors results in the development of APL-leukemia, although in this experimental setting it is not known what the target cell of the retrovirus would be (Minucci et al. 2002). The concomitant generation of KO mice and cells, where the various X genes are inactivated by homologous recombination, has also been extremely informative in assessing the consequences of the reduction to heterozygosity or the complete inactivation of X gene function in TM harboring APL fusion proteins, and in elucidating the normal function of these genes.

3
X-RARα Proteins Are Necessary but Not Sufficient to Cause Leukemia and Represent Biologically Distinct RARα Mutants

Characterization of PML-RARα, PLZF-RARα, NPM-RARα, and NUMA-RARα TM in which the expression of the fusion gene is restricted to the promyelocytic compartment has revealed that the X-RARα fusion proteins play a critical causal role in leukemogenesis. PML-RARα and NuMA-RARα TM develop, in fact, APL leukemia, NPM-RARα develops a myelo-monocytic acute leukemia, while PLZF-RARα TM develop a myeloproliferative disorder reminiscent of human chronic myelogenous leukemia (CML) rather than of human APL (Grisolano et al. 1997; Brown et al. 1997; He et al. 1997, 1998; Sukhai et al. 2004; Rego et al. 2006). In addition, X-RARα molecules dictate sensitivity to RA treatment. For example, PLZF-RARα mice develop RA-resistant, while PML-RARα mice develop RA-responsive leukemia (Grisolano et al. 1997; He et al. 1997, 1998). Taken together, these observations indicate that X-RARα molecules act as bona fide oncogenes, but do not represent identical RARα mutants, strongly suggesting that the X-moiety lends the X-RARα fusion proteins distinct biological properties. Furthermore, TM harboring a PML-RARα mutant (M4) that can no longer bind RA develop an APL-like RA-resistant leukemia. This observation indicates that ligand-dependent transactivation by the PML-RARα fusion protein is not required for leukemogenesis and lends further support to the suggestion that the X-moiety of the APL fusion proteins exerts a critical leukemogenic function (Kogan et al. 2000; Matsushita et al. 2006).

4
RARα-X Proteins Do Play a Critical Role in APL Leukemogenesis, but Are Not Sufficient for Full-Blown Transformation

Comparative characterization of RARα-X TM has determined that these molecules do not display transforming ability per se but do display an important cooperative role with the X-RARα molecules in APL leukemogenesis.

RARα-PML and RARα-PLZF TM do not develop full-blown leukemia but instead a myeloproliferative disorder without an apparent block in myeloid differentiation (Pollock et al. 1999; He et al. 2000). In PML-RARα/RARα-PML double TM, the RARα-PML transgene increases the penetrance and the onset of leukemia, thus acting as a classic tumor modifier (Pollock et al. 1999). Interestingly, in PLZF-RARα/RARα-PLZF double TM, RARα-PLZF metamorphoses the CML phenotype observed in single PLZF-RARα TM into an APL-like acute leukemia (He et al. 2000). Leukemia onset in double TM is still preceded by a long preleukemic phase (Pollock et al. 1999; He et al. 2000), which suggests that other cooperative genetic events are still needed for full-blown transformation. RARα-X plays therefore an important role in APL leukemogenesis acting as a tumor modifier (RARα-PML), tumor metamorphoser (RARα-PLZF), or both. When these molecules are not expressed in human APL, as it is the case in 30% of t(15;17) APL and very rarely in t(11;17) APL, their function could be substituted by additional, yet unknown, genetic events. These findings in turn underscore the "qualitative nature" of the multistep leukemogenesis process in APL. In fact, the phenotype observed in the PLZF-RARα/RARα-PLZF double TM is not the result of the simple addition of the phenotypes observed in single TM. Neither of these mutants in fact displays the distinctive promyelocytic block of differentiation, which is only observed in double TM. The phenotype is instead a qualitatively novel biological outcome due to the aberrant molecular activities of at least two molecules (He et al. 2000).

5
Multiple Genetic Hits in APL Pathogenesis

The long latency observed in the various mouse models of APL strongly suggests that additional genetic events may cooperate with the APL-specific fusion proteins toward leukemogenesis. The same events could contribute to the pathogenesis of human APL. The identification of such mutated/deregulated genes will further improve our understanding of the genetics and molecular basis underlying APL leukemogenesis and will allow the identification of novel therapeutic targets. Several technological approaches are now available that render the identification of these additional genetic hits possible both in human and murine leukemic cells. For example, spectral karyotyping (SKY), a more sensitive karyological technique, has already determined that leukemic cells from PML-RARα and PLZF-RARα TM do indeed harbor multiple recurrent chromosomal abnormalities (Zimonjic et al. 2000; Le Beau et al. 2002, 2003; P.P. Scaglioni, H. Matsushita, and P.P. Pandolfi, unpublished results). As an example, these studies indicated that an interstitial deletion of chromosome 2 is one of the most common recurrent chromosomal abnormalities in murine APL models. Genetic characterization of this region led to the discovery that loss of one copy of PU.1, a master regulator of hematopoietic development, increases APL penetrance in mice expressing PML-RARα (Walter et al. 2005). These findings suggest that PU.1 functional loss may contribute to human APL leukemogenesis and provide the rationale for the validation and identification of such cooperative genetic events in primary human APL samples.

6
X Molecules Are Involved in the Control of the Cell Mitogenic and Survival Signals, and of Genomic Stability

Analysis of $X^{-/-}$ mice and cells has, in the last few years, corroborated the notion that the blockade or the interference with pathways normally regulated by these molecules can indeed play a critical role in APL pathogenesis. While the main outcome resulting from X gene heterozygosity and the interference of the fusion protein with the function of the remaining normal X allele product was originally proposed to lend a proliferative and survival advantage to the leukemic cells, more recent data indicate that these events may also cause an underlying genomic instability that could greatly contribute to APL multistep leukemogenesis. Analysis of PML, PLZF, and NPM KO mice is currently ongoing and has been instrumental in reaching these conclusions. Primary PML KO cells such as mouse embryonic fibroblasts (MEFs) or primary thymocytes display a marked proliferative advantage (Wang et al. 1998a). Furthermore, $PML^{-/-}$ cells of various histological origins including hematopoietic cells and $PML^{-/-}$ mice are protected from multiple apoptotic stimuli such as ionizing radiation (Wang et al. 1998b; Quignon et al. 1998). In this respect, PML has been found to modulate both p53-dependent (Fogal et al. 2000; Guo et al. 2000) and p53-independent (Torii et al. 1999; Zhong et al. 2000) apoptotic pathways. PML inactivation markedly impairs cellular senescence induced by oncogenic Ras, as well as by transforming growth factor (TGF)-β (Pearson et al. 2000; Ferbeyre et al. 2000; Lin et al. 2004). In addition, cytoplasmic forms of PML have also been found to modulate the tumor-growth tumor suppressive role of TGF-β, while PML-RARα can oppose the function of PML toward TGF-β (Lin et al. 2004). Finally, $PML^{-/-}$ mice are more susceptible to tumorigenesis when challenged with carcinogens as well as spontaneously (Wang et al. 1998a; Trotman et al. 2006). Analysis of $PLZF^{-/-}$ mice and cells revealed that the inactivation of this gene also results in a proliferative and survival advantage throughout embryonic development in various cellular compartments (Barna et al. 2000; Costoya et al. 2004).

Analysis of NPM$^{-/-}$ cells and embryos has more recently allowed us to determine that NPM heterozygosity results in genomic instability as a consequence of aberrant centrosome amplification (Grisendi et al. 2005; Grisendi et al. in press). PML inactivation has been previously shown to cause an increased rate of sister-chromatid exchange (SCE), which also underlies genetic instability (Zhong et al. 1999b). Thus, it is reasonable to propose that X gene haploinsufficiency and/or the interference of the X-RARα and RARα-X fusion proteins with their functions may result in genomic instability, hence favoring the accumulation of additional genetic hits toward overt leukemogenesis.

Furthermore, characterization of PLZF$^{-/-}$ mutants indicates that X genes may exert a key role in stem cell biology and maintenance (Costoya et al. 2004; Piazza et al. 2004). It remains to be seen if the same is true for the other X genes and if this is of relevance to the pathogenesis of APL.

X gene inactivation in the mouse is therefore uncovering functional commonalities among the partners of RARα involved in the various APL-associated chromosomal translocations. These functions may be deregulated in APL as a consequence of aberrant fusion protein activity.

7
The Crosstalk Between X and RAR/RXR Pathways

Analysis of X$^{-/-}$ mice and cells has also revealed that the X and RARα pathways could functionally interact. This in turn suggests that the X-RARα and RARα-X fusion proteins by interfering with the X pathway affect the RARα pathway and vice versa. It was shown that PML is required for the differentiating and growth inhibitory activities of RA. Induction of myeloid differentiation and the ability of RA to induce growth arrest in MEFs are impaired in PML$^{-/-}$ cells and mice (Wang et al. 1998a). Subsequently, PML was found to act as a ligand-dependent coactivator of RXRα/RARα through its ability to interact with the Tif1α and CREB-binding protein (CBP) transcriptional cofactors. In PML$^{-/-}$ cells, the RA-dependent induction of genes such as *RARβ2* and the ability of Tif1α and CBP to act as transcriptional coactivators upon RA are in turn impaired (Zhong et al. 1999a). Taken together, these data demonstrate that the PML and RARα pathways crosstalk and that PML-RARα can in principle disrupt the RA-dependent activity of a tumor-growth suppressive transcription complex in a DN manner at multiple levels (both on DNA and in the absence of a direct DNA binding activity through heterodimerization with PML), resulting in growth advantage and RA unresponsiveness. It remains to be determined whether this is also true for the other X-RARα fusion proteins, their reciprocal products, or a combination of the two.

8
X Haploinsufficiency and Functional Interference of X-RARα and RARα-X with X-Regulated Pathways Is Critical for APL Leukemogenesis

In vivo analysis of APL transgenic mice has provided genetic evidence that the various X-RARα proteins can interfere with X pathways. It is now becoming apparent that this property is also shared by the RARα-X fusion proteins. For instance, RARα-PLZF can bind the PLZF DNA responsive element through seven out of the nine zinc-fingers of the Krüppel type that constitute the PLZF DNA binding domain. This mutant, however, is devoid of the transcriptional repressive ability of PLZF because in RARα-PLZF the POZ domain (responsible for PLZF transcriptional repression) is replaced by one of the transacting domain of RARα. Thus, having lost the transcriptional repressive ability of PLZF, RARα-PLZF can act as a putative DN PLZF mutant (He et al. 2000).

Furthermore, in the human APL blast cells, the oncogenic function of the various fusion proteins can be, in principle, greatly facilitated by the reduction to heterozygosity of the X and RARα genes caused by the APL chromosomal translocations. This hypothesis is being tested through the use of $X^{-/-}$ and $RAR\alpha^{-/-}$ mutants. If this is indeed the case, the reduction to heterozygosity or the inactivation of the X or RARα genes should accelerate/exacerbate leukemogenesis in APL mouse models. Indeed, crosses of PML-RARα TM with $PML^{-/-}$ mice or PLZF-RARα TM with $PLZF^{-/-}$ mice have been extremely informative, fully supporting this notion. The progressive reduction of the dose of PML resulted, in fact, in a dramatic increase in the incidence of leukemia, and in an acceleration of leukemia onset in PML-RARα TM. Furthermore, PML loss resulted in impaired response to differentiating agents such as RA and vitamin D_3 as well as in a marked survival advantage upon pro-apoptotic stimuli in hematopoietic cells from PML-RARα TM. These results in turn proved that PML acts in vivo as an APL suppressor by rendering the cells sensitive to pro-apoptotic and differentiating stimuli and that the functional impairment of PML by PML-RARα is a critical event in APL pathogenesis (Rego et al. 2001). Comparative analysis of PLZF-RARα TM/$PLZF^{-/-}$ mutants and PLZF-RARα/RARα-PLZF double TM also supports in full the notion that RARα-PLZF can act as a DN RARα mutant and that PLZF haploinsufficiency is critical for APL pathogenesis. In fact, $PLZF^{-/-}$/PLZF-RARα mutants develop APL-like leukemia indistinguishable from the one observed in PLZF-RARα/RARα-PLZF double TM (He et al. 2000).

9
The X Moiety Lends to the X-RARα Fusion Protein Distinct Gain-of-Function Proteins

The RARα gene is invariably involved in the APL-associated chromosomal translocations. Thus, alteration of the RARα pathway and transcriptional function has been thought to be central in APL pathogenesis. X-RARα fusion proteins robustly and constitutively recruit transcriptional corepressors, suggesting that DN blockade of the RARα pathway and transcriptional repression of canonical retinoic acid responsive element (RARE) sites are crucial events for APL leukemogenesis. However, several lines of evidence have challenged this hypothesis. For example, histone deacetylase 1-dependent DN blockade of RARα function is neither sufficient to cause leukemia nor to block myeloid differentiation in vivo, while PML-RARαM4, a fusion protein, containing an RA-resistant RARα moiety retains the ability to induce APL (Matsushita et al. 2006; Kogan et al. 2000). Furthermore, in transgenic mice, forced RARα dimerization/multimerization induces leukemogenesis at a much reduced frequency as compared to PML-RARα (Sternsdorf et al. 2006). These observations strongly suggest that blockade of RARα function may be necessary but not sufficient for leukemogenesis, lending further support to the notion that the X moiety-dependent ability of the fusion protein to interfere with the tumor suppressive function of the wildtype X gene products may be critical. These findings also suggest that the X-RARα fusion proteins may exert "gain of function" activities both at the transcriptional level and by interfering with signaling pathways (Lin et al. 2004). Indeed, it has been shown that through the PML moiety the PML-RARα fusion protein acquires aberrant gain-of-function DNA binding activities (Kamashev et al. 2004). In particular, PML-RARα homodimers can bind DNA consensus sites that are not preferentially recognized by a RARα/RXRα heterodimer (e.g., the RARE), allowing the PML-RARα oncoprotein to bind and potentially repress an expanded repertoire of genes normally not regulated by RARα (Kamashev et al. 2004).

Collectively, these observations support the notion that the various X-RARα and RARα-X fusion proteins may exert novel oncogenic functions that are not simply derived from their ability to interfere with the function of endogenous X and RARα genes.

10
Conclusions and Future Directions

In the last few years, important progress has been made in dissecting the genetics of APL in vivo in engineered mouse mutants as well as in vitro in cells derived from these animals. Altogether the data obtained from these analyses allow the proposal of a unified model by which the various X-RARα and RARα-X fusion proteins play a critical and cooperative role in APL leukemogenesis (Fig. 1). These molecules may exert their aberrant activities through the concomitant interference/disruption of crosstalking X and RARα pathways, but also through gain-of-function aberrant activities yet to be fully elucidated.

This analysis has also revealed that APL, as a clinical and biological entity, is much more heterogeneous than was originally anticipated and that distinct molecular lesions result in differential response to therapy. This notion will allow tailoring therapeutic intervention according to the molecular makeup of the APL blast.

While tremendous progress has been made resulting in effective treatment modalities already, APL will remain a fantastic model system to study human tumorigenesis at large in the future. In this respect, the identification of the target genes/pathways that mediate the leukemogenic activity of the various fusion proteins of APL, the identification of cooperative events toward full-blown leukemogenesis, and the elucidation of the function of the APL genes and their role in tumors other than APL will greatly contribute to this understanding.

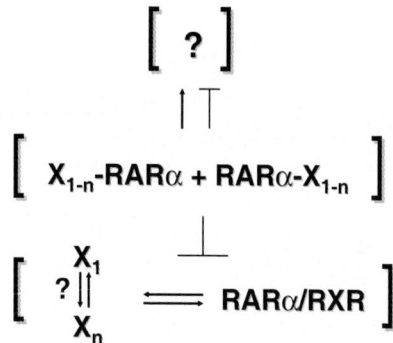

Fig. 1 A unified model for the molecular pathogenesis of APL. In vivo analysis of TM and KO mice supports a model by which the concomitant activity of X-RARα and RARα-X fusion proteins is essential in APL pathogenesis. The APL fusion proteins can deregulate X and RARα functions in a dominant-negative fashion. At the same time, the APL fusion proteins may exert novel gain-of-function properties. These activities may be necessary but not sufficient in APL leukemogenesis as suggested by the fact that cooperative genetic events occur toward overt full-blown transformation in mouse models of APL. X_1-n, the various RARα fusion partners; →, transcriptional activation; ⊣, transcriptional repression; ?, unknown target genes/molecular events

10.1
Identification and Validation of Cooperative Events and X-RARα and RARα Target Genes

Some of the critical biochemical properties of the X-RARα fusion protein have been recently elucidated, such as its ability to act as potent transcriptional repressor in view of an aberrant affinity for transcriptional corepressors and histone deacetylases and aberrant DNA binding activities (He et al. 1998; Grignani et al. 1998; Lin et al. 1998; Kamashev et al. 2004; Zhou et al. 2006). However, the biological implications of these findings are in some way limited by the fact that only very few bona fide X-RARα target genes have been identified so far. Furthermore, a distinct biological activity has been attributed only to a limited subset of them such as $p21^{WAF1/CIP1}$ and transglutaminase type II (Liu et al. 1996; Casini et al. 1999; Ruthardt et al. 1997). Thus, the identification and validation of RARα target genes and genes deregulated by the aberrant transcriptional activity of the X-RARα oncoprotein is a major and essential future undertaking.

Furthermore, concerning target gene identification, much can be learned by taking advantage of the fact that the X-RARα fusion proteins cause distinct hematological malignancies in TM. As the various fusion proteins are identical in their RARα moiety, their differential biological behavior has to be conferred by the X moiety. In this respect two models can be entertained: The X moiety confers a distinct DNA binding specificity to the fusion protein that could in turn deregulate distinct, albeit overlapping, gene sets. Alternatively, the various fusion proteins could deregulate the same set of genes, but their differential repressive/activating ability on distinct promoters could result in different biological outcomes. To address these open and important questions, microarray and chromatin immunoprecipitation (ChIP) on chip technology applied to transgenic models of APL will be of tremendous value.

Lastly, the characterization and validation, on a comparative basis, of the additional genetic events that cooperate with the fusion proteins toward leukemogenesis in vivo in the various TM will allow us to better understand the natural history of human APL and the identification of novel genes relevant to human tumorigenesis.

10.2
Beyond APL: A Role for the Genes of APL in Other Malignancies

APL-related research has so far already firmly implicated PML in the pathogenesis of cancer other than APL (e.g., in epithelial cancer tumorigenesis; see Salomoni and Pandolfi 2002; Gurrieri et al. 2004; Trotman et al. 2006).

The same is true in the case of NPM, whose loss and overexpression can participate in tumorigenesis at large (Grisendi et al. 2005, 2006). On this basis, a systematic analysis of the status of the genes and proteins of APL, their targets and their associated cooperative events in human cancers other than APL is therefore needed and warranted. In fact, it is likely that the X genes of APL have been selected by leukemogenic process precisely because of their ability to modulate critical oncogenic pathways and functions. Thus, research on the mechanisms, genetics, and therapy of this paradigmatic form of leukemia will undoubtedly continue to greatly contribute to our understanding of human cancer, and our fight against it, far beyond APL in the years to come.

Acknowledgements This work is supported by the NCI through the Mouse Models of Human Cancer Consortium (MMHCC), an NCI K08 grant to P.P.S. and NIH grants to P.P.P. We thank L. DiSantis for editing of the manuscript. We are indebted to all the past and present members of the Molecular and Developmental Biology (MADB) lab at Memorial Sloan-Kettering Cancer Center working on APL and related subjects.

References

Albertson DG, Ylstra B, Segraves R, Collins C, Dairkee SH, Kowbel D, Kuo WL, Gray JW, Pinkel D (2000) Quantitative mapping of amplicon structure by array CGH identifies CYP24 as a candidate oncogene. Nat Genet 25:144–146

Arnould C, Philippe C, Bourdon V, Gr goire MJ, Berger R, Jonveaux P (1999) The signal transducer and activator of transcription STAT5b gene is a new partner of retinoic acid receptor alpha in acute promyelocytic-like leukaemia. Hum Mol Genet 8:1741–1749

Bardwell VJ, Treisman R (1994) The POZ domain: a conserved protein-protein interaction motif. Genes Dev 8:1664–1677

Barna M, Hawe N, Niswander L, Pandolfi PP (2000) Plzf regulates limb and axial skeletal patterning. Nat Genet 25:166–172

Brown D, Kogan S, Lagasse E, Weissman I, Alcalay M, Pelicci PG, Atwater S Bishop JM (1997) A PMLRARα transgene initiates murine acute promyelocytic leukemia. Proc Natl Acad Sci U S A 94:2551–2556

Casini T, Pelicci PG (1999) A function of p21 during promyelocytic leukemia cell differentiation independent of CDK inhibition and cell cycle arrest. Oncogene 18:3235–3243

Chen Z, Brand NJ, Chen A, Chen SJ, Tong JH, Wang ZY, Waxman S, Zelent A (1993) Fusion between a novel Kruppel-like zinc finger gene and the retinoic acid receptor-alpha locus due to a variant translocation associated with acute promyelocytic leukaemia. EMBO J 12:1161–1167

Costoya JA, Hobbs RM, Barna M, Cattoretti G, Manova K, Sukhwani M, Orwig KE, Wolgemuth DJ, Pandolfi PP (2004) Essential role of Plzf in maintenance of spermatogonial stem cells. Nat Genet 36:653–659 de The H, Lavau C, Marchio A, Chomienne C, Degos L, Dejean A (1991) The PML-RAR alpha fusion mRNA generated by the t(15;17) translocation in acute promyelocytic leukemia encodes a functionally altered RAR. Cell 66:675–684

Early E, Moore MA, Kakizuka A, Nason-Burchenal K, Martin P, Evans RM, Dmitrovsky E (1996) Transgenic expression of PML/RARα impairs myelopoiesis. Proc Natl Acad Sci U S A 93:7900–7904

Ferbeyre G, de Stanchina E, Querido E, Baptiste N, Prives C Lowe SW (2000) PML is induced by oncogenic ras and promotes premature senescence. Genes Dev 14:2015–2027

Fogal V, Gostissa M, Sandy P, Zacvchi P, Sternsdorf K, Jensen K, Pandolfi PP, Will H, Schneider C, Del Sal G (2000) Regulation of p53 activity in nuclear bodies by a specific PML isoform. EMBO J 6:185–195

Goddard AD, Borrow J, Freemont PS, Solomon E (1991) Characterization of a zinc finger gene disrupted by the t(15;17) in acute promyelocytic leukemia. Science 254:1371–1374

Grignani F, De Matteis S, Nervi C, Tomassoni L, Gelmetti V, Cioce M, Fanelli M, Ruthardt M, Ferrara FF, Zamir I, Seiser C, Lazar MA, Minucci S, Pelicci PG (1998) Fusion proteins of the retinoic acid receptor-alpha recruit histone deacetylase in promyelocytic leukaemia. Nature 391:815–818

Grisendi S, Bernardi R, Rossi M, Cheng K, Khandker L, Manova K, Pandolfi PP (2005) Role of Npm in embryonic development and tumourigenesis. Nature 437:147–153

Grisendi S, Mecucci C, Falini B, Pandolfi PP (2006) Nucleophosmin and cancer. Nat Rev Cancer 6:493–505

Grisolano JL, Wesselschmidt RL, Pelicci PG, Ley TJ (1997) Altered myeloid development and acute leukemia in transgenic mice expressing PML-RARα under control of cathepsin G regulatory sequences. Blood 89:376–387

Guo A, Salomoni P, Juo J, Shih A, Zhong S, Gu W, Pandolfi PP (2000) The function of PML in p53-dependent apoptosis. Nat Cell Biol 2:730–736

Gurrieri C, Capodieci P, Bernardi R, Scaglioni PP, Nafa K, Rush LJ, Verbel DA, Cordon-Cardo C, Pandolfi PP (2004) Loss of the tumor suppressor PML in human cancers of multiple histologic origins. J Natl Cancer Inst 96:269–279

He LZ, Tribioli C, Rivi R, Peruzzi D, Pelicci PG, Soares V, Cattoretti G, Pandolfi PP (1997) Acute leukemia with promyelocytic features in PML/RARα transgenic mice. Proc Natl Acad Sci U S A 94:5302–5307

He LZ, Guidez F, Tribioli C, Peruzzi D, Ruthardt M, Zelent A Pandolfi PP (1998) Distinct interactions of PML-RARα and PLZF-RARα with co-repressors determine differential responses to RA in APL. Nat Genet 18:126–135

He LZ, Bhaumik M, Tribioli C, Rego EM, Ivins S, Zelent A, Pandolfi PP (2000) Two critical hits for promyelocytic leukemia. Mol Cell 6:1131–1141

Kakizuka A, Miller WH, Jr Umesono K, Warrell RP, Jr Frankel SR, Murty VV, Dmitrovsky E, Evans RM (1991) Chromosomal translocation t(15;17) in human acute promyelocytic leukemia fuses RARα with a novel putative transcription factor, PML. Cell 66:663–674

Kamashev D, Vitoux D, de Thé H (2004) PML-RARA-RXR oligomers mediate retinoid and rexinoid/cAMP cross-talk in acute promyelocytic leukemia cell differentiation. J Exp Med 199:1163–1174

Kogan SC, Hong SH, Shultz DB, Privalsky ML, Bishop JM (2000) Leukemia initiated by PMLRARα: the PML domain plays a critical role while retinoic acid-mediated transactivation is dispensable. Blood 95:1541–1550

Le Beau MM, Bitts S, Davis EM, Kogan SC (2002) Recurring chromosomal abnormalities in leukemia in PML-RARA transgenic mice parallel human acute promyelocytic leukemia. Blood 99:2985–2991

Le Beau MM, Davis EM, Patel B, Phan VT, Sohal J, Kogan SC (2003) Recurring chromosomal abnormalities in leukemia in PML-RARA transgenic mice identify cooperating events and genetic pathways to acute promyelocytic leukemia. Blood 102:1072–1074

Lin HJ, Bergmann S, Pandolfi PP (2004) Cytoplasmic PML function in TGF-β signaling. Nature 431:205–211

Lin RJ, Nagy L, Inoue S, Shao W, Miller WH Jr, Evans RM (1998) Clinical and molecular characterization of a rare syndrome of acute promyelocytic leukemia associated with translocation (11;17). Nature 391:811–814

Liu M, Iavarone A, Freedman LP (1996) Transcriptional activation of the human p21(WAF1/CIP1) gene by retinoic acid receptor. Correlation with retinoid induction of U937 cell differentiation. J Biol Chem 271:31723–31728

Liu QR, Chan PK (1991) Formation of nucleophosmin/B23 oligomers requires both the amino- and the carboxyl-terminal domains of the protein. Eur J Biochem 200:715–721

Matsushita H, Scaglioni PP, Bhaumik M, Rego EM, Cai LF, Majid SM, Miyachi H, Kakizuka A, Miller Jr WH, Pandolfi PP (2006) In vivo analysis of the role of aberrant HDAC recruitment and RARα blockade in the pathogenesis of APL. J Exp Med 203:821–828

Minucci S, Monestiroli S, Giavara S, Ronzoni S, Marchesi F, Insinga A, Diverio D, Gasparini P, Capillo M, Colombo E, Matteucci C, Contegno F, Lo-Coco F, Scanziani E, Gobbi A, Pelicci PG (2002) PML-RAR induces promyelocytic leukemias with high efficiency following retroviral gene transfer into purified murine hematopoietic progenitors. Blood 100:2989–2995

Pandolfi PP, Grignani F Alcalay M, Mencarelli A, Biondi A, LoCoco F, Pelicci PG (1991) Structure and origin of the acute promyelocytic leukemia myl/RAR alpha cDNA and characterization of its retinoid-binding and transactivation properties. Oncogene 6:1285–1292

Pearson M, Carbone R, Sebastiani C, Cioce M, Fagioli M, Saito S, Higashimoto Y, Appella E, Minucci S, Pandolfi PP, Pelicci PG (2000) PML regulates p53 acetylation and premature senescence induced by oncogenic Ras. Nature 406:207–210

Perez A, Kastner P, Sethi S, Lutz Y, Reibel C, Chambon P (1993) PMLRAR homodimers: distinct DNA binding properties and heteromeric interactions with RXR. EMBO J 12:3171–3182

Piazza F, Costoya JA, Merghoub T, Hobbs RM, Pandolfi PP (2004) Disruption of PLZF in mice leads to increased T-lymphocyte proliferation, cytokine producing and altered hematopoietic stem cell homeostasis. Mol Cell Biol 24:10456–10469

Pollock JL, Westervelt P, Kurichety AK, Pelicci PG, Grisolano JL, Ley TJ (1999) A bcr-3 isoform of RARalpha-PML potentiates the development of PML-RARα-driven acute promyelocytic leukemia. Proc Natl Acad Sci U S A 96:15103–15108

Quignon F, De Bels F, Koken M, Feunteun J, Ameisen JC, de The H (1998) PML induces a novel caspase-independent death process. Nat Genet 20:259–265

Redner RL, Rush EA, Faas S, Rudert WA, Corey SJ (1996) The t(5;17) variant of acute promyelocytic leukemia expresses a nucleophosmin-retinoic acid receptor fusion. Blood 87:882–886

Rego EM, Wang ZG, Peruzzi D, He LZ, Cordon-Cardo C, Pandolfi PP (2001) Role of promyelocytic leukemia (PML) protein in tumor suppression. J Exp Med 193:521–529

Rego EM, Ruggero D, Tribioli C, Cattoretti G, Kogan S, Redner RL, Pandolfi PP (2006) Leukemia with distinct phenotypes in transgenic mice expressing PML/RARα, PLZF/RARα or NPM/RARα. Oncogene 25:1974–1979

Ruthardt M, Testa U, Nervi C, Ferrucci PF, Grignani F, Puccetti E, Grignani F, Peschle C, Pelicci PG (1997) Opposite effects of the acute promyelocytic leukemia PML-retinoic acid receptor alpha (RAR alpha) and PLZF-RAR alpha fusion proteins on retinoic acid signalling. Mol Cell Biol 17:4859–4869

Salomoni P, Pandolfi PP (2002) The role of PML in tumor suppression. Cell 108:165–170

Sternsdorf T, Phan VT, Maunakea ML, Ocampo CB, Sohal J, Silletto A, Galimi F, Le Beau MM, Evans RM, Kogan SC (2006) Forced retinoic acid receptor alpha homodimers prime mice for APL-like leukemia. Cancer Cell 9:81–94

Sukhai MA, Wu X, Xuan Y, Zhang T, Reis PP, Dube K, Rego EM, Bhaumik M, Bailey DJ, Wells RA, Kamel-Reid S, Pandolfi PP (2004) Myeloid leukemia with promyelocytic features in transgenic mice expressing hCG-NuMA-RARα. Oncogene 23:665–678

Torii S, Egan DA, Evans RA, Reed JC (1999) Human Daxx regulates Fas-induced apoptosis from nuclear PML oncogenic domains (PODs). EMBO J 18:6037–6049

Trotman LC, Alimonti A, Scaglioni PP, Koutcher JA, Cordon-Cardo C, Pandolfi PP (2006) Identification of a tumour suppressor network opposing nuclear Akt function. Nature 441:523–527

Walter MJ, Park JS, Ries RE, Lau SK, McLellan M, Jaeger S, Wilson RK, Mardis ER, Ley TJ (2005) Reduced PU.1 expression causes myeloid progenitor expansion and increased leukemia penetrance in mice expressing PML-RARα. Proc Natl Acad Sci U S A 102:12513–12518

Wang ZG, Delva L, Gaboli M, Rivi R, Giorgio M, Cordon-Cardo C, Grosveld F, Pandolfi PP (1998a) Role of PML in cell growth and the retinoic acid pathway. Science 279:1547–1551

Wang ZG, Ruggero D, Ronchetti S, Zhong S, Gaboli M, Rivi R, Pandolfi PP (1998b) PML is essential for multiple apoptotic pathways. Nat Genet 20:266–272

Wells RA, Catzavelos C, Kamel-Reid S (1997) Fusion of retinoic acid receptor alpha to NuMA, the nuclear mitotic apparatus protein, by a variant translocation in acute promyelocytic leukaemia. Nat Genet 17:109–113

Zhong S, Delva L, Rachez C, Cenciarelli C, Gandini D, Zhang H, Kalantry S, Freedman LP, Pandolfi PP (1999a) A RA-dependent, tumour-growth suppressive transcription complex is the target of the PML-RARα and T18 oncoproteins. Nat Genet 23:287–295

Zhong S, Hu P, Ye TZ, Stan R, Ellis NA, Pandolfi PP (1999b) A role for PML and the nuclear body in genomic stability. Oncogene 18:7941–7947

Zhong S, Salomoni P, Ronchetti S, Guo A, Ruggero D, Pandolfi PP (2000) Promyelocytic leukemia protein (PML) and Daxx participate in a novel nuclear pathway for apoptosis. J Exp Med 191:631–640

Zhou J, Peres L, Honore N, Nasr R, Zhu J, de Thé H (2006) Dimerization-induced corepressor binding and relaxed DNA-binding specificity are critical for PML/RARA-induced immortalization. Proc Natl Acad Sci U S A 103:9238–9243

Zimonjic DB, Pollock JL, Westervelt P, Popescu NC, Ley TJ (2000) Acquired, non-random chromosomal abnormalities associated with the development of acute promyelocytic leukemia in transgenic mice. Proc Natl Acad Sci U S A 97:13306–13311

Treatment of Acute Promyelocytic Leukemia by Retinoids

P. Fenaux[1] (✉) · Z. Z. Wang[2] · L. Degos[3]

[1]Service d'Hématologie Clinique, Hôpital Avicenne, Paris 13 University, 93000 Bobigny, France
pierre.fenaux@avc.ap-hop-paris.fr
[2]Institute of Hematology, Shangai, China
[3]Institut d'Hématologie, Hôpital Saint Louis, Paris, France

1	Background: Results of Chemotherapy Alone in APL	103
1.1	Induction Chemotherapy	103
1.2	Optimal Management of Coagulopathy During Treatment with Chemotherapy Alone	103
1.3	Post-induction Chemotherapy	104
1.4	Prognostic Factors of Treatment with Chemotherapy Alone in APL	104
1.5	In Conclusion: Achievements and Limits of Chemotherapy Alone in APL	104
2	First Results Obtained with ATRA Alone in APL	105
3	ATRA Combined to Intensive Chemotherapy in Newly Diagnosed APL	106
3.1	Randomized Studies Demonstrate the Superiority of ATRA Chemotherapy Combinations over Chemotherapy Alone	106
3.2	CR Rates Obtained with ATRA Combined to Chemotherapy	106
4	Consolidation and Maintenance Treatment with ATRA in APL	107
5	Prognostic Factors in Patients Treated with ATRA and Chemotherapy	108
5.1	Prognostic Factors of CR Achievement	108
5.2	Prognostic Factors of Relapse	109
5.2.1	Pretreatment Factors	109
5.2.2	Monitoring of Minimal Residual Disease	110
5.3	Extramedullary Relapses	110
6	Unresolved Issues in the ATRA and Chemotherapy Combination Treatment of Newly Diagnosed APL	111
6.1	Duration and Dosing of ATRA During Induction Treatment	111
6.2	Scheduling of ATRA and Chemotherapy in APL	111
6.3	Role of AraC in the Chemotherapy of APL	112
7	Role of Retinoids in the Treatment of Relapsing APL	113
7.1	Retreatment with ATRA	113
7.2	Other Forms of Retinoids	114

8	APL Differentiation Syndrome (ATRA Syndrome) and Other Side Effects of ATRA	114
8.1	APL Differentiation Syndrome (ATRA syndrome)	115
8.1.1	Incidence and Clinical Signs	115
8.1.2	Pathophysiology of Hyperleukocytosis and ATRA Syndrome	115
8.1.3	Prophylaxis and Treatment	116
8.2	Coagulopathy and Thrombosis	117
8.3	Other Side Effects of ATRA	117

References ... 118

Abstract We review the role of all-*trans* retinoic acid (ATRA) in the treatment of acute promyelocytic leukemia (APL). The combination of ATRA and conventional anthracycline-ARA-C chemotherapy (CT) has clearly demonstrated its superiority over CT alone (in terms of relapse and survival) in newly diagnosed APL. Combination treatment probably also reduces the incidence of initial failures, and complete remission (CR) rates greater than 90% are now regularly reported in large multi-center trials. Some randomized studies strongly suggest that prolonged maintenance treatment (for 1 or 2 years) with ATRA and low-dose CT, and possibly very early introduction of anthracycline CT during induction treatment, may reduce the incidence of relapse. With those treatments, the relapse risk appears to be only 10%–15%, although it remains greater in patients who initially have high white blood cell counts (often associated with variant M_3 morphology, short bcr_3 isoform, etc.) and patients with residual disease detectable by RT-PCR at the end of consolidation courses. In those patients, addition of arsenic derivatives to induction or consolidation treatment (or both treatments together) may prove useful and is currently being tested. ATRA syndrome (now generally called APL differentiation syndrome, as it is also seen with arsenic derivatives) remains the major side effect of ATRA treatment. It occurs in 10%–15% of patients and is currently fatal in at least 10% of them. Rapid onset of CT or high dose steroids (or both) should improve its outcome. A sizeable proportion of APL patients who relapse after ATRA and CT can be durably salvaged by the same treatment followed by allogeneic or autologous stem cell transplantation, provided the transplant (in the autologous setting) is RT-PCR-negative. However, in relapsing APL arsenic derivatives (mainly arsenic trioxide) are now considered to be the reference treatment. Some of the current issues with ATRA treatment in newly diagnosed APL include whether ATRA has a role during consolidation treatment and whether arabinoside (AraC) is required in addition to anthracyclines in the chemotherapy combined to ATRA.

Acute promyelocytic leukemia (APL) is a specific type of acute myeloid leukemia (AML) characterized by the morphology of blast cells (M_3 in the French–American–British classification of AML) [1, 2], the t(15;17) translocation [3] that fuses the PML gene on chromosome 15 to the retinoic acid receptor (RAR) alpha gene on chromosome 17 [4, 5], and a specific type of coagulopathy [6, 7]. Until the late 1980s, intensive cytoreductive chemotherapy (CT), usually combining an anthracycline and cytosine arabinoside (AraC), was the only effective treatment of APL. Over the last 15 years, the advent of all-*trans* retinoic acid (ATRA), and more recently of arsenic trioxide, have greatly improved the therapeutic approach of APL.

1
Background: Results of Chemotherapy Alone in APL

1.1
Induction Chemotherapy

With anthracycline AraC regimens, complete remission (CR) rates of only 50%–60% had generally been reported in the 1970s, but results subsequently improved, and CR rates of 70%–0% were reported in the 1980s [8–13]. Failure to achieve CR was due, in early reports, to CNS bleeding during the first days of treatment in at least two-thirds of the cases. Sepsis during the phase of aplasia accounted for the majority of other failures. By contrast, resistant leukemia was generally seen in less than 10% of the patients, probably reflecting the high sensitivity of APL cells to anthracyclines. Several studies, including recent ones, have shown that total induction doses of daunorubicin (DNR) greater than 200 mg/m^2–250 mg/m^2 were required to obtain these results [8, 14, 15]. In addition, both in randomized and nonrandomized studies, there was no evidence that anthracycline–AraC combinations were superior to anthracyclines alone if the latter were given at high dose (e.g., at least 300 mg/m^2 during induction for DNR [16]). Idarubicin appeared to be at least as effective as DNR in APL.

Other induction drugs (6 thioguanine, VP 16) do not seem to bring any benefit during induction CT in APL. High-dose AraC has been suggested to improve results over conventional dose AraC in one study [19], but gave poorer results due to increased toxicity in other studies [16, 20].

1.2
Optimal Management of Coagulopathy During Treatment
with Chemotherapy Alone

The bleeding diathesis in APL results from a combination of disseminated intravascular coagulation (DIC) due to the release of procoagulants from abnormal promyelocytes and also from excessive fibrinolysis and proteolysis, as blast cells also contain plasminogen activators and liposomal neutrophil enzymes that may be released during cell lysis, and are able to cleave various substrates, including fibrinogen [6, 7].

Significant coagulopathy, present at diagnosis in 80% of cases of APL, is worsened (or triggered in the remaining patients) by the onset of CT. Intensive platelet support during CT, aiming at maintaining platelet counts above 50,000/mm^3, is crucial in the management of coagulopathy of APL, especially in patients presenting with hyperleukocytosis, who have an increased risk of early death due to bleeding whereas the role of other treatments, including heparin, antifibrinolytic agents, and fibrinogen concentrates, is unproven [23].

1.3
Post-induction Chemotherapy

Once CR has been achieved, APL, even when treated with CT alone, is associated with a lower risk of relapse than other types of AML treated identically [12, 16]. However, the optimal post-induction therapy remains controversial in APL. In AML as a whole, it has been shown that intensive consolidation CT, without maintenance, was at least equal or superior to milder consolidation courses followed by prolonged maintenance therapy. However, in APL, two studies have suggested that prolonged maintenance CT with 6 mercaptopurine (6MP) and methotrexate (MTX) could prolong remissions when compared to shorter consolidation regimens [15, 23], although those results were not confirmed in a large randomized GIMEMA (Gruppo Italiano Malattie Ematologiche dell'Adulto) trial [17].

1.4
Prognostic Factors of Treatment with Chemotherapy Alone in APL

In newly diagnosed APL treated with CT alone, patients older than 50 [15, 23] with hyperleukocytosis at diagnosis or major thrombocytopenia [23] had a higher risk of early death.

Shorter remissions were seen in patients with hyperleukocytosis [12] and in patients with a microgranular APL variant [15].

1.5
In Conclusion: Achievements and Limits of Chemotherapy Alone in APL

Published data suggest that anthracycline–AraC regimens with sufficient anthracycline dosage, associated to intensive platelet support during induction, yielded CR in 75%–80% of newly diagnosed APL patients, with a risk of early death due to bleeding of about 10%–15%. With anthracycline-based consolidation and possibly maintenance CT, median CR duration ranged from 11 to 25 months so that, overall, only 35%–45% of the patients could be cured by CT alone. Patients presenting with high leukocyte counts, which account for 15%–20% of APL cases, had a particularly poor prognosis with CT alone, as their CR rate was only 50%–60%, and the risk of relapse was high.

2
First Results Obtained with ATRA Alone in APL

Discovery of the activity of ATRA in APL was made by Chinese investigators, especially the Shanghai group [25], and the drug was subsequently used in France and other Western countries. In the first reports of ATRA therapy published by the Shanghai group [25], the French group [26, 27], and then by other groups [28, 29], CR rates of about 90% were reported in newly diagnosed and first-relapse APL, generally with a 45 mg/m^2 daily dose of ATRA. The presence of Auer rods in neutrophils, the absence of aplasia, and the study of X chromosome-linked polymorphisms, in particular, showed that response was not obtained by cytotoxicity but by differentiation of APL blasts into neutrophils, leading to progressive replacement of leukemic hematopoiesis by normal polyclonal hematopoiesis [25, 26,29–32]. Rapid improvement of coagulopathy, instead of the initial worsening observed with conventional CT, was also seen.

These first reports, however, drew attention to two major drawbacks of ATRA treatment. The first was that, mainly in newly diagnosed APL, a rapid rise in leukocytes was seen in one-third to one-half of the patients, accompanied by clinical signs of "ATRA syndrome" which proved fatal in some patients [26, 33, 34]. Low-dose CT (with hydroxyurea or low dose AraC) did not succeed in lowering leukocyte counts and preventing the fatal outcome, whereas more intensive anthracycline-AraC CT was able to reduce leukocyte counts and allowed most patients to enter CR [33]. It was also shown that high-dose dexamethasone also had a favorable effect on "ATRA syndrome," now often called "APL differentiation syndrome." The second drawback of ATRA therapy was the development of resistance to this drug: patients who achieved CR with ATRA and received either ATRA alone or low-dose CT for maintenance therapy generally relapsed within a few months of CR achievement [26, 27, 32]. These findings prompted clinicians to administer treatment combining ATRA and intensive CT in APL.

3
ATRA Combined to Intensive Chemotherapy in Newly Diagnosed APL

Many studies including two randomized trials (the European APL 91 trial and a U.S. Intergroup study) have clearly demonstrated the superiority of combined treatment with ATRA and intensive CT over intensive CT alone in newly diagnosed APL.

3.1
Randomized Studies Demonstrate the Superiority of ATRA Chemotherapy Combinations over Chemotherapy Alone

The European trial (APL 91) compared CT alone (three intensive courses of DNR and AraC) and ATRA followed by the same CT in newly diagnosed APL between 1991 and 1992. In the ATRA group, the first CT course was rapidly added to ATRA if WBC counts were greater than 5,000/mm^3 at diagnosis, or increased during treatment. The trial was prematurely stopped after 18 months because event free survival (EFS) was significantly better in the ATRA group [36, 37]. The last interim analysis, performed 73 months after closing date of the study, confirmed the significantly higher actuarial EFS, lower relapse rate, and better survival in the ATRA group [38]. This trial also confirmed that the combination of ATRA and CT reduced the incidence of early relapses, occurring within 18 months of diagnosis, without increasing the incidence of later relapses by comparison with CT alone. The U.S. Intergroup study, randomizing ATRA followed by CT and CT alone in newly diagnosed APL, was performed between 1992 and 1995. Patients who achieved CR were further randomized between no maintenance and ATRA maintenance (see Sect. 4). The CR rate did not differ between patients who received ATRA for induction and those that did not. However, the incidence of relapse was significantly reduced in patients who received ATRA during induction compared to those who received CT alone, and those differences translated into survival differences [39, 41]. Also of note was that fewer relapses occurred with CT followed by ATRA, as compared to CT alone. All subsequent cooperative group studies have also shown superiority of ATRA CT combination over CT alone (47,109).

3.2
CR Rates Obtained with ATRA Combined to Chemotherapy

Although the above-mentioned randomized trials did not show significant differences in CR rates between patients treated with ATRA combined to CT compared to CT alone, it appears that the addition of ATRA to CT, in recent experiences, has somewhat increased CR rates. Indeed, results of several recent European trials of ATRA combined to CT in newly diagnosed APL, which has included more than 1,500 evaluable patients, showed CR rates between of 92% and 91% [40]. These results, obtained on a multicenter basis, show that with better knowledge of the utilization of ATRA (and especially of the prophylaxis of its major side effect, i.e., ATRA syndrome) by clinicians, very high CR rates, above 90%, can be achieved by combining this drug to CT in newly diagnosed APL. By contrast, CR rates above 80% have rarely been reported in newly diagnosed APL treated with CT alone.

4
Consolidation and Maintenance Treatment with ATRA in APL

Two randomized studies strongly suggest a beneficial role for maintenance treatment in newly diagnosed APL treated with ATRA and consolidation CT. The U.S. Intergroup trial randomized patients who had received ATRA followed by three DNR-AraC courses to continuous maintenance with ATRA (45 mg/m^2 per day) during 1 year or no maintenance. The incidence of relapse was significantly lower in patients who received maintenance ATRA (10 of 46 cases) than in patients who received no maintenance (21 of 54 patients). Liver toxicity of the treatment was, however, relatively important. A benefit for ATRA maintenance was also found in patients who had received no ATRA during induction therapy. In addition, patients who received CT alone followed by maintenance with ATRA had a similar outcome to patients who received ATRA followed by CT, but no maintenance ATRA [39].

The European APL group (APL 93 trial) randomized patients who had achieved CR with a combination of ATRA and CT to receive no maintenance, maintenance with ATRA (45 mg/m^2 per day) 15 days every 3 months, continuous low-dose CT with 6MP and MTX or both during 2 years using a 2-by-2 factorial design [40]. The rationale for intermittent rather than continuous ATRA for maintenance was based on pharmacokinetic studies showing a progressive decrease of serum peak levels of ATRA after a few weeks of treatment, due to hypercatabolism of the drug [49–52], those studies showed that this hypercatabolism was reversible after a few weeks of drug discontinuation [51]. The rationale for low-dose maintenance CT was based on two nonrandomized studies (see previous paragraph). The incidence of relapse after 2 years was 25% in patients who received no maintenance ATRA vs 13% in those who received maintenance ATRA ($p = 0.02$), and 27% in patients who received no maintenance CT vs 11% in those who received maintenance CT ($p = 0.0003$). Furthermore, an additive effect of intermittent ATRA and low-dose CT in reducing the risk of relapse was seen. Regarding survival, the effect was significant for maintenance with CT, but was only borderline for ATRA, at least with the current follow-up. In addition, patients presenting with WBC counts exceeding 10,000/mm^3, who remain at higher risk of relapse after ATRA and intensive CT, seemed to benefit particularly from maintenance with both CT and ATRA. Finally, liver toxicity (and other toxicities) was moderate with intermittent ATRA.

Those results have led most groups to use ATRA for maintenance treatment generally in combination with low-dose CT, especially MTX and 6MP. Long-term results of the APL 93 trial suggest that this type of maintenance treatment should be administered during at least 1 year. Indeed, in that trial, where maintenance treatment was scheduled for 2 years, the incidence of relapse was 45% in patients who discontinued treatment after less than 1 year (for reasons other than relapse) as compared to 16% in patients who received it during more than 1 year.

ATRA may also play a role when administered during consolidation courses, in combination with anthracycline-based CT. In the PETHEMA (Programa para el Tratamiento de Hemopatías Malignas) experience, reduction in the relapse rate was observed between the LPA (Leucemia Promielocitica Aguda) 96 and LPA 99 trials by addition of 15 days of ATRA during the three consolidation courses in the high- and intermediate-risk patients [52]. However, the addition of ATRA during consolidation courses in the LPA 99 trial was not randomized. It was also associated with an increase in the cumulative dose of anthracyclines, by comparison with the LPA 96 trial, rendering any straightforward explanation difficult.

5
Prognostic Factors in Patients Treated with ATRA and Chemotherapy

In spite of the improvement of outcome seen with the combination of ATRA and CT, some patients with newly diagnosed APL still do not achieve CR, and others still relapse.

5.1
Prognostic Factors of CR Achievement

Of APL patients, 5%–10% fail to achieve CR with ATRA and CT, almost exclusively due to early death, as resistance to ATRA is exceptional (probably less than 1/500) in cytogenetically t(15;17) or molecularly (PML-RAR alpha rearrangement) confirmed APL [40]. The three major causes of early death are CNS bleeding, ATRA syndrome, and sepsis, the latter usually occurring later, during the phase of aplasia induced by CT. High WBC counts and older age appear to be the main risk factors of early death in APL.

5.2
Prognostic Factors of Relapse

With a combination of ATRA and CT followed by maintenance treatment, about 10%–15% of APL cases still relapse. Prognostic factors of relapse include pretreatment factors, and monitoring of minimal residual disease (mrd) by reverse transcriptase (RT)-PCR analysis of PML-RAR alpha rearrangement.

5.2.1
Pretreatment Factors

High WBC counts remain a risk factor of relapse in all reports [53], even if, as seen above, results of the European APL group suggest that maintenance treatment may particularly reduce the risk of relapse in this population [40]. Some of the other risk factors found in most studies—including morphological M3 variant, low platelet count, and expression of CD34 or CD2 on blast surface Fms-like tyrosine kinase 3 (FLT3) duplication—are generally correlated to high WBC counts [54–56]. On the other hand, a meta-analysis of GIMEMA and PETHEMA protocols in APL (both of which included maintenance with ATRA and low-dose CT) showed that WBC and platelet counts had independent prognostic value for relapse. Disease-free survival (DFS) at 4 years was 98% in patients with WBC counts less than 10,000/mm^3 and platelets greater than 40,000/mm^3, 90% in patients with platelets less than 40,000/mm^3 but WBC less than 10,000/mm^3, and only 68% in patients with WBC greater than 10,000/mm^3 [47].

Other factors independent of the WBC count, including CD13 and CD56 [57] expression, were associated with an increased risk of relapse in some studies, whereas cytogenetic abnormalities in addition to t(15;17) did not confer a higher relapse risk. Regarding the PML-RAR alpha breakpoint, the short isoform (S isoform or bcr$_3$) and possibly the rare bcr$_2$ (or V) breakpoint have poorer prognosis than bcr$_1$ (or L breakpoint); they are also usually correlated with high WBC counts and may not carry a poor prognostic value per se. The degree and rapidity of in vitro differentiation of APL blasts with ATRA may also have prognostic value [58].

5.2.2
Monitoring of Minimal Residual Disease

A clear correlation has been found in APL between detectable disease by RT-PCR and the risk of relapse. Patients with detectable PML-RAR alpha fusion messenger RNA (mRNA) by RT-PCR at the end of consolidation and perhaps, more importantly, patients with positive findings after a phase of negative results are at high risk of relapse [59–63]. It should be noted, however, that for unknown reasons, the PML-RAR fusion transcript appears to be easily degraded in bone marrow samples, often making results uninterpretable. In addition, in spite of consensus meetings [64], there may be a certain interlaboratory variation in the sensitivity of RT-PCR, especially due to the fact that some laboratories perform one-round PCR, and others two-round PCR. Therefore, comparison between successive samples rather than interpretation of one given sample is advised.

U.S. and Italian investigators have used an assay with consistent but only moderate sensitivity but close to 100% specificity [59, 60]. With this assay, a negative result had good but not perfect predictive value, whereas a positive test ("molecular relapse") was considered sufficiently reliable to institute treatment, including toxic treatment with autologous stem cell transplantation [59, 60].

Quantitative PCR techniques, especially with TaqMan probes, determine for each patient at a given point a quantity of fusion PML-RAR mRNA. This allows better analysis of an increase or decrease in successive samples, and should improve clinical interpretation of results and therapeutic decisions [61, 63].

5.3
Extramedullary Relapses

A relatively large number of cases of extramedullary relapses have been reported in APL treated with ATRA and CT, generally as single case reports [65]. Extramedullary sites were seen in 13 of the 97 relapses in a GIMEMA group study and 10 of the 169 relapses seen by the European APL 93, LPA 96, and LPA 99 trials [40, 65]. Sites of extramedullary relapse in those three studies mainly included the CNS and less often the skin or other organs. CNS relapse was associated with marrow relapse in 8 of our 10 cases; it was only molecular, however, in half of those cases.

Although it was initially suggested that the use of ATRA could increase the incidence of extramedullary relapses in APL, this was not confirmed by subsequent studies. The latter in fact strongly supported the fact that it was the prognostic improvement brought by ATRA that increased the number of surviving patients potentially at risk of extramedullary disease.

6 Unresolved Issues in the ATRA and Chemotherapy Combination Treatment of Newly Diagnosed APL

6.1 Duration and Dosing of ATRA During Induction Treatment

The optimal duration of ATRA during induction treatment of APL is not known. Most centers administer ATRA until achievement of hematological CR, which usually occurs after 40–60 days if ATRA is used alone and after less than 30 days if CT is combined to ATRA from the onset. A British Medical Research Council (MRC) randomized study compared a short course (5 days) of ATRA followed by CT to a long course of ATRA (until CR achievement) combined to the same CT in newly diagnosed APL. A better outcome was seen in the latter group, demonstrating that longer administration of ATRA during induction is required [43]. It is, however, unknown if discontinuation of ATRA before CR achievement (e.g., after 15 to 20 days of treatment) is sufficient to achieve full activity of the drug, in particular in terms of reduction of the incidence of relapses. Analysis of the outcome of patients who had early discontinuation of ATRA may be difficult to interpret in this context, as early discontinuation is generally due to the occurrence of ATRA syndrome, which may be per se a risk factor of relapse in APL [44].

Although ATRA is generally used at the dose of 45 mg/m^2 per day, it has been shown that lower doses, i.e., 25 mg/m^2 per day, gave similar CR results [45]. Those lower doses are often applied in children when severe headache, due to ATRA, develops [46]. It is not certain, however, if the additive or synergistic effect obtained with ATRA, at 45 mg/m^2 per day, and CT on reducing the incidence of relapses in APL would persist completely with lower doses of ATRA.

6.2 Scheduling of ATRA and Chemotherapy in APL

Most cooperative groups initially treated APL patients by ATRA alone, until CR achievement, and then introduced CT. The European group (APL 93 trial) randomized newly diagnosed APL patients with WBC counts 5,000/mm^3 between ATRA followed by CT (ATRACT) and ATRA plus CT (ATRA+CT, where CT was started on day 3 of ATRA treatment). The CR rate was similar in the two groups, but relapses at 2 years were significantly less frequent in the ATRA+CT group [40]. This suggested that the "additive" or "synergistic" effect of ATRA and CT on reducing the incidence of relapse in APL was optimal when the two treatment modalities were administered together. In addition, there was a lower incidence of APL differentiation syndrome in the ATRA+CT group, as compared to the ATRA followed by CT group (see below).

6.3
Role of AraC in the Chemotherapy of APL

As previously seen, when APL is treated with CT alone, it is unclear if AraC has a beneficial role in addition to an anthracycline in the treatment of APL. When CT is combined to ATRA, this is also debated. Sanz et al. [47] treated, in the LPA 96 trial, newly diagnosed APL with ATRA and four successive courses of CT with idarubicin or mitoxantrone alone, followed by maintenance treatment with intermittent ATRA and low-dose continuous 6MP and MTX. The CR rate was 89% and the 4-year incidence of relapse was 79%. After the end of CT, 93% of the patients had converted to PCR-negative. Furthermore, consolidation CT courses were associated with no mortality, limited morbidity, and very few days in hospital. Those results were recently confirmed in the LPA 99 trial [52]. The low mortality in CR was in contrast with the 3.5% mortality (when unrelated causes of death in CR were excluded) observed by the European APL group after consolidation CT with two DNR-AraC courses [40]. Estey et al. [48] also obtained favorable results in APL using ATRA followed by idarubicin without AraC in 43 patients. However, the European APL group performed a study randomizing newly diagnosed APL patients with an initial WBC count of less than 10,000/mm^3 between treatment with ATRA+DNR and treatment with ATRA+DNR+AraC. All patients received maintenance treatment with continuous 6MP+MTX and intermittent ATRA. Early termination of the trial was made due to significantly higher relapse rates in patients treated without AraC. Differences with the (nonrandomized) Spanish LPA 96 and LAP 99 trials are difficult to explain. They may be due to the higher cumulative dose of anthracyclines used in the Spanish studies, to a possible superiority of idarubicin over daunorubicin in APL or to the fact that, as seen above, the addition of ATRA during consolidation courses may reduce the incidence of relapses.

The role of AraC in addition to ATRA and anthracycline therefore remains debated, at least concerning patients with no high pretreatment WBC counts. Indeed, in patients with WBC counts greater than 10,000/mm^3, the relapse rate was 23% in LPA 96 and 99, without AraC, whereas it was only 8% in the French APL 2000 trials, where patients received AraC (including high-dose

AraC). The GIMEMA group's results, although they were not randomized, also strongly supported a role for AraC in reducing the relapse rate in APL with WBC counts greater than 10,000/mm^3 [67]. Results of the German APL group also support those findings [68]. Therefore, in APL with high WBC counts, where the risk of relapse remains relatively important, the main issue may not be so much the role of AraC, which appears justified, but a possible interest of adding arsenic derivatives during consolidation courses.

7
Role of Retinoids in the Treatment of Relapsing APL

7.1
Retreatment with ATRA

In patients who relapse shortly after discontinuation of ATRA no response to ATRA, even at higher doses, is generally observed [32, 69, 70]. Pharmacokinetic studies have indeed shown that prolonged use of ATRA was associated with hypercatabolism of the drug through cytochrome P450 mechanisms, with dramatic reduction of the serum peak levels of ATRA [50, 51].

On the other hand, in the APL 91 European trial, all the 10 patients initially treated with ATRA who relapsed and were retreated with ATRA achieved a second CR. An explanation could be that all relapses, in patients initially treated with ATRA and intensive CT in this trial, occurred more than 6 months after CR achievement (i.e., more than 6 months after discontinuation of ATRA). Pharmacokinetic studies indeed suggest that the hypercatabolism of ATRA induced by treatment with this drug is reversible after a few weeks of ATRA discontinuation [52, 70]. Another reason is that in some of those patients, CT was relatively rapidly added to ATRA, generally due to increasing WBC counts, and that this possibly overcame partial resistance to ATRA. Recently, the European APL group completed a study of ATRA followed by intensive CT in 50 APL patients in first relapse who had received ATRA during their first line treatment. Of the 50, 45 achieved CR [71]. When performed after this intensive salvage treatment, autologous stem cell transplantation gave very favorable results if (this was generally the case) stem cells were collected in molecular CR. By contrast, allogeneic stem cell transplantation (SCT) after such an intensive regimen give a high incidence of toxic mortality [72]. These findings further support a role for arsenic trioxide, a nonmyelosuppressive agent capable of inducing molecular CR after two courses in most relapsing patients, as the first-line treatment of relapsing APL.

7.2
Other Forms of Retinoids

Another argument supporting the systematic use of arsenic derivatives in the first-line treatment of relapsing APL is that maintenance treatment with ATRA is used more often by clinical cooperative groups. Therefore a large proportion of first relapses now concern patients who are receiving or have recently received ATRA, and will probably show resistance to this drug. In addition, in some patients, resistance to ATRA is not due to hypercatabolism of the drug, but to the occurrence of point mutations in the DNA-binding domain of the RAR alpha gene [73]. Those mutations are associated to irreversible resistance to ATRA.

In those situations of resistance to ATRA, preliminary studies suggest that liposomal ATRA can still induce some responses [74]. One reason is that this mode of administration of ATRA does not seem to induce hypercatabolism of the drug and reduction of its plasma levels [48, 75]. Because it interacts with both RXR and RAR receptors, 9-*cis* retinoic acid (RA), does not induce its own catabolism to the same extent as ATRA. Favorable preliminary results with 9-*cis* RA have been published, but responses were seen in relapsing patients that were possibly not resistant to conventional ATRA [76, 77]. A synthetic retinoid Am80, approximately 10 times more potent than ATRA as an in vitro differentiation inducer, has been used in a cohort of relapsing APL patients and 58% achieved CR [78]. However, because all those patients had discontinued ATRA for at least 18 months, it is also unclear whether Am80 was superior to ATRA in this situation, and whether it was able to overcome resistance to ATRA.

8
APL Differentiation Syndrome (ATRA Syndrome) and Other Side Effects of ATRA

ATRA therapy is usually well-tolerated and its side effects moderate. ATRA has a few major side effects, however, dominated by ATRA syndrome (now rather called APL differentiation syndrome, as it can also be observed during treatment with arsenic derivatives).

8.1
APL Differentiation Syndrome (ATRA syndrome)

8.1.1
Incidence and Clinical Signs

A progressive and symptomless rise in WBC counts is frequently seen with ATRA treatment, but our group [26, 33] reported in some cases a rapid rise of WBC counts associated with cardiopulmonary and renal failure. Frankel et al. (1992) [34] then precisely described clinical symptoms of this "ATRA syndrome," and several large series of cases of this syndrome have been published [44, 108]. Clinical signs of ATRA syndrome combine fever, respiratory distress, weight gain, lower extremity edema, pleural or pericardial effusions, hypotension, and sometimes renal failure. These signs are preceded by increasing WBC counts in the majority of case, but some patients develop symptoms at normal WBC counts [69]. Of note is that some cases of ATRA syndrome can occur upon recovery from aplasia in patients who have received early CT and are still receiving ATRA [44].

ATRA syndrome occurred in 6%–27% of the patients in previous reports, and mortality of the syndrome ranged from 8%–15% [34, 37, 39, 109, 110]. In the European APL 93 trial, patients who survived ATRA syndrome had a higher risk of bone marrow relapse than patients who had no ATRA syndrome (32% vs 15% at 2 years). In another study, the occurrence of ATRA syndrome was associated with a possibly higher risk of subsequent extramedullary relapse [111]. Finally, of note is that ATRA syndrome has not been reported during maintenance treatment with ATRA. Therefore, patients who experience tretinoin syndrome during induction treatment may safety receive tretinoin for maintenance.

8.1.2
Pathophysiology of Hyperleukocytosis and ATRA Syndrome

The pathophysiology of hyperleukocytosis and ATRA syndrome is still not completely understood. ATRA syndrome is not due to leukostasis or thrombosis (or both) [34], and because its clinical signs are reminiscent of those observed in endotoxic shock and in adult respiratory distress syndrome (ARDS), a possible stimulatory effect of ATRA on cytokine expression by APL cells has been envisaged. Induction of interleukin (IL)-1 alpha and granulocyte colony-stimulating factor (G-CSF) secretion by APL cells under ATRA may contribute to hyperleukocytosis in vivo. On the other hand, the secretion of IL-1 alpha, IL-6, tumor necrosis factor (TNF) alpha, and IL-8—which are involved in leukocyte activation and adherence, and are implicated in the development of ARDS—could have a pathogenetic role in ATRA syndrome [112, 113].

More recently, it has been shown that ATRA induced aggregation of NB4 cells (an APL cell line). This process was mediated by the adhesion molecules lymphocyte function-associated antigen (LFA)1 and intercellular adhesion molecule (ICAM)2 and was reversed by addition of methylprednisolone [114]. These findings suggest that modification of the adhesive properties of APL cells by ATRA could play a role in ATRA syndrome.

8.1.3
Prophylaxis and Treatment

Once ATRA syndrome has developed, addition of low-dose CT is ineffective in lowering WBC counts, and leukapheresis is unable to reverse symptoms. Two different approaches aimed at preventing or treating early ATRA syndrome are proposed. One of them, mainly used by the European and Japanese groups [33, 37, 109], consists of adding CT from the onset of ATRA in patients presenting with high WBC counts (WBC greater than 5,000/mm^3 in the European trial, or greater than 3,000/mm^3 in the Japanese trials) or when increases in the WBC counts are seen with ATRA. This approach has been associated with a low incidence of fatal ATRA syndrome. A disadvantage of this approach is that about two-thirds of the patients treated with ATRA also received early CT. However, several reports have shown that the period of neutropenia and thrombocytopenia is significantly shorter in patients who receive CT while already on ATRA, by comparison with CT alone [37, 115]. Furthermore, intensive CT, if not administered early, would have to be administered later on, as consolidation treatment. The possibility, suggested by the European APL 93 trial, that early onset of CT (ATRA+CT) reduces the incidence of relapse, by comparison to ATRA followed by CT (ATRA CT), could be an additional argument for the early onset CT, even in the absence of high WBC counts. This attitude is now a standard approach for the Spanish PETHEMA and Italian GIMEMA groups. Also, of note is that, in APL 93 trial, there were significantly fewer cases of ATRA syndrome in patients who received ATRA+CT as compared to those treated by ATRA CT (y%) [44, 116].

By contrast, the usual U.S. approach is to prevent ATRA syndrome by high-dose intravenous corticosteroids (dexamethasone, 10 mg IV twice daily for 3 days or more) as soon as the first symptoms occur. This attitude proved effective in the U.S. Intergroup study, both for preventing ATRA syndrome and reducing its mortality [39].

Finally, there is a consensus concerning the fact that patients presenting with high WBC counts (e.g., more than 15,000–20,000/mm^3) will very often develop severe ATRA syndrome with ATRA alone, and require CT and intravenous dexamethasone from the onset of treatment. Some of these patients even present with symptoms analogous to those of ATRA syndrome at diagnosis [117]. The same recommendations that apply to ATRA syndrome during treatment with ATRA apply to the similar syndrome observed after treatment with arsenic derivatives.

8.2
Coagulopathy and Thrombosis

Because the release of leukemic cell components during ATRA treatment is slow when compared to massive cell death induced by CT, no exacerbation of the bleeding tendency is observed in APL patients undergoing ATRA therapy. In the European APL 91 trial, median time to disappearance of significant coagulopathy was 6 days after CT alone and 3 days in the ATRA group ($p = 0.001$) [37]. ATRA therapy may be especially important in reducing the severity of the bleeding tendency in hyperleukocytic APL patients, a population still at a relatively high risk of early death with CT alone [6, 7, 118].

In APL patients treated with ATRA alone, primary fibrinogenolysis disappears during the first 5 days of treatment, while DIC and leukocyte-mediated proteolysis seem to persist during the first 2 or 3 weeks of ATRA therapy. This could lead to a transient period of hypercoagulability, which could explain the few well-documented cases of thromboembolic events in APL patients treated with ATRA [119–121].

8.3
Other Side Effects of ATRA

Dryness of lips and mucosae are usual but are reversible with symptomatic treatment. Increases in transaminases and triglycerides are common, but they have never required treatment discontinuation in our experience. Headache, due to intracranial hypertension, is generally moderate in adults but may be severe in children, and associated with signs of pseudotumor cerebri [46]. Lower ATRA doses (25 mg/m^2 per day) reduce this side effect in children and seem as effective as conventional doses of 45 mg/m^2 per day in inducing CR [46]. Isolated fever frequently develops in the absence of other signs of ATRA syndrome (or infection) and is reversible within 48 h of ATRA discontinuation [37, 109].

Other side effects, including bone marrow necrosis [11], hypercalcemia [122], erythema nodosum [123], marked basophilia [124, 125], severe myositis [126], Sweet syndrome [127, 128], Fournier's gangrene (necrotizing fasciitis of the penis and scrotum) [129, 130], thrombocytosis [131], and necrotizing vasculitis [132] have rarely been reported with ATRA treatment.

References

1. Bennett JM, Catovsky D, Daniel MT, Flandrin G, Galton DA, Gralnick HR, Sultan C (1976) Proposals for the classification of the acute leukaemias. French-American-British (FAB) co-operative group. Br J Haematol 33:451–458
2. Bennett JM, Catovsky D, Daniel MT, Flandrin G, Galton DA, Gralnick HR, Sultan C (1980) A variant form of hypergranular promyelocytic leukemia (M3). Ann Intern Med 92:261
3. Larson RA, Kondo K, Vardiman JW, Butler AE, Golomb HM, Rowley JD (1984) Evidence for a 15;17 translocation in every patient with acute promyelocytic leukemia. Am J Med 76:827–841
4. de The H, Lavau C, Marchio A, Chomienne C, Degos L, Dejean A (1991) The PML-RAR alpha fusion mRNA generated by the t(15;17) translocation in acute promyelocytic leukemia encodes a functionally altered RAR. Cell 66:675–684
5. Kakizuka A, Miller WH Jr, Umesono K, Warrell RP Jr, Frankel SR, Murty VV, Dmitrovsky E, Evans RM (1991) Chromosomal translocation t(15;17) in human acute promyelocytic leukemia fuses RAR alpha with a novel putative transcription factor, PML. Cell 66:663–674
6. Tallman MS, Brenner B, Serna JdL, Dombret H, Falanga A, Kwaan HC, Liebman H, Raffoux E, Rickles FR (2005) Meeting report. Acute promyelocytic leukemia-associated coagulopathy, 21 January 2004, London, United Kingdom. Leuk Res 29:347–351
7. Tallman MS (1999) The thrombophilic state in acute promyelocytic leukemia. Semin Thromb Hemost 25:209–215
8. Bernard J, Weil M, Boiron M, Jacquillat C, Flandrin G, Gemon MF (1973) Acute promyelocytic leukemia: results of treatment by daunorubicin. Blood 41:489–496
9. Goldberg MA, Ginsburg D, Mayer RJ, Stone RM, Maguire M, Rosenthal DS, Antin JH (1987) Is heparin administration necessary during induction chemotherapy for patients with acute promyelocytic leukemia? Blood 69:187–191
10. Hoyle CF, Swirsky DM, Freedman L, Hayhoe FG (1988) Beneficial effect of heparin in the management of patients with APL. Br J Haematol 68:283–289
11. Sanz MA, Jarque I, Martin G, Lorenzo I, Martinez J, Rafecas J, Pastor E, Sayas MJ, Sanz G, Gomis F (1988) Acute promyelocytic leukemia. Therapy results and prognostic factors. Cancer 61:7–13
12. Cunningham I, Gee TS, Reich LM, Kempin SJ, Naval AN, Clarkson BD (1989) Acute promyelocytic leukemia: treatment results during a decade at Memorial Hospital. Blood 73:1116–1122
13. Fenaux P, Tertian G, Castaigne S, Tilly H, Leverger G, Guy H, Bordessoule D, Leblay R, Le Gall E, Colombat P, et al (1991) A randomized trial of amsacrine and rubidazone in 39 patients with acute promyelocytic leukemia. J Clin Oncol 9:1556–1561
14. Fenaux P, Degos L (1991) Treatment of acute promyelocytic leukemia with all-trans retinoic acid. Leuk Res 15:655–657
15. Marty M, Ganem G, Fischer J, Flandrin G, Berger R, Schaison G, Degos L, Boiron M (1984) Acute promyelocytic leukemia: retrospective study of 119 patients treated with daunorubicin (in French). Nouv Rev Fr Hematol 26:371–378

16. Head DR, Kopecky KJ, Weick J, Files FC, Ryan D, Foucar K, Montiel Bickers J, Fishleder A, Miller M, et al (1995) Effect of aggressive daunomycin therapy on survival in acute promyelocytic leukemia. Blood 86:1717–1728
17. Avvisatti G, Petti MC, Lo-Coco F, et al (2002) Induction therapy with idarubicin alone significantly influences event-free survival duration in patients with newly diagnosed hypergranular acute promyelocytic leukemia: final results of the GIMEMA randomized study LAP 0389 with 7 years of minimal follow-up. Blood 100:3141–3146
18. Arlin Z, Kempin S, Mertelsmann R, Gee T, Higgins C, Jhanwar S, Chaganti RS, Clarkson B (1984) Primary therapy of acute promyelocytic leukemia: results of amsacrine- and daunorubicin-based therapy. Blood 63:211–212
19. Lengfelder E, Reichert A, Hehlmann R (1997) Effect of high dose AraCX in APL. Blood 92 Suppl
20. Bassan R, Battista R, Viero P, d'Emilio A, Buelli M, Montaldi A, Rambaldi A, Tremul L, Dini E, Barbui T (1995) Short-term treatment for adult hypergranular and microgranular acute promyelocytic leukemia. Leukemia 9:238–243
21. Reference deleted in proof
22. Cordonnier C, Vernant JP, Brun B, Heilmann MG, Kuentz M, Bierling P, Farcet JP, Rodet M, Duedari N, Imbert M, et al (1985) Acute promyelocytic leukemia in 57 previously untreated patients. Cancer 55:18–25
23. Kantarjian HM, Keating MJ, Walters RS, Estey EH, McCredie KB, Smith TL, Dalton WT Jr, Cork A, Trujillo JM, Freireich EJ (1986) Acute promyelocytic leukemia. MD Anderson Hospital experience. Am J Med 80:789–797
24. Fenaux P, Pollet J, Vandebossche L, et al (1991) Treatment of acute promyelocytic leukemia: a report of 70 cases. Leuk Lymphoma 4:249–256
25. Huang ME, Ye YC, Chen SR, Chai JR, Lu JX, Zhoa L, Gu LJ, Wang ZY (1988) Use of all-trans retinoic acid in the treatment of acute promyelocytic leukemia. Blood 72:567–572
26. Castaigne S, Chomienne C, Daniel MT, Ballerini P, Berger R, Fenaux P, Degos L (1990) All-trans retinoic acid as a differentiation therapy for acute promyelocytic leukemia. I. Clinical results. Blood 76:1704–1709
27. Degos L, Chomienne C, Daniel MT, Berger R, Dombret H, Fenaux P, Castaigne S (1990) Treatment of first relapse in acute promyelocytic leukaemia with all-trans retinoic acid. Lancet 336:1440–1441
28. Chen ZX, Xue YQ, Zhang R, Tao RF, Xia XM, Li C, Wang W, Zu WY, Yao XZ, Ling BJ (1991) A clinical and experimental study on all-trans retinoic acid-treated acute promyelocytic leukemia patients. Blood 78:1413–1419
29. Warrell RP Jr, Frankel SR, Miller WH Jr, Scheinberg DA, Itri LM, Hittelman WN, Vyas R, Andreeff M, Tafuri A, Jakubowski A, et al (1991) Differentiation therapy of acute promyelocytic leukemia with tretinoin (all-trans-retinoic acid). N Engl J Med 324:1385–1393
30. Chomienne C, Ballerini P, Balitrand N, Daniel MT, Fenaux P, Castaigne S, Degos L (1990) All-trans retinoic acid in acute promyelocytic leukemias. II. In vitro studies: structure-function relationship. Blood 76:1710–1717

31. Elliott S, Taylor K, White S, Rodwell R, Marlton P, Meagher D, Wiley J, Taylor D, Wright S, Timms P (1992) Proof of differentiative mode of action of all-trans retinoic acid in acute promyelocytic leukemia using X-linked clonal analysis. Blood 79:1916–1919
32. Ohashi H, Ichikawa A, Takagi N, Hotta T, Naoe T, Ohno R, Saito H (1992) Remission induction of acute promyelocytic leukemia by all-trans-retinoic acid: molecular evidence of restoration of normal hematopoiesis after differentiation and subsequent extinction of leukemic clone. Leukemia 6:859–862
33. Fenaux P, Castaigne S, Dombret H, Archimbaud E, Duarte M, Morel P, Lamy T, Tilly H, Guerci A, Maloisel F, et al (1992) All-transretinoic acid followed by intensive chemotherapy gives a high complete remission rate and may prolong remissions in newly diagnosed acute promyelocytic leukemia: a pilot study on 26 cases. Blood 80:2176–2181
34. Frankel SR, Eardley A, Lauwers G, Weiss M, Warrell RP Jr (1992) The "retinoic acid syndrome" in acute promyelocytic leukemia. Ann Intern Med 117:292–296
35. Fenaux P, Degos L (1996) Treatment of acute promyelocytic leukaemia. Baillieres Clin Haematol 9:107–128
36. Fenaux P, Wattel E, Archimbaud E, Sanz M, Hecquet B, Fegueux N, Guerci A, Link H, Fey M, Castaigne S, et al (1994) Prolonged follow-up confirms that all-trans retinoic acid followed by chemotherapy reduces the risk of relapse in newly diagnosed acute promyelocytic leukemia. The French APL Group. Blood 84:666–667
37. Fenaux P, Le Deley MC, Castaigne S, Archimbaud E, Chomienne C, Link H, Guerci A, Duarte M, Daniel MT, Bowen D, et al (1993) Effect of all transretinoic acid in newly diagnosed acute promyelocytic leukemia. Results of a multicenter randomized trial. European APL 91 Group. Blood 82:3241–3249
38. Fenaux P, Chevret S, Guerci A, Fegueux N, Dombret H, Thomas X, Sanz M, Link H, Maloisel F, Gardin C, Bordessoule D, Stoppa AM, Sadoun A, Muus P, Wandt H, Mineur P, Whittaker JA, Fey M, Daniel MT, Castaigne S, Degos L (2000) Long-term follow-up confirms the benefit of all-trans retinoic acid in acute promyelocytic leukemia. European APL group. Leukemia 14:1371–1377
39. Tallman MS, Andersen JW, Schiffer CA, Appelbaum FR, Feusner JH, Ogden A, Shepherd L, Willman C, Bloomfield CD, Rowe JM, Wiernik PH (1997) All-transretinoic acid in acute promyelocytic leukemia. N Engl J Med 337:1021–1028
40. Fenaux P, Chastang C, Chevret S, Sanz M, Dombret H, Archimbaud E, Fey M, Rayon C, Huguet F, Sotto JJ, Gardin C, Makhoul PC, Travade P, Solary E, Fegueux N, Bordessoule D, Miguel JS, Link H, Desablens B, Stamatoullas A, Deconinck E, Maloisel F, Castaigne S, Preudhomme C, Degos L (1999) A randomized comparison of all transretinoic acid (ATRA) followed by chemotherapy and ATRA plus chemotherapy and the role of maintenance therapy in newly diagnosed acute promyelocytic leukemia. The European APL Group. Blood 94:1192–1200
41. Tallman MS, Andersen JW, Schiffer CA, Appelbaum FR, Feusner JH, Woods WG, Ogden A, Weinstein H, Shepherd L, Willman C, Bloomfield CD, Rowe JM, Wiernik PH (2002) All-trans retinoic acid in acute promyelocytic leukemia: long-term outcome and prognostic factor analysis from the North American Intergroup protocol. Blood 100:4298–4302

42. Girmenia C, Latagliata R, Tosti S, Morano SG, Celesti F, Coppola L, Spadea A, Breccia M, Battistini R, Tafuri A, Cimino G, Mandelli F, Alimena G (1999) Outpatient management of acute promyelocytic leukemia after consolidation chemotherapy. Leukemia 13:514–517
43. Burnett AK, Grimwade D, Solomon E, Wheatley K, Goldstone AH (1999) Presenting white blood cell count and kinetics of molecular remission predict prognosis in acute promyelocytic leukemia treated with all-trans retinoic acid: result of the Randomized MRC Trial. Blood 93:4131–4143
44. De Botton S, Dombret H, Sanz M, Miguel JS, Caillot D, Zittoun R, Gardembas M, Stamatoulas A, Conde E, Guerci A, Gardin C, Geiser K, Makhoul DC, Reman O, de la Serna J, Lefrere F, Chomienne C, Chastang C, Degos L, Fenaux P (1998) Incidence, clinical features, and outcome of all trans-retinoic acid syndrome in 413 cases of newly diagnosed acute promyelocytic leukemia. The European APL Group. Blood 92:2712–2718
45. Castaigne S, Lefebvre P, Chomienne C, Suc E, Rigal-Huguet F, Gardin C, Delmer A, Archimbaud E, Tilly H, Janvier M, et al (1993) Effectiveness and pharmacokinetics of low-dose all-trans retinoic acid (25 mg/m^2) in acute promyelocytic leukemia. Blood 82:3560–3563
46. Mahmoud HH, Hurwitz CA, Roberts WM, Santana VM, Ribeiro RC, Krance RA (1993) Tretinoin toxicity in children with acute promyelocytic leukaemia. Lancet 342:1394–1395
47. Sanz MA, Lo-Coco F (2000) Definition of relapse risk and role of nonanthracycline drugs for consolidation in patients with acute promyelocytic leukemia: a joint study of the PETHEMA and GIMEMA cooperative groups. Blood 96:1247–1253
48. Estey E, Thall PF, Pierce S, Kantarjian H, Keating M (1997) Treatment of newly diagnosed acute promyelocytic leukemia without cytarabine. J Clin Oncol 15:483–490
49. Cornic M, Delva L, Guidez F, Balitrand N, Degos L, Chomienne C (1992) Induction of retinoic acid-binding protein in normal and malignant human myeloid cells by retinoic acid in acute promyelocytic leukemia patients. Cancer Res 52:3329–3334
50. Muindi J, Frankel SR, Miller WH Jr, Jakubowski A, Scheinberg DA, Young CW, Dmitrovsky E, Warrell RP Jr (1992) Continuous treatment with all-trans retinoic acid causes a progressive reduction in plasma drug concentrations: implications for relapse and retinoid "resistance" in patients with acute promyelocytic leukemia. Blood 79:299–303
51. Adamson PC, Bailey J, Pluda J, Poplack DG, Bauza S, Murphy RF, Yarchoan R, Balis FM (1995) Pharmacokinetics of all-trans-retinoic acid administered on an intermittent schedule. J Clin Oncol 13:1238–1241
52. Sanz A, Martin G, Gonzalez M, et al (2004) Risk-adapted treatment of acute promyelocytic leukemia with all-trans-retinoic acid and anthracycline monochemotherapy: a multicenter study par the PETHEMA group. Blood 103:1237–1243

53. Asou N, Adachi K, Tamura J, Kanamaru A, Kageyama S, Hiraoka A, Omoto E, Akiyama H, Tsubaki K, Saito K, Kuriyama K, Oh H, Kitano K, Miyawaki S, Takeyama K, Yamada O, Nishikawa K, Takahashi M, Matsuda S, Ohtake S, Suzushima H, Emi N, Ohno R (1998) Analysis of prognostic factors in newly diagnosed acute promyelocytic leukemia treated with all-trans retinoic acid and chemotherapy. Japan Adult Leukemia Study Group. J Clin Oncol 16:78–85
54. Claxton DF, Reading CL, Nagarajan L, Tsujimoto Y, Andersson BS, Estey E, Cork A, Huh YO, Trujillo J, Deisseroth AB (1992) Correlation of CD2 expression with PML gene breakpoints in patients with acute promyelocytic leukemia. Blood 80:582–586
55. Paietta E, Andersen J, Gallagher R, Bennett J, Yunis J, Cassileth P, Rowe J, Wiernik PH (1994) The immunophenotype of acute promyelocytic leukemia (APL): an ECOG study. Leukemia 8:1108–1112
56. Guglielmi C, Martelli MP, Diverio D, Fenu S, Vegna ML, Cantu-Rajnoldi A, Biondi A, Cocito MG, Del Vecchio L, Tabilio A, Avvisati G, Basso G, Lo Coco F (1998) Immunophenotype of adult and childhood acute promyelocytic leukaemia: correlation with morphology, type of PML gene breakpoint and clinical outcome. A cooperative Italian study on 196 cases. Br J Haematol 102:1035–1041
57. Murray CK, Estey E, Paietta E, Howard RS, Edenfield WJ, Pierce S, Mann KP, Bolan C, Byrd JC (1999) CD56 expression in acute promyelocytic leukemia: a possible indicator of poor treatment outcome? J Clin Oncol 17:293–297
58. Cassinat B, Chevret S, Zassadowski F, Balitrand N, Guillemot I, Menot ML, Degos L, et al (2001) In vitro all-trans retinoic acid sensitivity of acute promyelocytic leukemia blasts: a novel indicator of poor patient outcome. Blood 98:2862–2864
59. Jurcic JG, Nimer SD, Scheinberg DA, DeBlasio T, Warrell RP Jr, Miller WH Jr (2001) Prognostic significance of minimal residual disease detection and PML/RAR- isoform type: long-term follow-up in acute promyelocytic leukemia. Blood 98:2651–2656
60. Diverio D, Rossi V, Avvisati G, De Santis S, Pistilli A, Pane F, Saglio G, Martinelli G, Petti MC, Santoro A, Pelicci PG, Mandelli F, Biondi A, Lo Coco F (1998) Early detection of relapse by prospective reverse transcriptase-polymerase chain reaction analysis of the PML/RARalpha fusion gene in patients with acute promyelocytic leukemia enrolled in the GIMEMA-AIEOP multicenter "AIDA" trial. GIMEMA-AIEOP Multicenter "AIDA" Trial. Blood 92:784–789
61. Cassinat B, Zassadowski F, Balitrand N, Barbey C, Rain JD, Fenaux P, Degos L, Vidaud M, Chomienne C (2000) Quantitation of minimal residual disease in acute promyelocytic leukemia patients with t(15;17) translocation using real-time RT-PCR. Leukemia 14:324
62. Visani G, Buonamici S, Malagola M, Isidori A, Piccaluga PP, Martin G, Ottaviani E, Grafone T, Baccarani M, Tura S (2000) Pulsed ATRA as single therapy restores long-term remission PML-RARalpha-positive acute promyelocytic leukemia patient real time quantification of minimal residual disease. A pilot study. Leukemia 15:1696–1700
63. Gallagher RE, Yeap BY, Bi W, et al (2003) Quantitative real-time RT-PCR analysis of PML-RAR alpha mRNA in acute promyelocytic leukemia: assessment of prognostic significance in adult patients from intergroup protocol 0129. Blood 101:2521–2528

64. Bolufer P, Barragan E, Sanz MA, Martin G, Bornstein R, Colomer D, Delgado MD, Gonzalez M, Marugan I, Roman J, Gomez MT, Anguita E, Diverio D, Chomienne C, Briz M (1998) Preliminary experience in external quality control of RT-PCR PML-RAR alpha detection in promyelocytic leukemia. Leukemia 12:2024–2028
65. Evans GD, Grimwade DJ (1999) Extramedullary disease in acute promyelocytic leukemia. Leuk Lymphoma 33:219–229
66. de Botton S, Sanz M, Chevret S, et al (2006) Extramedullary relapse in acute promyelocytic leukemia treated with all-trans retinoic acid and chemotherapy. Leukemia 20:35–41
67. Lo-Coco F, Vignetti M, Avvisatti G, et al (2004) Front-line treatment of acute promyelocytic leukemia with AIDA induction followed by risk-adapted consolidation: results of the AIDA-2000 trial of the Italian GIMEMA group. Blood 104 Suppl 1 Abstr 392
68. Lengfelder E, Reichert A, Schoch C, et al (2000) Double induction strategy including high dose cytarabine in combination with all-trans retinoic acid: effects in patients with newly diagnosed acute promyelocytic leukemia. German AML Cooperative Group. Leukemia 14:1362–1370
69. Warrell RP Jr, Maslak P, Eardley A, Heller G, Miller WH Jr, Frankel SR (1994) Treatment of acute promyelocytic leukemia with all-trans retinoic acid: an update of the New York experience. Leukemia 8:929–933
70. Delva L, Cornic M, Balitrand N, Guidez F, Miclea JM, Delmer A, Teillet F, Fenaux P, Castaigne S, Degos L, et al (1993) Resistance to all-trans retinoic acid (ATRA) therapy in relapsing acute promyelocytic leukemia: study of in vitro ATRA sensitivity and cellular retinoic acid binding protein levels in leukemic cells. Blood 82:2175–2181
71. Thomas X, Dombret H, Cordonnier C, Pigneux A, Gardin C, Guerci A, Vekhoff A, Sadoun A, Stamatoullas A, Fegueux N, Maloisel F, Cahn JY, Reman O, Gratecos N, Berthou C, Huguet F, Kotoucek P, Travade P, Buzyn A, de Revel T, Vilque JP, Naccache P, Chomienne C, Degos L, Fenaux P (2000) Treatment of relapsing acute promyelocytic leukemia by all-trans retinoic acid therapy followed by timed sequential chemotherapy and stem cell transplantation. APL Study Group. Acute promyelocytic leukemia. Leukemia 14:1006–1013
72. de Botton S, Fawaz A, Chevret S, et al (2005) Autologous and allogeneic stem-cell transplantation as salvage treatment of acute promyelocytic leukemia initially treated with all-trans-retinoic acid: a retrospective analysis of the European acute promyelocytic leukemia group. J Clin Oncol 23:120–126
73. Ding W, Li YP, Nobile LM, Grills G, Carrera I, Paietta E, Tallman MS, Wiernik PH, Gallagher RE (1998) Leukemic cellular retinoic acid resistance and missense mutations in the PML-RARalpha fusion gene after relapse of acute promyelocytic leukemia from treatment with all-trans retinoic acid and intensive chemotherapy. Blood 92:1172–1183
74. Douer D, Estey E, Santillana S, Bennett JM, Lopez-Bernstein G, et al (2001) Treatment of newly diagnosed and relapsed acute promyelocytic leukemia with intravenous liposomal all-trans retinoic acid. Blood 97:73–80
75. Mehta K, Sadeghi T, McQueen T, Lopez-Berestein G (1994) Liposome encapsulation circumvents the hepatic clearance mechanisms of all-trans-retinoic acid. Leuk Res 18:587–596

76. Soignet SL, Benedetti F, Fleischauer A, Parker BA, Truglia JA, Ra Crisp M, Warrell RP Jr (1998) Clinical study of 9-cis retinoic acid (LGD1057) in acute promyelocytic leukemia. Leukemia 12:1518–1521
77. Miller WH, Jakubowski A, Tong WP, Miller VA, Rigas JR, Benedetti F, Gill GM, Truglia JA, Ulm E, Shirley M (1995) 9-cis retinoic acid induces complete remission but does not reverse clinically acquired retinoid resistance in acute promyelocytic leukemia. Blood 85:3021
78. Tobita T, Takeshita A, Kitamura K, Ohnishi K, Yanagi M, Hiraoka A, Karasuno T, Takeuchi M, Miyawaki S, Ueda R, Naoe T, Ohno R (1997) Treatment with a new synthetic retinoid, Am80, of acute promyelocytic leukemia relapsed from complete remission induced by all-trans retinoic acid. Blood 90:967–973
79. Warrell RP Jr, He LZ, Richon V, Calleja E, Pandolfi PP (1998) Therapeutic targeting of transcription in acute promyelocytic leukemia by use of an inhibitor of histone deacetylase. J Natl Cancer Inst 90:1621–1625
80. Kosugi H, Towatari M, Hatano S, Kitamura K, Kiyoi H, Kinoshita T, Tanimoto M, Murate T, Kawashima K, Saito H, Naoe T (1999) Histone deacetylase inhibitors are the potent inducer/enhancer of differentiation in acute myeloid leukemia: a new approach to anti-leukemia therapy. Leukemia 13:1316–1324
81. Jurcic JG, DeBlasio T, Dumont L, Yao TJ, Scheinberg DA (2000) Molecular remission induction with retinoic acid and anti-CD33 monoclonal antibody HuM195 in acute promyelocytic leukemia. Clin Cancer Res 6:372–380
82. Petti MC, Pinazzi MB, Diverio D, Romano A, Petrucci MT, De Santis S, Meloni G, Tafuri A, Mandelli F, Lo Coco F (2001) Prolonged molecular remission in advanced acute promyelocytic leukaemia after treatment with gemtuzumab ozogamicin (Mylotarg CMA-676). Br J Haematol 115:63–65
83. Yang Y, Liu T, Liang Y, Qin P, Yuan S (1994) Study on anti-leukemic effect of tanshinone IIA in vitro and in vivo to acute promyelocytic leukemia. Blood 94 Suppl 1
84. Shen ZX, Chen GQ, Ni JH, Li XS, Xiong SM, Qiu QY, Zhu J, Tang W, Sun GL, Yang KQ, Chen Y, Zhou L, Fang ZW, Wang YT, Ma J, Zhang P, Zhang TD, Chen SJ, Chen Z, Wang ZY (1997) Use of arsenic trioxide (As2O3) in the treatment of acute promyelocytic leukemia (APL). II. Clinical efficacy and pharmacokinetics in relapsed patients. Blood 89:3354–3360
85. Soignet SL, Maslak P, Wang ZG, Jhanwar S, Calleja E, Dardashti LJ, Corso D, DeBlasio A, Gabrilove J, Scheinberg DA, Pandolfi PP, Warrell RP Jr (1998) Complete remission after treatment of acute promyelocytic leukemia with arsenic trioxide. N Engl J Med 339:1341–1348
86. Niu C, Yan H, Yu T, Sun HP, Liu JX, Li XS, Wu W, Zhang FQ, Chen Y, Zhou L, Li JM, Zeng XY, Yang RR, Yuan MM, Ren MY, Gu FY, Cao Q, Gu BW, Su XY, Chen GQ, Xiong SM, Zhang T, Waxman S, Wang ZY, Chen SJ, et al (1999) Studies on treatment of acute promyelocytic leukemia with arsenic trioxide: remission induction, follow-up, and molecular monitoring in 11 newly diagnosed and 47 relapsed acute promyelocytic leukemia patients. Blood 94:3315–3324
87. Soignet SL, Frankel SR, Douer D, Tallman MS, Kantarjian H, Calleja E, Stone RM, Kalaycio M, Scheinberg DA, Steinherz P, Sievers EL, Coutre S, Dahlberg S, Ellison R, Warrell RP Jr (2001) United States multicenter study of arsenic trioxide in relapsed acute promyelocytic leukemia. J Clin Oncol 19:3852–3860

88. Leoni F, Gianfaldoni G, Annunziata M, Fanci R, Ciolli S, Nozzoli C, Ferrara F (2002) Arsenic trioxide therapy for relapsed acute promyelocytic leukemia: a bridge to transplantation. Haematologica 87:485–489
89. Ohnishi K, Yoshida H, Shigeno K, Nakamura S, Fujisawa S, Naito K, Shinjo K, Fujita Y, Matsui H, Takeshita A, Sugiyama S, Satoh H, Terada H, Ohno R (2000) Prolongation of the QT interval and ventricular tachycardia in patients treated with arsenic trioxide for acute promyelocytic leukemia. Ann Intern Med 133:881–885
90. Westervelt P, Brown RA, Adkins DR, Khoury H, Curtin P, Hurd D, Luger SM, Ma MK, Ley TJ, DiPersio JF (2001) Sudden death among patients with acute promyelocytic leukemia treated with arsenic trioxide. Blood 98:266–271
91. Kwong YL, Au WY, Chim CS, Pang A, Suen C, Liang R (2001) Arsenic trioxide- and idarubicin-induced remissions in relapsed acute promyelocytic leukaemia: clinicopathological and molecular features of a pilot study. Am J Hematol 66:274–279
92. Shen Y, Shen ZX, Yan H, Chen J, Zeng XY, Li JM, Li XS, Wu W, Xiong SM, Zhao WL, Tang W, Wu F, Liu YF, Niu C, Wang ZY, Chen SJ, Chen Z (2001) Studies on the clinical efficacy and pharmacokinetics of low-dose arsenic trioxide in the treatment of relapsed acute promyelocytic leukemia: a comparison with conventional dosage. Leukemia 15:735–741
93. Roberts TF, Sprague K, Schenkein D, Miller KB, Relias V (2000) Hyperleukocytosis during induction therapy with arsenic trioxide for relapsed acute promyelocytic leukemia associated with central nervous system infarction. Blood 96:4000–4001
94. Camacho LH, Soignet SL, Chanel S, Ho R, Heller G, Scheinberg DA, Ellison R, Warrell RP Jr (2000) Leukocytosis and the retinoic acid syndrome in patients with acute promyelocytic leukemia treated with arsenic trioxide. J Clin Oncol 18:2620–2625
95. Che-Pin L, Huang MJ, Chang IY, Lin WY, Sheu YT (2000) Retinoic acid syndrome induced by arsenic trioxide in treating recurrent all-trans retinoic acid resistant acute promyelocytic leukemia. Leuk Lymphoma 38:195–198
96. Unnikrishnan D, Dutcher JP, Varshneya N, Lucariello R, Api M, Garl S, Wiernik PH, Chiaramida S (2001) Torsades de pointes in 3 patients with leukemia treated with arsenic trioxide. Blood 97:1514–1516
97. Yip SF, Yeung YM, Tsui EY (2002) Severe neurotoxicity following arsenic therapy for acute promyelocytic leukemia: potentiation by thiamine deficiency. Blood 99:3481–3482
98. Lu DP, Qiu JY, Jiang B, Wang Q, Liu KY, Liu YR, Chen SS (2002) Tetra-arsenic tetra-sulfide for the treatment of acute promyelocytic leukemia: a pilot report. Blood 99:3136–3143
99. Jing Y, Wang L, Xia L, Chen GQ, Chen Z, Miller WH, Waxman S (2001) Combined effect of all-trans retinoic acid and arsenic trioxide in acute promyelocytic leukemia cells in vitro and in vivo. Blood 97:264–269
100. Au WY, Chim CS, Lie AK, Liang R, Kwong YL (2002) Combined arsenic trioxide and all-trans retinoic acid treatment for acute promyelocytic leukaemia recurring from previous relapses successfully treated using arsenic trioxide. Br J Haematol 117:130–132

101. Marasca R, Zucchini P, Galimberti S, Leonardi G, Vaccari P, Donelli A, Luppi M, Petrini M, Torelli G (1999) Missense mutations in the PML/RARalpha ligand binding domain in ATRA-resistant As(2)O(3) sensitive relapsed acute promyelocytic leukemia. Haematologica 84:963–968
102. Wang ZG, Rivi R, Delva L, Konig A, Scheinberg DA, Gambacorti-Passerini C, Gabrilove JL, Warrell RP Jr, Pandolfi PP (1998) Arsenic trioxide and melarsoprol induce programmed cell death in myeloid leukemia cell lines and function in a PML and PML-RARalpha independent manner. Blood 92:1497–1504
103. Jing Y, Dai J, Chalmers-Redman RM, Tatton WG, Waxman S (1999) Arsenic trioxide selectively induces acute promyelocytic leukemia cell apoptosis via a hydrogen peroxide-dependent pathway. Blood 94:2102–2111
104. Davison K, Mann KK, Miller WH Jr (2002) Arsenic trioxide: mechanisms of action. Semin Hematol 39:3–7
105. Hong SH, Yang Z, Privalsky ML (2001) Arsenic trioxide is a potent inhibitor of the interaction of SMRT corepressor with its transcription factor partners, including the PML-retinoic acid receptor alpha oncoprotein found in human acute promyelocytic leukemia. Mol Cell Biol 21:7172–7182
106. Roboz GJ, Dias S, Lam G, Lane WJ, Soignet SL, Warrell RP Jr, Rafii S (2000) Arsenic trioxide induces dose- and time-dependent apoptosis of endothelium and may exert an antileukemic effect via inhibition of angiogenesis. Blood 96:1525–1530
107. Chen GQ, Shi XG, Tang W, Xiong SM, Zhu J, Cai X, Han ZG, Ni JH, Shi GY, Jia PM, Liu MM, He KL, Niu C, Ma J, Zhang P, Zhang TD, Paul P, Naoe T, Kitamura K, Miller W, Waxman S, Wang ZY, de The H, Chen SJ, Chen Z (1997) Use of arsenic trioxide (As2O3) in the treatment of acute promyelocytic leukemia (APL). I. As2O3 exerts dose-dependent dual effects on APL cells. Blood 89:3345–3353
108. Tallman MS, Andersen JW, Schiffer CA, Appelbaum FR, Feusner JH, Ogden A, Shepherd L, Rowe JM, Francois C, Larson RS, Wiernik PH (2000) Clinical description of 44 patients with acute promyelocytic leukemia who developed the retinoic acid syndrome. Blood 95:90–95
109. Kanamaru A, Takemoto Y, Tanimoto M, Murakami H, Asou N, Kobayashi T, Kuriyama K, Ohmoto E, Sakamaki H, Tsubaki K, et al (1995) All-trans retinoic acid for the treatment of newly diagnosed acute promyelocytic leukemia. Japan Adult Leukemia Study Group. Blood 85:1202–1206
110. Vahdat L, Maslak P, Miller WH Jr, Eardley A, Heller G, Scheinberg DA, Warrell RP Jr (1994) Early mortality and the retinoic acid syndrome in acute promyelocytic leukemia: impact of leukocytosis, low-dose chemotherapy, PMN/RAR-alpha isoform, and CD13 expression in patients treated with all-trans retinoic acid. Blood 84:3843–3849
111. Ko BS, Tang JL, Chen YC, Yao M, Wang CH, Shen MC, Tien HF (1999) Extramedullary relapse after all-trans retinoic acid treatment in acute promyelocytic leukemia—the occurrence of retinoic acid syndrome is a risk factor. Leukemia 13:1406–1408
112. Dubois C, Schlageter MH, de Gentile A, Balitrand N, Toubert ME, Krawice I, Fenaux P, Castaigne S, Najean Y, Degos L, et al (1994) Modulation of IL-8, IL-1 beta, and G-CSF secretion by all-trans retinoic acid in acute promyelocytic leukemia. Leukemia 8:1750–1757

113. Dubois C, Schlageter MH, de Gentile A, Guidez F, Balitrand N, Toubert ME, Krawice I, Fenaux P, Castaigne S, Najean Y, et al (1994) Hematopoietic growth factor expression and ATRA sensitivity in acute promyelocytic blast cells. Blood 83:3264–3270
114. Larson RS, Brown DC, Sklar LA (1997) Retinoic acid induces aggregation of the acute promyelocytic leukemia cell line NB-4 by utilization of LFA-1 and ICAM-2. Blood 90:2747–2756
115. Visani G, Tosi P, Cenacchi A, Manfroi S, Gamberi B, Ottaviani E, Tura S (1994) Pre-treatment with all-trans retinoic acid accelerates polymorphonuclear recovery after chemotherapy in patients with acute promyelocytic leukemia. Leuk Lymphoma 15:143–147
116. De Botton S, Coitteux V, Chevret S, Dombret H, Sanz M, San Miguel J, Caillot D, et al (2001) Early onset chemotherapy can reduce the incidence of ATRA syndrome in newly diagnosed acute promyelocytic leukemia (APL). Results of a randomized study. Blood 98:766a
117. Stadler M, Ganser A, Hoelzer D (1994) Acute promyelocytic leukemia. N Engl J Med 330:140–141
118. Tapiovaara H, Matikainen S, Hurme M, Vaheri A (1994) Induction of differentiation of promyelocytic NB4 cells by retinoic acid is associated with rapid increase in urokinase activity subsequently downregulated by production of inhibitors. Blood 83:1883–1891
119. de Lacerda JF, do Carmo JA, Guerra ML, Geraldes J, de Lacerda JM (1993) Multiple thrombosis in acute promyelocytic leukaemia after tretinoin. Lancet 342:114–115
120. Hashimoto S, Koike T, Tatewaki W, Seki Y, Sato N, Azegami T, Tsukada N, Takahashi H, Kimura H, Ueno M, et al (1994) Fatal thromboembolism in acute promyelocytic leukemia during all-trans retinoic acid therapy combined with antifibrinolytic therapy for prophylaxis of hemorrhage. Leukemia 8:1113–1115
121. Torromeo C, Latagliata R, Avvisati G, Petti MC, Mandelli F (1999) Coronaric thrombotic events in acute promyelocytic leukemia during all-trans retinoic acid treatment: a role for adhesion molecules overexpression? Leukemia 13:312–313
122. Akiyama H, Nakamura N, Nagasaka S, Sakamaki H, Onozawa Y (1992) Hypercalcaemia due to all-trans retinoic acid. Lancet 339:308–309
123. Hakimian D, Tallman MS, Zugerman C, Caro WA (1993) Erythema nodosum associated with all-trans-retinoic acid in the treatment of acute promyelocytic leukemia. Leukemia 7:758–759
124. Koike T, Tatewaki W, Aoki A, Yoshimoto H, Yagisawa K, Hashimoto S, Furukawa T, Saitoh H, Takahashi M, Yang LB, et al (1992) Brief report: severe symptoms of hyperhistaminemia after the treatment of acute promyelocytic leukemia with tretinoin (all-trans-retinoic acid). N Engl J Med 327:385–387
125. Iwakiri R, Inokuchi K, Dan K, Nomura T (1994) Marked basophilia in acute promyelocytic leukaemia treated with all-trans retinoic acid: molecular analysis of the cell origin of the basophils. Br J Haematol 86:870–872
126. Miranda N, Oliveira P, Frade MJ, Melo J, Marques MS, Parreira A (1994) Myositis with tretinoin. Lancet 344:1096
127. Tomas JF, Escudero A, Fernandez-Ranada JM (1994) All-trans retinoic acid treatment and Sweet syndrome. Leukemia 8:1596

128. Arun B, Berberian B, Azumi N, Frankel SR, Luksenburg H, Freter C (1998) Sweet's syndrome during treatment with all-trans retinoic acid in a patient with acute promyelocytic leukemia. Leuk Lymphoma 31:613–615
129. Levy V, Jaffarbey J, Aouad K, Zittoun R (1998) Fournier's gangrene during induction treatment of acute promyelocytic leukemia, a case report. Ann Hematol 76:91–92
130. Mori A, Tamura S, Katsuno T, Nishimura Y, Itoh T, Saheki K, Takatsuka H, Wada H, Fujimori Y, Okamoto T, Takemoto Y, Kakishita E (1999) Scrotal ulcer occurring in patients with acute promyelocytic leukemia during treatment with all-trans retinoic acid. Oncol Rep 6:55–58
131. Kentos A, Le Moine F, Crenier L, Capel P, Meyer S, Muus P, Mandelli F, Feremans W (1997) All-trans retinoic acid induced thrombocytosis in a patient with acute promyelocytic leukaemia. Br J Haematol 97:685
132. Paydas S, Sahin B, Zorludemir S, Hazar B (1998) All trans retinoic acid as the possible cause of necrotizing vasculitis. Leuk Res 22:655–657

Arsenic Trioxide and Acute Promyelocytic Leukemia: Clinical and Biological

Z. Chen[1] (✉) · W.-L. Zhao[1] · Z.-X. Shen[1] · J.-M. Li[1] · S.-J. Chen[1] · J. Zhu[1,2] ·
V. Lallemand-Breittenbach[2] · J. Zhou[1,2] · M.-C. Guillemin[2] · D. Vitoux[2] ·
H. de Thé[2]

[1] Shanghai Institute of Hematology, Rui Jin Hospital, School of Medicine,
Shanghai Jiao Tong University,
197 Rui Jin Road II, 200025 Shanghai, People's Republic of China
zchen@stn.sh.cn

[2] CNRS UMR 7151 Université de Paris VII, Hôpital St. Louis, 1 Av. C. Vellefaux 75475, Paris, France

1	As_2O_3 as Single Treatment in Remission Induction	130
2	Dosage and Pharmacokinetics	130
3	As_2O_3 as Combined Treatment with ATRA in Remission Induction	133
4	Adverse Effects	134
5	Postremission Treatment and Survival Time	135
6	Molecular Mechanisms of Arsenic Action	136
7	Perspectives	139
	References	140

Abstract Arsenic has recently been identified as an effective drug in the treatment of newly diagnosed and relapsed acute promyelocytic leukemia. Indeed, arsenic trioxide combined with all-*trans* retinoic acid shows a synergistic effect. Mechanistically, arsenic targets the key leukemogenic protein PML-RARα, setting up a new example of molecular target-based cancer therapy.

Arsenic is a natural substance that has been used as a drug for over 2,000 years in both traditional Chinese medicine and the Western world (Zhu et al. 2002a). However, in the early twentieth century, arsenic disappeared in medical history, due to its low effect compared to modern chemo- and radiotherapy and concerns about its toxicity and potential carcinogenicity. Until recently, this old remedy has been revived thanks to the discovery that it is specifically effective and remarkably safe in the treatment of acute promyelocytic leukemia (APL) (Chen et al. 1996a; Shen et al. 1997; Sun et al. 1992). Acting on the PML-retinoic acid receptor (RAR)α fusion protein, arsenic trioxide (As_2O_3) represents a promising example of molecular target-based cancer therapies, and a new approach in leukemia treatment (Chen Z et al. 1997; Zhou et al. 2005; see also below).

1
As_2O_3 as Single Treatment in Remission Induction

The application of arsenic compounds to APL treatment can be traced back to the early 1970s when white arsenic, containing essentially As_2O_3, was used by a group from Harbin Medical University in China, and its therapeutic effects were identified in some human cancers such as esophageal carcinoma, lymphoma, and leukemia. In 1992, the same group reported, for the first time, the administration of Ailin-1 (anticancer-1) solution, containing 1% As_2O_3 and a trace amount of mercury chloride by the intravenous route, for the treatment of APL. Of 32 cases treated, a complete remission (CR) rate of 65.6% was achieved, with the 5- and 10-year survival rates of 50.0% and 18.8%, respectively (Sun et al. 1992). In 1996, two groups in China, one from Harbin and the other from Shanghai Institute of Hematology, started to treat APL patients with pure 1% As_2O_3. Zhang et al. reported a CR rate of 73.3% in 30 primarily diagnosed patients, and 52.4% in 42 relapsed or refractory cases (Zhang et al. 1996), whereas our group obtained a CR rate of 93.3% in 15 relapsed patients (Chen et al. 1996b; Shen et al. 1997). Hence, As_2O_3 is an effective therapy not only in newly diagnosed APL patients, but also in relapsed ones who obtained CR with all-*trans* retinoic acid (ATRA)/chemotherapy. These results have gradually been confirmed by reports of larger trials in China and then in Western countries (Niu et al. 1999; Soignet et al. 2001; Zhang et al. 2000). Table 1 summarizes the CR rate in APL treated with As_2O_3.

2
Dosage and Pharmacokinetics

The 10% solution of As_2O_3 can be diluted in 250–500 ml of 5% glucose normal solution and administered by intravenous drip for 2–3 h. The standard dosage of 0.16 mg/kg per day over a course of 28–42 days is usually required to induce CR. Importantly, treating APL with low doses of As_2O_3 (0.08 mg/kg per day) can yield similar CR rate (80%) to that attained with a conventional dosage. In

Table 1 Clinical efficacy and side effects of As_2O_3 in APL

Report	Reagent	Disease	n	CR	Time to CR (days)	Side effects (percentage)	Post-remission therapy	Survival
Shen et al. 1997	As_2O_3	Relapse	15	93.3%	38	Skin (26.7%), GI (26.7%), liver (13.3%), heart (13.3%), leukocytosis (13.3%), headache (6.7%)	–	–
Niu et al. 1999	As_2O_3	De novo	11	72.7%	35	Leukocytosis (58.6%), liver (37.9%), skin (25.9%), GI (24.1%), heart (15.5%), neuropathy (10.3%)	$As_2O_3 \pm$ chemo	All in CR 8–20 (median 12) months
		Relapse	47	85.1%	30–39		$As_2O \pm$ chemo	2-year DFS 41.6%[A] 2-year OS 50.2%[A]
Zhang et al. 2000	As_2O_3	De novo + relapse + refractory	242	74.8%	–	Leukocytosis (75.6%), GI (24.0%), skin (22.7%), liver (14.1%)	$As_2O_3 \pm$ chemo	5-year OS 92.0% 7-year OS 76.7%
Soignet et al. 2001	As_2O_3	Relapse + refractory	40	85%	35	GI (75%), cough (65%), fatigue (63%), fever (63%), headache (60%), heart (55%), leukocytosis (50%), hypokalemia (50%), hyperglycemia (45%), skin (43%), neuropathy (43%), liver (25%), RA syndrome (25%)	As_2O_3/HSCT	18-month RFS 56%[A] 18-month OS 66%[A]
Mathews et al. 2002	As_2O_3	De novo	11	91%	52.3	Leukocytosis (63.6%), skin (54.5%), neuropathy (36.4%), fluid retention (27.3%), GI (18.2%), liver (18.2%), RA syndrome (9.1%)	As_2O_3	All in CR 2–33 (median 15) months

Table 1 (continued)

Report	Reagent	Disease	n	CR	Time to CR (days)	Side effects (percentage)	Post-remission therapy	Survival
Au et al. 2003	As$_2$O$_3$ (oral)	Relapse	8	100%	37	Liver (38.5%), leukocytosis (30.8%), skin (30.8%), headache (15.4%)	Chemo	7 in CR 6–18 (median 14 months)[A]
	As$_2$O$_3$+ATRA (oral)	Relapse	5	80%	31		As$_2$O$_3$+ATRA	4 in CR 14–19 (median 17 months)[A]
Lazo et al. 2003	As$_2$O$_3$	Relapse	12	100%	52	Headache (41.7%), skin (33.3%), fatigue (25.0%), fluid retention (16.7%), GI (16.7%), neuropathy (16.7%)	As$_2$O$_3$± chemo/ ATRA± chemo	8 in CR 37–181 (median 98 weeks)[A]
Raffoux et al. 2003	As$_2$O$_3$+ATRA	Relapse	10	80%	42	Fluid retention (60%), liver (50%), hypokalemia (40%), hyperglycemia (30%), heart (30%), leukocytosis (30%), RA syndrome (20%), GI (20%), headache (10%)	As$_2$O$_3$± ATRA/ HSCT	2-year OS 59%[A]
Shen et al. 2004	As$_2$O$_3$	De novo	20	90%	31	Leukocytosis (66.7%), liver (55%), mouth dryness (11.1%), GI (5.6%), headache (5.6%)	As$_2$O$_3$+ ATRA+ chemo	2-year DFS 85%
	As$_2$O$_3$+ATRA	De novo	21	95.2%	25.5	Leukocytosis (70%), liver (61.9%), mouth dryness (60%), headache (10%), skin (10%), GI (5%)		2-year DFS 100%

As$_2$O$_3$, arsenic trioxide; APL, acute promyelocytic leukemia; ATRA, all-*trans* retinoic acid; CR, complete remission; DFS, disease-free survival; GI, gastrointestinal; HSCT, hematopoietic stem cell transplantation; OS, overall survival; RA, retinoic acid; RFS, relapse-free survival; [A] After relapse the low-dose group, among 14 relapsed patients followed-up for 7–33 months after CR, the estimated disease-free survival (DFS) rates and overall survival (OS) at 2 years were 42±10% and 50±10%, respectively, which were similar to the results obtained among 33 relapsed patients followed up for 7 to 48 months in the standard-dose group (49±15% and 62±16%, respectively; Niu et al. 1999). Hence, low-dose As_2O_3 treatment was proved equally effective in APL patients, although a larger scale randomized study must be launched in order to reach a firm conclusion (Shen et al. 2001).

Pharmacokinetic studies showed that plasma arsenic concentration rapidly reached the peak level, with the mean C_{pmax} at 6.85 µmol/l (5.54–7.30 µmol/l), $t_{1/2\alpha}$ 0.89±0.29 h and $t_{1/2\beta}$ 12.13±3.31 h (Shen et al. 1997). In patients given 0.08 mg/kg As_2O_3, the mean C_{pmax} fell to 2.45 µmol/l (1.54–2.81 µmol/l), and the ranges of $t_{1/2\alpha}$ and $t_{1/2\beta}$ were 1.2–2.7 h (median 1.4 h) and 6.23–14.9 h (median 9.4 h), respectively (Shen et al. 2001). Although the mean C_{pmax} occurred in nearly the half of the results with standard dose, the plasma concentration was maintained in the range of 0.1–0.5 µmol/l, which is the level of in vitro differentiation.

Urinary arsenic content increased during drug administration, and the total amount of arsenic excreted daily in the urine accounted for 1%–8% of the daily dose. A temporary increase of arsenic in hair and nails was documented, with peak levels at 2.5–2.7 µg/g tissues, and a decline of arsenic was observed soon after withdrawal of arsenic therapy (Shen et al. 1997).

3
As_2O_3 as Combined Treatment with ATRA in Remission Induction

In accordance with the synergistic effect of As_2O_3 and ATRA supported in experimental studies (Jing et al. 2001; Lallemand-Breitenbach et al. 1999; Rego et al. 2000), clinical application of As_2O_3 combined with ATRA demonstrated a significant improvement on disease control in newly diagnosed APL patients (Shen et al. 2004). Dual treatment induced remission faster than treatment with ATRA or As_2O_3 alone. With the CR rate remaining high (>90%), the median time to achieve CR in patients treated with As_2O_3 and ATRA [25.5 days (range 18–35 days)] was significantly decreased as compared to those of patients treated with ATRA [40.5 days (range 25–65 days)] or As_2O_3 alone [31 days (range 28–38 days)]. Correspondingly, earlier recovery of normal platelets counts (>100×10^9/l) was observed in combined therapy vs monotherapy.

The reverse transcriptase polymerase chain reaction (RT-PCR) system for examining PML-RARα fusion gene transcripts, apart from its value for diagnosis, offers a reliable tool for the detection of minimal residual disease. After CR, evaluation by quantitative real-time RT-PCR for PML-RARα transcripts confirmed that the combined therapy achieved a more profound molecular response than monotherapy, with the median fold reduction of PML-RARα fusion transcript copies as 118.9 (As_2O_3 and ATRA), 32.1 (As_2O_3), and 6.7 (ATRA), respectively. Further decrease of this fold reduction was found after consolidation chemotherapy, indicating that this beneficial effect in reducing tumor burden by combination therapy is persistent (Shen et al. 2004).

Integrated study using complementary DNA (cDNA) microarray, 2D gel electrophoresis with mass spectrometry (MS), and methods of computational biology revealed that the co-treatment with As_2O_3 and ATRA induced synergistic impact at the transcriptome and proteome levels, including a co-ordinated regulation of an array of transcription factors and cofactors, activation of calcium signaling, stimulating of interferon pathway, activation of the ubiquitin-proteasome system, induction of cell growth arrest, gain of apoptotic potential, and degradation of the PML-RARα fusion protein (Zheng et al. 2005). The latter is in accordance with our previous finding that the more degradation of the PML-RARα occurs, the better is recovery from the disease (Shen et al. 2004).

In relapsed patients, As_2O_3 and ATRA combination failed to show any superiority in the clinical outcome compared with As_2O_3 monotherapy, probably because most relapsed cases lost sensitivity to ATRA due to previous exposure, and so the synergism between As_2O_3 and ATRA could not be fully expected (Raffoux et al. 2003).

4
Adverse Effects

There is no bone marrow depression during As_2O_3 treatment, and no significant changes of hemoglobin and platelet levels were observed. However, an increase in the white blood cell count was observed in more than 50% of cases in most studies, but hyperleukocytosis with signs similar to retinoic acid syndrome was relatively infrequent and most cases responded to dexamethasone treatment.

Main adverse effects include skin reaction, gastrointestinal disturbances, peripheral neuropathy, and electrocardiographic changes. Mild to moderate increases of hepatic enzyme were observed, which was transient and responded well to either dose modification or concomitant hepatic protection therapy.

Other less frequent adverse effects include enlargement of salivary gland, enlarged thyroid gland without hyperthyroidism, oral ulcer, toothache, and gingival or nose bleeding. These side effects could disappear with symptomatic treatment, and the withdrawal of the drug is of no necessity during remission induction.

Some of the side effects seem to be less frequent in patients treated with low-dose As_2O_3 vs the standard dose; these include gastrointestinal disturbance, facial edema, and cardiac toxicity (Shen et al. 2001). In combination therapy with As_2O_3 and ATRA, no evidence of increased adverse effects was observed (Shen et al. 2004).

5
Postremission Treatment and Survival Time

For patients achieving CR and receiving As_2O_3, chemotherapy, or both as maintenance therapy in our previous study, 33 relapsed APL patients were followed for 8 to 48 months and the estimated DFS rates and OS rates at 2 years were 41.6% and 50.2%, respectively (Niu et al. 1999). Zhang et al. reported in 136 cases that the 5- and 7-year OS rates were 92.0% and 76.7%, respectively (Zhang et al. 2000). In the U.S. multicenter study, when As_2O_3 was used in relapsed cases, among 32 patients achieving CR, 18 received additional As_2O_3 treatment and 11 underwent allogeneic or autologous bone marrow transplantation. The estimated 18-month OS and relapse-free survival rates were 66% and 56%, respectively (Soignet et al. 2001). Mathews et al. reported that 10 of 11 newly diagnosed APL patients treated with As_2O_3 and achieving CR remained in CR at a median follow-up of 15 months (Mathews et al. 2002). Therefore, it seems likely that As_2O_3 appropriately used in postremission therapy could prevent recurrence and achieve a longer survival time.

Recently, we developed a protocol for newly diagnosed APL with a combination of As_2O_3 and ATRA as front-line therapy followed by consolidation chemotherapy and maintenance with sequential use of ATRA, As_2O_3, and low-dose chemotherapy (Table 2; Shen et al. 2004). A total of 43 patients who have completed the whole treatment process have been followed up in a median time of 37 months (range 27–46 months) and only two patients relapsed. The first patient experienced central nervous system (CNS) leukemia and a subsequent bone marrow relapse and the second patient experienced a CNS relapse. Both patients presented a prior molecular relapse after an interval of about 6 months by regular and quantitative RT-PCR and achieved the second remission using the same protocol. These data suggested that, with the current ATRA+As_2O_3+chemotherapy protocol, the relapse rate remains low

Table 2 As_2O_3/ATRA combination treatment in newly diagnosed APL (Shen et al. 2004)

Induction therapy[A]	ATRA orally 25 mg/m^2 per day until CR
	As_2O_3 intravenously 0.16 mg/kg per day until CR[B]
Consolidation therapy	Three consecutive regimens
	DA regimen
	Daunorubicin 45 mg/m^2 per day for 3 days
	Ara-C 100 mg/m^2 per day for 7 days
	Ara-C "pulse" regimen
	Ara-C 1.5–2.5 g/m^2 per day for 3 days
	HA regimen
	Homoharringtonine 2–3mg/m^2 per day for 3 days
	Ara-C 100 mg/m^2 per day for 7 days
Maintenance therapy	Five cycles of three regimens
	ATRA orally 25 mg/m^2 per day for 30 days
	As_2O_3 intravenously 0.16 mg/kg per day for 30 days
	6-Mercaptopurine 100 mg/day for 30 days or 15 mg of methotrexate once a week for 4 weeks

As_2O_3, arsenic trioxide; APL, acute promyelocytic leukemia; ATRA, all-trans retinoic acid; CR, complete remission

[A] Hydroxyurea (daily doses of 20–40 mg/kg) or IA regimen (idarubicin: 6 mg/m^2 per day for 3 days, Ara-c: 100 mg/m^2 per day for 3–5 days) when peripheral white blood cell counts were over 10×10^9/l

[B] As_2O_3 decreased to 0.08 mg/kg per day for patients with grade 0–1 liver dysfunction, and withdrawn in those of grade 2–4, according to Miller et al. (1981)

with prolonged follow-up; however, CNS involvement should be watched for, as close molecular monitoring was informative in predicting the potential of relapse.

6
Molecular Mechanisms of Arsenic Action

At the molecular level, APL is characterized by a chromosomal translocation t(15 ;17), which fuses the RARα on chromosome 17 to the PML gene on chromosome 15 (de Thé et al. 1990, 1991; see other chapters in this volume). The PML-RARα fusion gene and its protein product PML-RAR are thought to be responsible for APL pathogenesis. In the now classic model of APL leukemogenesis, PML-RAR homodimers, by tightly binding to the transcription co-repressor NcoR or SMRT, repress the expression of master genes of myeloid cell differentiation (Lin and Evans 2000; Minucci et al. 2000). Only a pharmacological RA concentration will release repressors, recruit activators, and allow myeloid differentiation. The nature of the complex which contains PML-RARα is still poorly characterized, although it seems to be very large (Nervi et al. 1992). Several piece of evidence suggest that the DNA-binding specificity of PML-RARα is considerably relaxed with respect to that of RARα, identifying a major gain of function of the fusion protein (Jansen et al. 1995; Kamashev et al. 2004; Perez et al. 1993). The precise molecular bases of repression are still the subject of intense research and involve both histone deacetylation and DNA methylation (Di Croce et al. 2002; Grignani et al. 1998; He et al. 1998; Lin et al. 1998; see below).

PML belongs to a so-called RBCC/TRIM protein family, which is basically composed by one RING finger, two B boxes and a coiled-coil dimerization domain (Reymond et al. 2001). The RING-finger motif in other protein families has been reported to be involved in ubiquitin conjugation; its exact role in PML remains unclear. PML knockout mice are viable but susceptible to various infections and tumor development (Wang et al. 1998a, b). In contrast to the PML-null cells, which are resistant to apoptosis triggered by different stimuli, PML overexpression could induce cell growth arrest, senescence, and apoptosis (Quignon et al. 1998). One of the most characteristic features of PML is so-called PML nuclear bodies (NBs) (Salomoni and Pandolfi 2002). PML is the organizer of these nuclear matrix-associated multiprotein complexes, which include many key regulators such as Sp100, CBP, and Daxx. Although the physiological function of PML NBs is far from clear, disruption of these structures has been observed in a variety of disease processes, for instance, neurodegenerative disorders, virus infections, and APL (Seeler and Dejean 2001).

PML can be covalently modified by a small peptide, SUMO (small ubiquitin-like modifier)(Duprez et al. 1999; Kamitani et al. 1998a; Kamitani et al. 1998b; Lallemand-Breitenbach et al. 2001; Muller et al. 1998). Sumoylation has also been reported for many other proteins, such as, Sp100, IκBα, RanGAP1, and a variety of transcription factors. In contrast to ubiquitination, which usually targets the modified proteins for proteasome dependent degradation, sumoylation is thought to regulate the subcellular localization, stability, and transcription activity of its target proteins (Seeler and Dejean 2001). For instance, RanGAP1 sumoylation triggers its binding to the nuclear pore complex, while unsumoylated ones are cytoplasmic. In the case of IκBα, SUMO competes with ubiquitin for the same target lysine, which stabilizes IκBα by inhibiting its ubiquitin-proteasome degradation. PML has three SUMO modification sites, K65, K160, and K490 (Kamitani et al. 1998a). While it has been proposed that sumoylation of PML is required for PML NB formation (Muller et al. 1998), we demonstrated that PML sumoylation is dispensable for the organization of the primary PML NBs and is only required for the maturation of NBs and the recruitment of other partners (Lallemand-Breitenbach et al. 2001). Furthermore, we demonstrated that only K160 sumoylation is critical for the partners' recruitment (Lallemand-Breitenbach et al. 2001; Zhu et al. 2005), identifying a critical asymmetry in the function of the two major PML sumoylation sites.

Before the discovery of its sensitivity to arsenic, APL was already a model disease for both differentiation therapy and oncogene-targeted treatment (Warrell et al. 1993). Retinoic acid targeting of the PML-RARα fusion involves a number of distinct steps whose contribution to APL cell differentiation are still unclear. Those involve disruption of corepressor/RARα binding, coactivator recruitment, and PML-RARα degradation. The molecular details of this degradation pathway have been well described (Zhu et al. 2001). ATRA activates the RARα through its activation function 2 (AF2) transactivation domain and induces the polyubiquitination-19S proteasome-dependent catabolism of fusion protein (Zhu et al. 1999). It was also shown that ATRA triggers caspases that cleave PML-RARα (Nervi et al. 1998).

While the molecular mechanism of ATRA treatment has been extensively studied and well-elucidated, that of arsenic therapy is still under debate (Miller et al. 2002; Zhu et al. 2002a). The cellular mechanisms of arsenic therapy was first proposed by our group (Chen et al. 1996a). Based on ex vivo experiments with the human APL cell line NB4, we found the major effect of arsenic is to trigger cell apoptosis at high concentration, while it also triggers a partial differentiation at low concentration. Of note, when APL cells were exposed to both As_2O_3 and cyclic AMP (cAMP), a terminal differentiation could be achieved (Zhu et al. 2002b). Interestingly, in an in vivo setting, arsenic had a dominant differentiation effect, with modest apoptotic effect in APL transgenic mice (Lallemand-Breitenbach et al. 1999). In 1997, we found that in striking similarity to ATRA, As_2O_3 degrades PML-RARα (Quignon et al. 1997; Zhu et al. 1997, 2001). In contrast to ATRA, which targets the RARα moiety of the fusion, As_2O_3 targets its PML part, since it degrades either PML or PML-RARα. More specifically, As_2O_3 induces the targeting of the nucleoplasmic fraction of PML onto the matrix-bound NB, where PML is degraded (Zhu et al. 1997). Intriguingly, As_2O_3 did not affect the localization (nor the abundance) of PML (or PML-RAR) in transiently transfected COS or CHO cells. This observation could suggest that As_2O_3 does not act directly on the protein, but on a rate-limiting posttranslational modification implicated in the NB/matrix association of the protein. The latter might be phosphorylation, as arsenicals are well known to inhibit phosphatases. Recently this hypothesis was supported by the observation that As_2O_3 treatment induces phosphorylation of the PML protein, through a mitogen-activated protein (MAP) kinase pathway. Increased PML phosphorylation is associated with increased sumoylation of PML (Hayakawa and Privalsky 2004). Using MAP kinase cascade inhibitors, or the introducing of phosphorylation or sumoylation-defective mutations of PML, As_2O_3-mediated apoptosis could be impaired by PML.

In a recently published paper, the functions of two informative mutants of PML-RARα in hematopoietic progenitor cells, determined by retroviral transduction and transgenic mouse, were studied. We introduced into PML-RARα the specific mutant of the site of sumoylation, K160, which is implicated in the degradation induced by the As_2O_3 and the recruitment of the other proteins of nuclear bodies, in particular Daxx (Zhu et al. 2005). We believed that this transgene would lead to an As_2O_3-resistant APL. To our great surprise, PML-RARαK160R is no longer transformative ex vivo. Similarly, the expression of this mutant in transgenic mice only induced myeloid hyperplasia, which was never associated with a differentiation block, the characteristic feature of APL. These results show that the dimerization of PML-RARα is not sufficient to induce transformation, which was not expected by the current models for APL pathogenesis. Yet, RARα dimerization can be implied in the process of myeloid hyperplasia. What is the role of K160 sumoylation? It appears that the function lost upon mutation of this site is transcriptional repression. In addition, sumoylation of the K160 site in PML induces the recruitment of the repressor, Daxx. Fusion of Daxx to PML-RARαK160R restores leukemogenesis ex vivo, strongly suggesting that K160 is essential for transcriptional repression. These observations could explain why PML is the recurrent partner of RARα in APL. Could arsenic-induced modulation of the posttranslational modifications occurring on K160 affect the ability of PML-RARα to repress target gene? This could be an attractive hypothesis that, as in the case of ATRA and RARα, would couple depression to degradation. Indeed, arsenic is well-established to greatly enhance sumoylation of K160, specifically (Lallemand-Breitenbach et al. 2001). Should K160-recruitment of the putative repressor onto PML be dependent on another posttranslational modification, this would provide an attractive new model for arsenic response of APL cells (Zhu et al. 2005).

7
Perspectives

Although remarkable clinical achievements have already been obtained in the treatment of APL with arsenic, and the underlying mechanism of action has gradually been uncovered, further investigation must be performed. Clinically, the ATRA, As$_2$O$_3$, and chemotherapy triad needs further confirmation in larger studies and over longer follow-up periods. Biologically, further efforts should be made to elucidate the mechanisms of apoptosis and differentiation induced by As$_2$O$_3$. In addition, it will be interesting to see if we can broaden the indication of As$_2$O$_3$ therapy in malignancies other than APL, making arsenic a more beneficial drug in cancer therapy.

Acknowledgements This manuscript was supported in part by the Chinese National Key Program for Basic Research (973), Chinese High Tech Program (863), National Natural Science Foundation of China, Shanghai Commission for Science and Technology, Samuel Waxman Cancer Research Foundation. Work in the Paris laboratory is supported by Ligue contre le cancer, ARECA, the Lilly Foundation.

References

Chen GQ, Zhu J, Shi XG, Ni JH, Zhong HJ, Si GY, Jin XL, et al (1996a) In vitro studies on cellular and molecular mechanisms of arsenic trioxide (As$_2$O$_3$) in the treatment of acute promyelocytic leukemia. As$_2$O$_3$ induces NB4 cell apoptosis with downregulation of Bcl-2 expression and modulation of PML-RAR alpha/PML proteins. Blood 88:1052–1061

Chen GQ, Shen ZX, Wu F, Han JY, Miao JM, Zhong HJ, Li XS, Zhao JQ, Zhu J, et al (1996b) Pharmacokinetics and efficacy of low-dose all-trans retinoic acid in the treatment of acute promyelocytic leukemia. Leukemia 10:825–828

Chen Z, Wang ZY, Chen SJ (1997) Acute promyelocytic leukemia: cellular and molecular basis of differentiation and apoptosis. Pharmacol Ther 76:141–149

de Thé H, Chomienne C, Lanotte M, Degos L, Dejean A (1990) The t(15;17) translocation of acute promyelocytic leukemia fuses the retinoic acid receptor a gene to a novel transcribed locus. Nature 347:558–561

de Thé H, Lavau C, Marchio A, Chomienne C, Degos L, Dejean A (1991) The PML-RAR alpha fusion mRNA generated by the t(15;17) translocation in acute promyelocytic leukemia encodes a functionally altered RAR. Cell 66:675–684

Di Croce L, Raker VA, Corsaro M, Fazi F, Fanelli M, Faretta M, Fuks F, Coco FL, Kouzarides T, Nervi C, Minucci S, Pelicci PG (2002) Methyltransferase recruitment and DNA hypermethylation of target promoters by an oncogenic transcription factor. Science 295:1079–1082

Duprez E, Saurin AJ, Desterro JM, Lallemand-Breitenbach V, Howe K, Boddy MN, Solomon E, de Thé H, Hay RT, Freemont PS (1999) SUMO-1 modification of the acute promyelocytic leukaemia protein PML: implications for nuclear localisation. J Cell Sci 112:381–393

Grignani F, de Matteis S, Nervi C, Tomassoni L, Gelmetti V, Cioce M, Fanelli M, Ruthardt M, Ferrara FF, Zamir I, Seiser C, Grignani F, Lazar MA, Minucci S, Pelicci PG (1998) Fusion proteins of the retinoic acid receptor-alpha recruit histone deacetylase in promyelocytic leukaemia. Nature 391:815–818

Hayakawa F, Privalsky ML (2004) Phosphorylation of PML by mitogen-activated protein kinases plays a key role in arsenic trioxide-mediated apoptosis. Cancer Cell 5:389–401
He LZ, Guidez F, Tribioli C, Peruzzi D, Ruthardt M, Zelent A, Pandolfi PP (1998) Distinct interactions of PML-RARalpha and PLZF-RARalpha with co-repressors determine differential responses to RA in APL. Nat Genet 18:126–135
Jansen JH, Mahfoudi A, Rambaud S, Lavau C, Wahli W, Dejean A (1995) Multimeric complexes of the PML-retinoic acid receptor alpha fusion protein in acute promyelocytic leukemia cells and interference with retinoid and peroxisome-proliferator signaling pathways. Proc Natl Acad Sci USA 92:7401–7405
Jing Y, Wang L, Xia L, Chen G, Chen Z, Miller WH, Waxman S (2001) Combined effect of all-trans retinoic acid and arsenic trioxide in acute promyelocytic leukemia cells in vitro and in vivo. Blood 97:264–269
Kamashev DE, Vitoux D, De Thé H (2004) PML-RARA-RXR oligomers mediate retinoid and rexinoid/cAMP in APL cell differentiation. J Exp Med 199:1–13
Kamitani T, Kito K, Nguyen HP, Wada H, Fukuda-Kamitani T, Yeh ETH (1998a) Identification of three major sentrinization sites in PML. J Biol Chem 41:26675–26682
Kamitani T, Nguyen HP, Kito K, Fukuda-Kamitani T, Yeh ET (1998b) Covalent modification of PML by the sentrin family of ubiquitin-like proteins. J Biol Chem 273:3117–3120
Lallemand-Breitenbach V, Guillemin MC, Janin A, Daniel MT, Degos L, Kogan SC, Bishop JM, de Thé H (1999) Retinoic acid and arsenic synergize to eradicate leukemic cells in a mouse model of acute promyelocytic leukemia. J Exp Med 189:1043–1052
Lallemand-Breitenbach V, Zhu J, Puvion F, Koken M, Honore N, Doubeikovsky A, Duprez E, Pandolfi PP, Puvion E, Freemont P, de Thé H (2001) Role of promyelocytic leukemia (PML) sumolation in nuclear body formation, 11S proteasome recruitment, and As(2)O(3)-induced PML or PML/retinoic acid receptor alpha degradation. J Exp Med 193:1361–1372
Lazo G, Kantarjian H, Estey E, Thomas D, O'Brien S, Cortes J (2003) Use of arsenic trioxide (As_2O_3) in the treatment of patients with acute promyelocytic leukemia: the MD Anderson experience. Cancer 97:2218–2224
Lin R, Evans R (2000) Acquisition of oncogenic potential by RAR chimeras in acute promyelocytic leukemia through formation of homodimers. Mol Cell 5:821–830
Lin RJ, Nagy L, Inoue S, Shao WL, Miller WH, Evans RM (1998) Role of the histone deacetylase complex in acute promyelocytic leukaemia. Nature 391:811–814
Mathews V, Balasubramanian P, Shaji RV, George B, Chandy M, Srivastava A (2002) Arsenic trioxide in the treatment of newly diagnosed acute promyelocytic leukemia: a single center experience. Am J Hematol 70:292–299
Miller WH Jr, Schipper HM, Lee JS, Singer J, Waxman S (2002) Mechanisms of action of arsenic trioxide. Cancer Res 62:3893–3903
Minucci S, Maccarana M, Cioce M, De Luca P, Gelmetti V, Segalla S, Di Croce L, Giavara S, Matteucci C, Gobbi A, Bianchini A, Colombo E, Schiavoni I, Badaracco G, Hu X, Lazar MA, Landsberger N, Nervi C, Pelicci PG (2000) Oligomerization of RAR and AML1 transcription factors as a novel mechanism of oncogenic activation. Mol Cell 5:811–820

Muller S, Matunis MJ, Dejean A (1998) Conjugation with the ubiquitin-related modifier SUMO-1 regulates the partitioning of PML within the nucleus. EMBO J 17:61–70

Nervi C, Poindexter EC, Grignani F, Pandolfi PP, Lo Coco F, Avvisati G, Pelicci PG, Jetten AM (1992) Characterization of the PML-RAR alpha chimeric product of the acute promyelocytic leukemia-specific t(15; 17) translocation. Cancer Res 52:3687–3692

Nervi C, Ferrara FF, Fanelli M, Rippo MR, Tomassini B, Ferrucci PF, Ruthardt M, Gelmetti V, Gambacorti-Passerini C, Diverio D, Grignani F, Pelicci PG, Testi R (1998) Caspases mediate retinoic acid-induced degradation of the acute promyelocytic leukemia PML/RARalpha fusion protein. Blood 92:2244–2251

Niu C, Yan H, Yu T, Sun HP, Liu JX, et al (1999) Studies on treatment of acute promyelocytic leukemia with arsenic trioxide: remission induction, follow-up, and molecular monitoring in 11 newly diagnosed and 47 relapsed acute promyelocytic leukemia patients. Blood 94:3315–3324

Perez A, Kastner P, Sethi S, Lutz Y, Reibel C, Chambon P (1993) PML/RAR homodimers: distinct binding properties and heteromeric interactions with RXR. EMBO J 12:3171–3182

Quignon F, Chen Z, de Thé H (1997) Retinoic acid and arsenic: towards oncogene targeted treatments of acute promyelocytic leukaemia. Biochim Biophys Acta 1333:M53–M61

Quignon F, de Bels F, Koken M, Feunteun J, Ameisen JC, de Thé H (1998) PML induces a caspase-independent cell death process. Nat Genet 20:259–265

Raffoux E, Rousselot P, Poupon J, Daniel MT, Cassinat B, Delarue R, Taksin AL, Rea D, Buzyn A, Tibi A, Lebbe G, Cimerman P, Chomienne C, Fermand JP, de Thé H, Degos L, Hermine O, Dombret H (2003) Combined treatment with arsenic trioxide and all-trans-retinoic acid in patients with relapsed acute promyelocytic leukemia. J Clin Oncol 21:2326–2334

Rego EM, He LZ, Warrell RP Jr, Wang ZG, Pandolfi PP (2000) Retinoic acid (RA) and As_2O_3 treatment in transgenic models of acute promyelocytic leukemia (APL) unravel the distinct nature of the leukemogenic process induced by the PML-RARalpha and PLZF-RARalpha oncoproteins. Proc Natl Acad Sci U S A 97:10173–10178

Reymond A, Meroni G, Fantozzi A, Merla G, Cairo S, Luzi L, Riganelli D, Zanaria E, Messali S, Cainarca S, Guffanti A, Minucci S, Pelicci PG, Ballabio A (2001) The tripartite motif family identifies cell compartments. EMBO J 20:2140–2151

Salomoni P, Pandolfi PP (2002) The role of PML in tumor suppression. Cell 108:165–170

Seeler JS, Dejean A (2001) SUMO: of branched proteins and nuclear bodies. Oncogene 20:7243–7249

Shen Y, Shen ZX, Yan H, Chen J, Zeng XY, Li JM, Li XS, Wu W, Xiong SM, Zhao WL, Tang W, Wu F, Liu YF, Niu C, Wang ZY, Chen SJ, Chen Z (2001) Studies on the clinical efficacy and pharmacokinetics of low-dose arsenic trioxide in the treatment of relapsed acute promyelocytic leukemia: a comparison with conventional dosage. Leukemia 15:735–741

Shen ZX, Chen GQ, Ni JH, Li XS, Xiong SM, Qiu QY, Zhu J, Tang W, Sun GL, Yang KQ, Chen Y, Zhou L, Fang ZW, Wang YT, Ma J, Zhang P, Zhang TD, Chen SJ, Chen Z, Wang ZY (1997) Use of arsenic trioxide (As203) in the treatment of acute promyelocytic leukemia (APL). II. Clinical efficacy and pharmacokinetics in relapsed patients. Blood 89:3354–3360

Shen ZX, Shi ZZ, Fang J, Gu BW, Li JM, Zhu YM, Shi JY, Zheng PZ, Yan H, Liu YF, Chen Y, Shen Y, Wu W, Tang W, Waxman S, De The H, Wang ZY, Chen SJ, Chen Z (2004) All-trans retinoic acid/As_2O_3 combination yields a high quality remission and survival in newly diagnosed acute promyelocytic leukemia. Proc Natl Acad Sci U S A 101:5328–5335

Soignet SL, Frankel SR, Douer D, Tallman MS, Kantarjian H, Calleja E, Stone RM, Kalaycio M, Scheinberg DA, Steinherz P, Sievers EL, Coutre S, Dahlberg S, Ellison R, Warrell RP Jr (2001) United States multicenter study of arsenic trioxide in relapsed acute promyelocytic leukemia. J Clin Oncol 19:3852–3860

Sun HD, Ma L, Hu HX, Zhang TD (1992) Use of Ai-Ling n. 1 injection, combined with pattern identification theory of Chinese traditional medicine, in the treatment of acute promyelocytic leukemia: report from 32 patients. Zhongguo Zhong Xi Yi Jie He Za Zhi 12:170–171

Wang ZG, Ruggero D, Ronchetti S, Zhong S, Gaboli M, Rivi R, Pandolfi PP (1998a) PML is essential for multiple apoptotic pathways. Nat Genet 20:266–272

Wang ZG, Delva L, Gaboli M, Rivi R, Giorgio M, Cordon-Cardo C, Grosveld F, Pandolfi PP (1998b) Role of PML in cell growth and the retinoic acid pathway. Science 279:1547–1551

Warrell R, de Thé H, Wang Z, Degos L (1993) Acute promyelocytic leukemia. N Engl J Med 329:177–189

Zhang P, Wang SY, Hu XH, et al (1996) Arsenic trioxide-treated 72 cases of acute promyelocytic leukemia. Zhongguo Shi Yan Xue Ye Xue Za Zhi 17:58–60

Zhang P, Wang S, Hu L, Qiu F, Yang H, Xiao Y, Li X, Han X, Zhou J, Liu P (2000) Seven years' summary report on the treatment of acute promyelocytic leukemia with arsenic trioxide—an analysis of 242 cases (in Chinese). Zhonghua Xue Ye Xue Za Zhi 21:67–70

Zheng PZ, Wang KK, Zhang QY, Huang QH, Du YZ, Zhang QH, Xiao DK, Shen SH, Imbeaud S, Eveno E, Zhao CJ, Chen YL, Fan HY, Waxman S, Auffray C, Jin G, Chen SJ, Chen Z, Zhang J (2005) Systems analysis of transcriptome and proteome in retinoic acid/arsenic trioxide-induced cell differentiation/apoptosis of promyelocytic leukemia. Proc Natl Acad Sci U S A 102:7653–7658

Zhou GB, Zhao WL, Wang ZY, Chen SJ, Chen Z (2005) Retinoic acid and arsenic for treating acute promyelocytic leukemia. PLoS Med 2:12

Zhu J, Koken MHM, Quignon F, Chelbi-Alix MK, Degos L, Wang ZY, Chen Z, de Thé H (1997) Arsenic-induced PML targeting onto nuclear bodies: implications for the treatment of acute promyelocytic leukemia. Proc Natl Acad Sci USA 94:3978–3983

Zhu J, Gianni M, Kopf E, Honore N, Chelbi-Alix M, Koken M, Quignon F, Rochette-Egly C, de Thé H (1999) Retinoic acid induces proteasome-dependent degradation of retinoic acid receptor alpha (RAR alpha) and oncogenic RAR alpha fusion proteins. Proc Natl Acad Sci U S A 96:14807–14812

Zhu J, Lallemand-Breitenbach V, de Thé H (2001) Pathways of retinoic acid- or arsenic trioxide-induced PML/RARalpha catabolism, role of oncogene degradation in disease remission. Oncogene 20:7257–7265

Zhu J, Chen Z, Lallemand-Breitenbach V, de Thé H (2002a) How acute promyelocytic leukemia revived arsenic. Nat Rev Cancer 2:705–713

Zhu Q, Zhang JW, Zhu HQ, Shen YL, Flexor M, Jia PM, Yu Y, Cai X, Waxman S, Lanotte M, Chen SJ, Chen Z, Tong JH (2002b) Synergic effects of arsenic trioxide and cAMP during acute promyelocytic leukemia cell maturation subtends a novel signaling cross-talk. Blood 99:1014–1022

Zhu J, Zhou J, Peres L, Riaucoux F, Honore N, Kogan S, de Thé H (2005) A sumoylation site in PML/RARA is essential for leukemic transformation. Cancer Cell 7:143–153

Front Line Clinical Trials and Minimal Residual Disease Monitoring in Acute Promyelocytic Leukemia

F. Lo-Coco (✉) · E. Ammatuna

Dipartimento di Biopatologia e Diagnostica per Immagini,
Università Tor Vergata via Montpellier, 1-00133 Rome, Italy
francesco.lo.coco@uniroma2.it

1	Diagnostic Approach	146
2	Molecular Architecture of the t(15;17) and Definition of the RT-PCR Strategy	147
3	Technical Issues Related to RT-PCR Amplification	148
4	Strategies to Improve RT-PCR Monitoring and Quantitative Real-Time RT-PCR	149
5	Front-Line Therapy	150
References		153

Abstract In spite of the very high cure rate (70%–80%) achieved in APL with combinatorial all-*trans* retinoic acid (ATRA) and anthracycline-based chemotherapy regimens, a number of issues are still open for investigation in front-line therapy of this disease. These include, among others, improvements in early death rate, the role of arsenic trioxide (ATO) and maintenance treatment, and, finally, optimization of molecular monitoring to better identify patients at increased risk of relapse. The current consensus on the most appropriate induction therapy consists of the concomitant administration of ATRA and anthracycline-based chemotherapy. Although the antileukemic benefit provided by the addition of ATRA to consolidation therapy has not been demonstrated in randomized studies, historical comparisons of consecutive studies carried out by Spanish and Italian cooperative groups suggest that the combination of ATRA and chemotherapy for consolidation may also contribute to improving therapeutic results. While a variety of distinct treatments are being investigated for front-line therapy, most experts agree that a risk-adapted therapy represents the optimal approach, through the use of more intensive therapy in patients with initial hyperleukocytosis. Longitudinal RT-PCR of PML/RARα allows sensitive assessment of response to treatment and minimal residual disease (MRD) monitoring in APL. Achievement of negative PCR status or molecular remission at the end of consolidation is now universally accepted and recommended as a therapeutic objective in this disease. On the other hand, persistence of, or conversion to, PCR positive in the marrow during follow-up is associated with impending relapse. Preliminary studies on therapy of molecular relapse indicate a survival advantage as compared to administering salvage treatment at time of hematologic relapse. The more accurate and reproducible real-time PCR method to detect at quantitative levels the *PML/RARα* hybrid will likely provide better inter-laboratory standardization and trial results comparison in the near future.

1
Diagnostic Approach

Acute promyelocytic leukemia is a medical emergency requiring rapid diagnosis and prompt administration of specific therapy. In typical hypergranular cases, morphologic characteristics of APL blast cells allow easy recognition of this leukemic subtype, while some difficulties may be encountered in the morphologic identification of the less frequent hypogranular variant (Bennett et al. 1976, 1980; McKenna et al. 1982; Tallman et al. 1993). Early initiation of specific treatment with all-*trans* retinoic acid (ATRA) is of paramount importance because this agent ameliorates the life-threatening coagulopathy associated with the disease (Barbui et al. 1998). Hence, although confirmation of diagnosis by genetic tests is always required, it is highly recommended that treatment be started with no delay based on morphologic/clinical suspect of APL (Sanz et al. 2005). In addition to cytological features, a characteristic immunophenotypic profile is detectable in this leukemia that usually includes lack of the HLA-DR expression, and positivity for CD13, CD15, and CD33 (Guglielmi et al. 1998; Paietta 2003). The demonstration of the APL unique genetic lesion, which may be searched by clinicians even after treatment initiation, is strongly recommended in all cases including the morphologically typical ones. In fact, the specific t(15;17) and particularly the corresponding gene fusion *PML/RARα* predict ATRA responsiveness in 100% of cases (Miller et al. 1992). The APL-unique hybrid gene may be detected using RT-PCR or fluorescent in situ hybridization (FISH) methods (Lo-Coco et al. 1999; Reiter et al. 2004). For the purpose of rapidly initiating ATRA-containing therapy, the use of anti-PML antibodies also represents a valid approach. Anti-PML antibodies allow identification in t(15;17)-positive APL of a microspeckled distribution of the PML protein, as opposed to the speckled distribution of the wildtype PML that is observed in non-APL leukemias (Falini et al. 1997; Samoszuk et al. 1998; Villamor et al. 2000; Gomis et al. 2004). This technique should not, however, replace RT-PCR, because only this latter method identifies the type of *PML/RARα* isoform and the target for minimal residual disease (MRD) evaluation in the individual patient.

2
Molecular Architecture of the t(15;17) and Definition of the RT-PCR Strategy

Two fusion genes are formed as a consequence of the t(15;17) translocation on the 17q and 15q derivatives. Of these, the *RARα/PML* fusion gene is transcribed in about 70% of APLs, whereas the reciprocal *PML/RARα* is expressed in 100% of cases (Alcalay et al. 1992). Therefore, most laboratories have adopted the *PML/RARa* RT-PCR assay for rapid diagnosis and monitoring of residual disease (Lo-Coco et al. 1999; van Dongen et al. 1999; Reiter et al. 2004). On the 17q, breakpoints are located in RARα intron 2, while on the 15q derivative breakpoints may be located at three different sites of the PML gene i.e, intron 6, exon 6, and intron 3. Based on this variability and due to alternative splicing of *PML* exons, three different *PML/RARα* isoforms are formed (Pandolfi et al. 1992). Of these, the so-called bcr1 type, derived from breakpoints in PML intron 6, is detected in 55%–60% of cases; bcr3 transcript type derives from breakpoints in PML intron 3 and is found in 35%–40% of patients, and finally, the bcr2 isoform (also referred to as "variant" type) results from breakpoints in PML exon 6 and is identified in approximately 8% of cases (Fig. 1). Together, bcr1 and bcr2 isoforms are frequently referred to as the "long transcript," while the bcr3 type is referred to as the "short transcript" (Grignani et al. 1994; Chen et al. 1995; Warrell 1996; Fenaux et al. 1997). Primers for *PML/RARα* amplification are usually located on *PML* exon 3 (forward primer) and *RARα* exon 3 (reverse primer). Using the conventional nested RT-PCR approach, a single amplification band is visualized in cases with the short transcript isoform, and a multiple band pattern due to alternative splicings downstream of PML exon 3 is detected in cases bearing the long (bcr1–2) isoform (Pandolfi et al. 1992).

Following the design of RT-PCR assays for PML/RARa in the early 1990s, many studies have been carried out to investigate the value of minimal residual disease (MRD) monitoring in APL. In addition, a number of technical issues have been addressed in the literature on the advantages and drawbacks of this assay as well as on the optimal ways to adapt PCR monitoring to clinical protocols. As discussed in the following section, a consensus exists on the invaluable clinical information provided by PCR testing, such that the status of molecular remission is nowadays recognized as a target of treatment and a surrogate marker of improved survival in APL (Cheson et al. 2003). In fact, according to the results of the largest prospective monitoring studies reported so far (Diverio et al. 1998; Burnett et al. 1999; Jurcic et al. 2001) the achievement of PCR negativity at the end of consolidation correlates with sustained remission while the persistence or reappearance of a PCR-

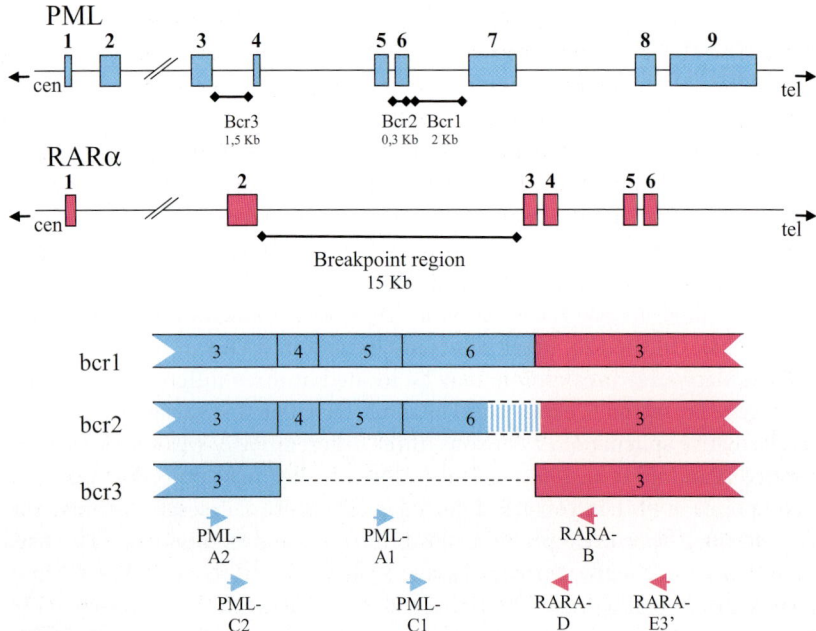

Fig. 1 Schematic representation of the *PML/RARα* cDNA hybrid with the distinct isoforms that are generated according to heterogeneous breakpoints in the PML gene. The *arrows* indicate the approximate location of primers used for PCR amplification of the fusion gene

positive test during follow-up is strongly associated with hematologic relapse (reviewed in Grimwade and Lo-Coco 2002).

3
Technical Issues Related to RT-PCR Amplification

The quality of RNA and efficiency of the reverse transcription (RT) step is one of the most important factors for successful RT-PCR amplification of PML/RARα. Assessment of RNA quality and choice of appropriate control genes in MRD experiments is crucial in order to avoid false-negative results. At diagnosis, APL is frequently characterized by low white blood cell count and activation of coagulation and proteolytic enzymes. Hence, obtaining sufficient RNA from the peripheral blood may be difficult. Improvement in the reverse transcription step has been reported using the so-called "hot start" method, which contributes to minimize primer misannealing and enhances sensitivity of the reaction (Seale et al. 1996; Lo-Coco et al. 1999b; Grimwade et al. 1999). As discussed above, the initial strategy should allow us to detect the *PML/RARα* isoform type and finally to resolve a single amplification fragment. Thus, the appropriate primer set will subsequently be adapted to the individual patient and be used after consolidation treatment for MRD monitoring. The precise characterization of cases with the bcr2 variant isoform requires sequencing of the breakpoint on PML exon 6.

4
Strategies to Improve RT-PCR Monitoring and Quantitative Real-Time RT-PCR

Although the standard RT-PCR-based approach is regarded as clinically relevant for response assessment and prognosis, several issues have to be considered for improving standardization and reliability of results. To define molecular relapse (i.e., conversion from PCR-negative to PCR-positive) some investigators have recommended confirming positivity of the test in two successive marrow samples before initiating salvage therapy (Lo-Coco et al. 1999; Estey et al. 1999). Moreover, the frequency of PCR testing in clinical trials may be adapted to the relapse risk. According to most of the recent trials in which ATRA and chemotherapy have been used, the majority of relapses occur within the first 6–8 months after the end of consolidation; therefore, a more stringent monitoring might be justified during this period. In addition, it seems reasonable to recommend more frequent sampling for monitoring studies in patients with hyperleukocytosis at presentation, as these patients have been shown in most trials to be at higher risk of relapse (Asou et all 1998; Fenaux et al. 1999; Mandelli et al. 1997; Sanz et al. 2004; Lengfelder et al. 2000; Tallman et al. 2002).

While it is commonly accepted that reduction of the *PML/RARα* transcript below the threshold detectable by standard RT-PCR is associated with long-term survival, the achievement of PCR-negative status is no guarantee of final cure. In fact, using assays with sensitivity thresholds of approximately 10^{-4}, a significant proportion of APL patients who ultimately relapse show no detectable residual disease after induction and consolidation therapy (Grimwade et al. 1996). Because of this, different approaches have been undertaken in order to better identify, at the molecular level, patients at higher relapse risk; these include attempts to increase the sensitivity level of the reaction, the analysis of the reciprocal RARα/*PML* fusion, and prolonged post-consolidation monitoring (Lo-Coco et al. 1999b; Grimwade et al. 1999).

The detection of reciprocal $RAR\alpha$-PML transcripts results in improved sensitivity (approximately 1 log) over the standard $PML/RAR\alpha$ assay. In APL patients enrolled in the Medical Research Council (MRC) group ATRA trial, the $RAR\alpha$-PML amplification led to the detection of residual disease in an additional 20% of patients who were in hematologic remission following induction or consolidation treatment (Burnett et al. 1999). This increased sensitivity did not, however, translate into better predictive value of MRD detection. In fact, most patients who relapsed in this study showed, at this time-point, levels of disease still below the detection limit of the more sensitive assay, whereas detection of $RAR\alpha$-PML transcripts was not necessarily indicative of impending relapse (Burnett et al. 1999).

Because the standard nested RT-PCR assays do not allow us to precisely quantitate the amount of residual disease, a comparison of MRD results in distinct clinical trials is imprecise. In light of this, for $PML/RARa$ monitoring some investigators have adopted the newly developed real-time PCR method (RQ-PCR), which holds promise for better interlaboratory standardization and interstudy comparison (Grimwade et al. 2002). This amplification system provides increased specificity and sensitivity, and it results in reduced risk of carry-over contamination due to the use of a closed vial system that avoids the need of nested PCR and the run of PCR products on an agarose gel electrophoresis. According to the largest RQ-PCR study reported so far in APL, this technology also allows for better monitoring in peripheral blood samples as compared to the conventional nested approach (Gallagher et al. 2003). This in turn would greatly improve clinicians' compliance for monitoring studies. The results of RQ-PCR monitoring in prospective studies on large patient cohorts are required to establish its value in guiding therapeutic decisions.

5
Front-Line Therapy

Anthracycline-based chemotherapy and ATRA are the mainstays of front-line treatment. Other agents that have recently proved to be highly effective in APL include arsenic trioxide (ATO) and anti-CD33 antibodies. These agents have been mainly used for relapsed patients, although their potential role in front-line therapy is currently under investigation (Estey et al. 2002; Shen et al. 2004). ATO and immunotherapy with anti-CD-33 antibodies are the subject of two dedicated chapters in this volume (see Z. Chen et al. and P.G. Maslak et al.).

The striking sensitivity of APL to anthracyclines was originally reported for daunorubicin by Bernard and colleagues in 1973 (Bernard et al. 1973), and confirmed successively by other European groups who extended this observation to other anthracyclines (Marty et al. 1984; Sanz et al. 1988; Avvisati et al. 1990). The reasons underlying such high sensitivity are unclear, but the absence of the multidrug resistance glycoprotein P170 on APL cells may be an important factor influencing the favorable response to anthracyclines (Paietta et al. 1994; Candoni et al. 2003).

Following the initial results on ATRA reported from China and confirmed by several groups worldwide, a number of multicenter trials were conducted in the 1990s to explore optimal ATRA and chemotherapy combination schedules (e.g., sequential vs simultaneous administration), the role of maintenance, and that of molecular monitoring (reviewed in Sanz et al. 2005). The main results of these studies may be summarized as follows:

1. The concomitant ATRA plus chemotherapy schedule provides better outcome results compared to the sequential (ATRA followed by chemotherapy) schedule, as demonstrated in a randomized comparison reported by the European APL 1993 study (Fenaux et al. 1999). In addition to better DFS rates, the simultaneous approach is more effective in diminishing the occurrence of overt ATRA syndrome (Fenaux et al. 1999).

2. The type and intensity of induction and consolidation chemotherapy varied considerably in the reported trials. In particular, polychemotherapy regimens including cytarabine have been used in most of the above studies (Asou et al. 1998; Burnett et al. 1999; Fenaux et al. 1999; Lengfelder et al. 2000; Tallman et al. 2002) while anthracycline-based chemotherapy has been used with ATRA for remission induction by the GIMEMA (Gruppo Italiano Malattie Ematologiche dell'Adulto) and PETHEMA (Programa para el Tratamiento de Hemopatías Malignas) groups. The GIMEMA and PETHEMA regimens also omitted nonintercalating agents from the consolidation phase, with no apparent reduction of therapeutic efficacy (Mandelli et al. 1997; Sanz et al. 1999). The PETHEMA study showed a substantial benefit of an anthracycline-based consolidation, due also to reduced toxicity (Sanz et al. 1999).

3. Two randomized trials showed the advantage of including ATRA-based maintenance (Tallman et al. 1997; Fenaux et al. 1999). The European APL 1993 study (Fenaux et al. 1999) suggested further benefit from maintenance with combined ATRA plus low-dose chemotherapy with methotrexate and 6-mercaptopurine. The role of maintenance was also investigated by the GIMEMA group, which adopted the same four randomization arms of the APL 1993 study (ATRA vs chemotherapy vs ATRA+chemotherapy vs observation; Mandelli et al. 1997). Updated results of the GIMEMA study do not seem to confirm a benefit from using maintenance in APL.

4. All studies reported the clinical relevance of longitudinal RT-PCR monitoring to assess response to therapy. Approximately 50% of patients receiving ATRA plus chemotherapy have detectable *PML/RARα* transcript in their marrow after completing induction. No correlations were found between the PCR status at the time of morphologic remission achievement and the relapse risk, whereas PCR status after consolidation is highly predictive of outcome (Diverio et al. 1998; Jurcic et al. 2001; Gallagher et al. 2003). After completion of consolidation, 90%–95% of cases tested PCR-negative in the GIMEMA, MRC, and PETHEMA studies (Burnett et al. 1999; Mandelli et al. 1997; Sanz et al. 1999).

As expected, a distinct kinetics of PML/RARα negativization was observed in the German AMLCG (Acute Myeloid Leukemia Cooperative Group) study, in which patients received a double-induction strategy including high-dose cytarabine (TAD/HAM regimen) in association with ATRA (Lengfelder et al. 2000). Up to 91% of patients studied after this induction tested negative by RT-PCR, corresponding to the fraction of molecular remission obtained after two chemotherapy courses in other trials.

In addition to the above multicenter trial results, investigators at the MD Anderson Cancer Center suggested that the liposomal ATRA formulation is more effective compared to orally administered ATRA, and that the amount of chemotherapy needed to cure the disease might be reduced if it were used in combination with liposomal ATRA (Estey et al. 1999). Unfortunately, this formulation is no longer available.

In spite of the dramatic improvement in patient outcome, the above studies left unsolved a number of issues that have been addressed in successive trials designed in 1999–2000, most of which are still ongoing. Investigational areas addressed in current trials are the role of cytarabine, the type and intensity of consolidation, the possibility to differentiate treatment according to the relapse risk, and the place of novel agents such as other retinoids and ATO. The main ongoing multicenter studies in untreated APL are summarized in Table 1.

At present, the results of the Spanish PETHEMA study have been reported (Sanz et al. 2004). According to the design of this trial, patients received after the AIDA (all-*trans* retinoic and idarubicin) induction distinct consolidation approaches based on a predefined relapse risk established at diagnosis (Sanz et al. 2000). The study reported low toxicity, a high degree of compliance, and high antileukemic efficacy, adding ATRA to anthracycline monochemotherapy during both induction and consolidation, with a considerably improved outcome for low- and intermediate-risk patients. As to the high-risk group, unpublished data of the GIMEMA group suggest this category of patients can

Table 1 Current multicenter trials in APL

Group	Induction	Consolidation	Maintenance
U.S. Intergroup	ATRA+DNR+AraC	ATRA+DNR±ATO	ATRA
JALSG	ATRA+IDA+AraC	Polychemotherapy	ATRA vs NO
European	ATRA+DNR±AraC	DNR±AraC	ATRA+CHT
UK MRC	AIDA vs ATRA+DAT	Pethema vs MRC	ATRA+CHT
GAMLCG	TAD/HAM+ATRA	TAD	CHT
GIMEMA	AIDA	Risk-adapted	ATRA+CHT
Pethema	AIDA	Risk-adapted	ATRA+CHT

AIDA, all-*trans* retinoic acid and idarubicin; AraC, cytosine arabinoside; ATO, arsenic trioxide; ATRA, all-*trans* retinoic acid; CHT, chemotherapy; DAT, daunorubicin, AraC, 6-thioguanine; DNR, daunorubicin; GAMLCG, German Acute Myeloid Leukemia Cooperative Group; GIMEMA, Gruppo Italiano Malattie Ematologiche dell'Adulto; IDA, idarubicin; JALSG, Japan Acute Leukemia Study Group; PETHEMA, Programa para el Tratamiento de Hemopatías Malignas; UK MRC, United Kingdom Medical Research Council

benefit from using a combination including both anthracycline and nonintercalating agents with high-dose cytarabine in addition to ATRA. While the results of other addressed issues are being awaited, these data suggest the importance of differentiating front-line treatment in APL patients by reducing the amount of chemotherapy in patients with low WBC, and by intensifying treatment or adding new therapies in hyperleukocytic patients.

References

Alcalay M, Zangrilli D, Fagioli M, et al (1992) Expression pattern of the RAR alpha-PML fusion gene in acute promyelocytic leukemia. Proc Natl Acad Sci U S A 89:4840–4844

Asou N, Adachi K, Tamura J, et al (1998) Analysis of prognostic factors in newly diagnosed acute promyelocytic leukemia treated with all-trans retinoic acid and chemotherapy. Japan Adult Leukemia Study Group. J Clin Oncol 16:78–85

Avvisati G (1999) Event-free survival (EFS) duration in newly diagnosed acute promyelocytic leukemia (APL) is favorably influenced by induction treatment with idarubicin alone: final results of the GIMEMA randomised study LAP0389 comparing IDA vs IDA+ARA-C in newly diagnosed APL. Blood 94 Suppl 1:505a

Avvisati G, Mandelli F, Petti MC, et al (1990) Idarubicin (4-demethoxidaunorubicin) as single agent for remission induction of previously untreated acute promyelocytic leukemia. A pilot study of the Italian cooperative group GIMEMA. Eur J Haematol 44:257–260

Barbui T, Finazzi G, Falanga A (1998) The impact of all-trans-retinoic acid on the coagulopathy of acute promyelocytic leukemia. Blood 91:3093–3102

Bennett JM, Catowsky D, Daniel MT, et al (1976) Proposal for the classification of the acute leukemias. Br J Haematol 33:451–458

Bennett JM, Catowsky D, Daniel MT, et al (1980) A variant form of hypergranular promyelocytic leukemia. Br J Haematol 44:169–170

Bernard J, Weil M, Boiron M, et al (1973) Acute promyelocytic leukemia. Results of treatment with daunorubicin. Blood 41:489–496

Burnett AK, Grimwade D, Solomon E, et al (1999) Presenting white blood cell count and kinetics of molecular remission predict prognosis in acute promyelocytic leukemia treated with all-trans retinoic acid: results of the randomized MRC trial. Blood 93:4131–4134

Candoni A, Damiani D, Michelutti A, et al (2003) Clinical characteristics, prognostic factors and multidrug-resistance related protein expression in 36 adult patients with acute promyelocytic leukemia. Eur J Haematol 71:1–8

Chen SJ, Wang ZY, Chen Z (1995) Acute promyelocytic leukaemia: from clinic to molecular biology. Stem Cells 13:22–31

Cheson BD, Bennett JM, Kopecky KJ, et al (2003) Revised recommendations of the International Working Group for Diagnosis, Standardization of Response Criteria, Treatment Outcomes, and Reporting Standards for Therapeutic Trials in Acute Myeloid Leukemia. J Clin Oncol 21:4642–4649

Diverio D, Pandolfi PP, Biondi A, et al (1993) Absence of RT-PCR detectable residual disease in acute promyelocytic leukemia in long term remission. Blood 85:3556–3559

Diverio D, Rossi V, Avvisati G, et al (1998) Early detection of relapse by prospective reverse transcriptase-polymerase chain reaction analysis of the PML/RARα fusion gene in patients with acute promyelocytic leukemia enrolled in the GIMEMA-AIEOP multicenter "AIDA" trial. Blood 92:784–789

Estey E, Thall PF, Mehta K, et al (1996) Alterations in tretinoin pharmacokinetics following administration of liposomal all-trans retinoic acid. Blood 87:3650–3654

Estey EH, Giles FJ, Beran M, et al (2002) Experience with gemtuzumab ozogamycin ("mylotarg") and all-trans retinoic acid in untreated acute promyelocytic leukemia. Blood 99:4222–4224

Falini B, Flenghi L, Fagioli M, et al (1997) Immunocytochemical diagnosis of acute promyelocytic leukemia (M3) with the monoclonal antibody PG-M3 (Anti-PML). Blood 90:4046–4053

Fenaux P, Chomienne C, Degos L (1997) Acute promyelocytic leukaemia: biology and treatment. Semin Oncol 24:92–102

Fenaux P, Chastang C, Chevret S, et al (1999) A randomized comparison of ATRA followed by chemotherapy and ATRA plus chemotherapy, and the role of maintenance therapy in newly diagnosed acute promyelocytic leukaemia. Blood 94:1192–1200

Gallagher RE, Yeap BY, Bi W, et al (2003) Quantitative real-time RT-PCR analysis of PML-RAR alpha mRNA in acute promyelocytic leukemia: assessment of prognostic significance in adult patients from intergroup protocol 0129. Blood 101:2521–2528

Gomis F, Sanz J, Sempere A, et al (2004) Immunofluorescent analysis with the anti-PML monoclonal antibody PG-M3 for rapid and accurate genetic diagnosis of acute promyelocytic leukemia. Ann Hematol 83:687–690

Grignani F, Fagioli M, Alcalay M, et al (1994) Acute promyelocytic leukaemia: from genetics to treatment. Blood 83:10–25

Grimwade D (1999) The pathogenesis of acute promyelocytic leukaemia: evaluation of the role of molecular diagnosis and monitoring in the management of the disease. Br J Haematol 106:591–613

Grimwade D, Lo-Coco F (2002) Acute promyelocytic leukemia: a model for the role of molecular diagnosis and residual disease monitoring in directing treatment approach in acute myeloid leukemia. Leukemia 16:1959–1973

Grimwade D, Howe K, Langabeer S, et al (1996) Minimal residual disease detection in acute promyelocytic leukemia by reverse-transcriptase PCR: evaluation of PML-RAR alpha and RAR alpha-PML assessment in patients who ultimately relapse. Leukemia 10:61–66

Guglielmi C, Martelli MP, Diverio D, et al (1998) Immunophenotype of adult and childhood acute promyelocytic leukaemia: correlation with morphology, type of PML gene breakpoint and clinical outcome. A cooperative Italian study on 196 cases. Br J Haematol 102:1035–1041

Jurcic JG, Nimer SD, Scheinberg DA, et al (2001) Prognostic significance of minimal residual disease detection and PML/RARα isoform type: long term follow-up in acute promyelocytic leukaemia. Blood 98:2651–2656

Lengfelder E, Reichert A, Schoch C, et al (2000) Double induction strategy including high dose cytarabine in combination with all-trans retinoic acid: effects in patients with newly diagnosed acute promyelocytic leukemia German AML Cooperative Group. Leukemia 14:1362–1370

Lo-Coco F, Diverio D, Avvisati G, et al (1999a) Therapy of molecular relapse in acute promyelocytic leukaemia. Blood 94:2225–2229

Lo-Coco F, Diverio D, Falini B, et al (1999b) Genetic diagnosis and molecular monitoring in the management of acute promyelocytic leukaemia. Blood 94:12–22

Mandelli F, Diverio D, Avvisati G, et al (1997) Molecular remission in PML/RARa positive acute promyelocytic leukemia by combined all-trans retinoic acid and idarubicin (AIDA) therapy. Blood 90:1014–1021

Marty M, Ganem G, Fischer J, et al (1984) Leucémie aigue promyélocitaire: étude retrospective de 119 malades traités par daunorubicine. Nouv Rev Fr Hematol 26:371–378

McKenna RW, Parkin J, Bloomfield CD, et al (1982) Acute promyelocytic leukemia a study of 39 cases with identification of a hyperbasophilic microgranular variant. Br J Haematol 50:201–214

Miller WH Jr, Kakizuka A, Frankel SR, et al (1992) Reverse transcription polymerase chain reaction for the rearranged retinoic acid receptor alpha clarifies diagnosis and detects minimal residual disease in acute promyelocytic leukemia. Proc Natl Acad Sci U S A 89:2694–2698

Paietta E (2003) Expression of cell-surface antigens in acute promyelocytic leukaemia. Best Pract Res Clin Haematol 16:369–385

Paietta E, Andersen J, Racevskis J, et al (1994) Significantly lower P-glycoprotein expression in acute promyelocytic leukemia than in other types of acute myeloid leukemia: immunological, molecular and functional analyses. Leukemia 8:968–973

Pandolfi PP, Alcalay A, Fagioli M, et al (1992) Genomic variability and alternative splicing generate multiple PML-RARα transcripts that encode aberrant PML proteins and PML-RARα isoforms in acute promyelocytic leukemia. EMBO J 11:1397–1407

Reiter A, Lengfelder E, Grimwade D (2004) Pathogenesis, diagnosis and monitoring of residual disease in acute promyelocytic leukaemia. Acta Haematol 112:55–67

Samoszuk MK, Tynan W, Sallash G, et al (1998) An immunofluorescent assay for acute promyelocytic leukemia. Am J Clin Pathol 109:205–210

Sanz M, Martin G, Gonzalez M, et al (2004) Risk-adapted treatment of acute promyelocytic leukemia with all-trans-retinoic acid and anthracycline monochemotherapy: a multicenter study by the PETHEMA group. Blood 103:1237–1243

Sanz MA, Jarque I, Martin G, et al (1988) Acute promyelocytic leukemia. Therapy results and prognostic factors. Cancer 61:7–13

Sanz MA, Martin G, Rayon C, et al (1999) A modified AIDA protocol with anthracycline-based consolidation results in high antileukemic efficacy and reduced toxicity in newly diagnosed PML/RARa positive acute promyelocytic leukemia. Blood 94:3015–3021

Sanz MA, Lo-Coco F, Martín G, et al (2000) Definition of relapse risk and role of non-anthracycline drugs for consolidation in patients with acute promyelocytic leukemia: a joint study of the PETHEMA and GIMEMA cooperative groups. Blood 96:1247–1253

Sanz MA, Tallman M, Lo-Coco F (2005) Tricks of the trade for the appropriate management of newly diagnosed acute promyelocytic leukemia. Blood 105:3019–3025

Seale JR, Varma S, Swirsky DM, et al (1996) Quantification of PML-RAR alpha transcripts in acute promyelocytic leukaemia: explanation for the lack of sensitivity of RT-PCR for the detection of minimal residual disease and induction of the leukaemia-specific mRNA by alpha interferon. Br J Haematol 95:95–101

Shen ZX, Shi ZZ, Fang J, et al (2004) All-trans retinoic acid/As2O3 combination yields a high quality remission and survival in newly diagnosed acute promyelocytic leukemia. Proc Natl Acad Sci USA 101:5328–5335

Tallman MS, Hakimian D, Snower D, et al (1993) Basophilic differentiation in acute promyelocytic leukemia. Leukemia 7:521–526

Tallman MS, Andersen JW, Schiffer CA, et al (2002) All-trans retinoic acid in acute promyelocytic leukemia: long-term outcome and prognostic factor analysis from the North American Intergroup protocol. Blood 100:4298–4302

van Dongen JJ, Macintyre EA, Gabert JA, et al (1999) Standardized RT-PCR analysis of fusion gene transcripts from chromosome aberrations in acute leukemia for detection of minimal residual disease. Report of the BIOMED-1 Concerted Action: investigation of minimal residual disease in acute leukemia. Leukemia 13:1901–1928

Villamor N, Costa D, Aymerich M, et al (2000) Rapid diagnosis of acute promyelocytic leukemia by analyzing the immunocytochemical pattern of the PML protein with the monoclonal antibody PG-M3. Am J Clin Pathol 114:786–792

Warrell RP Jr (1996) Pathogenesis and management of acute promyelocytic leukaemia. Annu Rev Med 47:555–565

Histone Deacetylase Inhibitors in APL and Beyond

K. Petrie · N. Prodromou · A. Zelent (✉)

Section of Haemato-Oncology, Institute of Cancer Research, Chester Beatty Laboratories, 237 Fulham Road, London SW3 6JB, UK
arthur.zelent@icr.ac.uk

1	Cancer Epigenetics and Histone Acetylation	158
2	The Histone Deacetylase Family	161
2.1	The Biological Roles of Histone Deacetylases	163
2.2	Regulation of Histone Deacetylase Activities	165
3	Histone Deacetylase Inhibitors	167
3.1	Hydroxamic Acids	168
3.2	Short Chain Fatty Acids	170
3.3	Benzamides	173
3.4	Cyclic Peptides	174
3.5	Molecular Mechanisms Underlying Biological Effects of HDACi	175
3.6	Combination Therapy	177
4	Future Directions	177
	References	182

Abstract In recent years the study of chemical modifications to chromatin and their effects on cellular processes has become increasingly important in the field of cancer research. Disruptions to the normal epigenetic pattern of the cell can serve as biomarkers and are important determinants of cancer progression. Accordingly, drugs that inhibit the enzymes responsible for modulating these epigenetic markers, in particular histone deacetylases, are the focus of intense research and development. In this chapter we provide an overview of class I and II histone deacetylases as well as a guide to the diverse types of histone deacetylase inhibitors and their activities in the context of APL. We also discuss the rationale for the use of histone deacetylase inhibitors in combination therapy for the treatment of cancer and the current status of clinical trials.

In the 18 years since all-*trans*-retinoic acid (ATRA) was first used against PML-RARα-associated acute promyelocytic leukaemia (APL) [109], combined treatment with chemotherapy has proved to be very successful and the prognosis for most patients is good [232, 254]. The relative simplicity of the molecular biology underlying APL arising from the t(15;17) translocation as a cancer model was able to provide a scientific rationale for the remarkable results of differentiation therapy using ATRA. Further studies have revealed that amongst fusion oncoproteins involving RARα and others, a common mechanism exists whereby a key transcriptional activator is rendered a constitutive repressor by acquisition of co-repressor/histone deacetylase binding domains from the fused sequences encoded by the translocation partner gene [160, 297, 298]. An important aspect of this research, which has great therapeutic potential, was the discovery that agents capable of inhibiting enzymatic components of the co-repressor complexes could revert the differentiation blocks imposed by such fusion proteins.

1
Cancer Epigenetics and Histone Acetylation

Although genetics have played a dominant role in cancer, in recent years the importance of epigenetic regulation of chromatin states through specific modifications to DNA or histones has become widely recognized [62, 284]. The term epigenetic is derived from the Greek for upon, *epi*, and can be viewed as a secondary level of cellular information, in addition to the genomic DNA sequence, that may be passed on during cell division. There are three conduits through which epigenetic information has thus far been shown to be conveyed: via genomic DNA methylation, histone modification and silencing of genes on parent-of-origin-specific alleles by genomic imprinting. Many of the enzymes responsible for the establishment of specific epigenetic modifications have been identified to date and some have been shown to directly associate with leukaemogenic fusion proteins, such as t(15;17)-associated PML-RARα in APL [164]. An important characteristic of these epigenetic modifications is their potential reversibility, and molecular therapies that target the underlying processes responsible for their deposition have been the focus of intense research [59].

Epigenetic modification of genomic DNA is characterized by methylation of cytosine and is important for gene repression in mammals and plants, although it does not occur in a number of eukaryotes including *Saccharomyces cerevisiae* and *Caenorhabditis elegans* [16]. In animal genomes, the cytosine residues of cytosine-guanine pairs (CpG) are often methylated [183], a reaction catalysed by members of the DNA methyltransferase (DNMT) family. Methylation can occur as part of a maintenance mechanism during DNA replication and repair, carried out by Dnmt1, as well as through de novo methylation by Dnmt3a or Dnmt3b [15]. Between 60% and 80% of all CpG dinucleotides are methylated in animal genomes and approximately 60% of genes have promoters containing dense regions of CpGs, called CpG islands, which in contrast to other CpG dinucleotides, are often unmethylated [5, 16]. In normal cells, the majority of CpG methylation occurs in heterochromatic DNA and is generally considered to facilitate static long-term gene silencing, and also to confer genome stability through repression of transposons and repetitive DNA elements [289]. Where methylation of CpG islands does occur, it leads to gene repression as evidenced by the silencing of tumour-suppressor genes during cancer progression, a process accompanied by genomic global hypomethylation [62]. Although the extent to which aberrant promoter hypermethylation plays a role in cancer initiation remains unresolved [11], there is some evidence for a "CpG island methylator phenotype" in some cell types [118].

The other central tenet of the epigenetic control of gene expression is the histone code [248, 261], which provides a means whereby input signals can be interpreted by a cell and translated into a heritable pattern of gene expression that defines a particular cellular output state or states (for a recent review see Margueron et al. [171]). Although it is clear that information encoded by histones is transmissible to daughter cells, the underlying mechanisms by which this occurs are not yet well understood [262]. The histone code itself is a combinatorial array of post-translational modifications (acetylation, phosphorylation, methylation, ubiquitination, sumoylation, for example) of N-terminal tails of core histone and to a lesser degree their globular domains. Probably the most studied component of this code, both in terms of the residues affected and the consequences for transcriptional activity, is histone acetylation. Multiple lysines on each of the core histones can be dynamically modified by reversible acetylation [58]. The acetylation reaction is catalysed by histone acetyltransferases, which modify the ε-amino group of histone lysine residues in an acetyl-CoA dependent reaction, whilst removal of acetyl group is catalysed by histone deacetylases. Hyperacetylated histones are stably associated with transcriptionally active domains and more accessible chromatin structure, whereas hypo-acetylated histones are enriched in regions that are transcriptionally silent [95]. Over the past few years, the complexity of cross-talk between different histone modifications, which can involve both same and different histones in the nucleosome, as well as between histones and DNA methylation, has begun to emerge [69]. For example, in mammalian cells, various degrees of histone H3 Lys^9 methylation and histone hypoacetylation are usually associated with methylated DNA, heterochromatin and gene silencing. Histone hyperacetylation and methylation of H3 Lys^4, on the other hand, are associated with unmethylated DNA, euchromatin and gene expression [139, 164]. Various DNA or histone markers that constitute active or inactive chromatin states, together with details of the cross-talk between them and the enzymes responsible for their deposition are shown in Fig. 1.

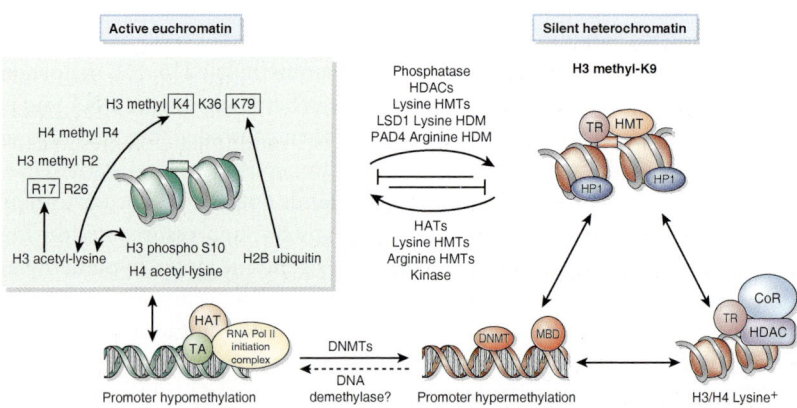

Fig. 1 Markers of active and inactive chromatin states. *Active euchromatin*: various biochemical markers found on the core histones are *boxed in green*. *Reciprocal arrows* indicate where a particular marker can influence the acquisition of another. *Single arrows* reflect a situation where the deposition of a marker enhances or has been demonstrated to be necessary for the acquisition of another. The *reciprocal arrows* in between promoter hypomethylation and euchromatic histone markers refer to the reinforcement of the active state that occurs as a result of HATs, for example, gaining access to 'open' chromatin and depositing acetyl lysine markers that, in turn, provide anchorage sites for coactivators and components of the transcription initiation complex. *TA* denotes a transcriptional activator. *Silent heterochromatin*: various proteins associated with transcriptionally inactive chromatin are indicated. *Lysine+* refers to positively charged, unacetylated histone H3 or H4. Recent evidence suggests that each epigenetic modification (histone acetylation, DNA methylation, histone methylation) can influence the acquisition of the other two (indicated by *reciprocal arrows*). Initiation of the heterochromatic state may occur through sequence-specific DNA binding proteins (*TR*) that promote either histone methylation or histone deacetylation, and subsequent recruitment of specific co-repressors and the general silencing machinery. DNMTs may also be recruited in this manner. Gene silencing and formation of heterochromatin may proceed through changing the balance of dynamic processes, e.g. histone acetylation/deacetylation, or deposition of long-term markers such as DNA or histone methylation. Maintenance of the repressive heterochromatic state is achieved through binding of proteins to specific histone modules (for example HP1α for methylated H3 Lys^9); or to methylated CpG dinucleotide sequences [methylDNA binding proteins (*MBD*)]. The enzymes responsible for the transition between the active and silent chromatin states are indicated. DNA demethylase activity is represented by a *dashed line* because, although an active DNA demethylase has been postulated [253], its existence remains to be established

Although many aspects of the mechanisms that are responsible for establishing pathological epigenetic changes remain to be elucidated, two non-exclusive models have emerged over the past years. In a stochastic model, overexpression of a given component of the machinery responsible for writing epigenetic code may increase probability of its mistargeting and causing deregulated expression of a gene important for tumourigenesis (tumour suppressor or oncogene) [62]. This is consistent with experimental findings indicating over-expression of some histone and DNA-modifying enzymes in cancer [32, 61, 133, 244]. In the other scenario, as mentioned above, chromatin-modifying complexes are inappropriately targeted to regulatory regions of specific genes by AML-associated fusion oncoproteins such as PML-retinoic acid receptor α (RARα) or PLZF-RARα [54, 160, 297, 298].

2
The Histone Deacetylase Family

Whilst it has not been demonstrated that alterations to histone deacetylase (HDAC) genes play a causative role in human cancer, recruitment of histone deacetylase activity by fusion oncoproteins [160, 297, 298] and abnormally expressed HDAC partner proteins such as BCL6 [196] is well known in haematological malignancies. Another important way in which, HDACs plays a role in the pathogenesis of cancer is based on their recruitment to hypermethylated CpG island-associated promoters by both DNMTs and methylCpG DNA-binding proteins [70, 124].

The breakthrough in the identification of mammalian histone deacetylases came with the isolation and cloning of HDAC1 by Stuart Schreiber's group in 1996 [255]. An affinity matrix containing trapoxin (a compound previously shown to inhibit histone deacetylation in vivo) was able to specifically bind HDAC1, and subsequent sequence analysis showed that HDAC1 shared homology with RPD3, a protein known to be regulator of gene expression in *S. cerevisiae* [271]. Histone deacetylases may represent the catalytic components of the large multi-protein complexes that make up part of the general transcriptional silencing machinery, or act as part of smaller, discrete protein complexes that perform diverse cellular functions in terms of gene-specific transcriptional regulation or activities against non-histone substrates. Eleven HDACs that share homology through their deacetylase domains have been characterized and may be broadly divided into two classes on the basis of homology to the *S. cerevisiae* HDACs: RPD3 (class I) and HDA1 (class IIa and IIb) [92] (Fig. 2). There also exists a third class of nicotinamide adenine dinucleotide $(NAD)^+$-dependent class III deacetylases, known as the sirtuins, but they will not be discussed in detail in this chapter. This family of proteins comprises seven members related to *S. cerevisiae* sirtuin, SIR2, but their catalytic domains do not share homology with the "classical" HDAC family, and core histones do not appear to be their main physiological substrates [192].

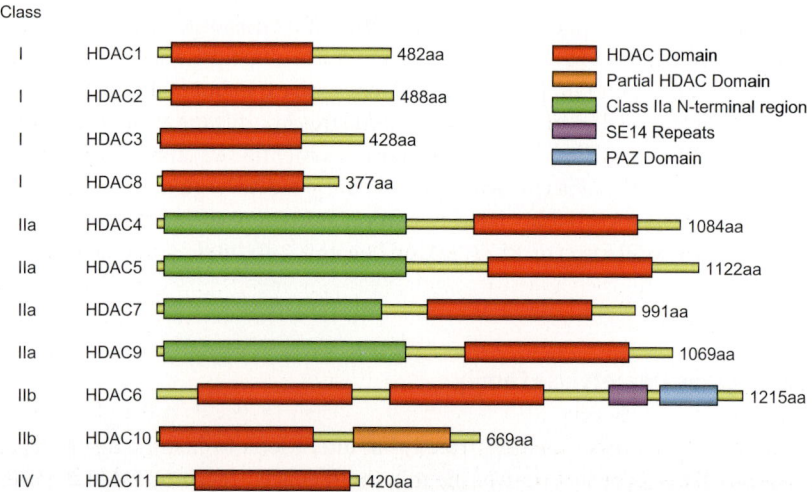

Fig. 2 The human histone deacetylase family. The eleven human HDACs are shown together with their length in amino acid residues and classification. Deacetylase domains are indicated in *red* and the common N-terminal region associated with class IIa HDACs is shown in *green*. The polyubiquitin-associated zinc finger (PAZ) and SE14 repeat domains of HDAC6 are indicated in *blue* and *purple*, respectively. The partial HDAC domain located in the C-terminal region of HDAC10 is shown in *orange*

HDAC1 and HDAC2 are closely related enzymes found together within well-characterized multi-protein complexes, such as the Sin3, NuRD and CoREST complexes [121]. In addition to interacting with chromatin-associated factors and transcriptional repressors through these complexes, HDAC1 and HDAC2 can also bind directly to many DNA-binding proteins that mediate their recruitment to a particular chromatin domain or gene promoter [46]. HDAC3 is present in a separate protein complex that contains SMRT (silencing mediator of retinoic and thyroid hormone receptors) or NCoR (nuclear receptor co-repressor) [121], which are two distinct, but highly related, co-repressor proteins sharing similar domain structure and function. HDAC3 also interacts directly with the class IIa HDACs [66, 287]. HDAC8 shares the least homology with the other class I HDACs, and in contrast to other class I HDACs, which are widely expressed in normal tissues, its expression is restricted to differentiated smooth muscle cells [272]. Moreover, endogenous HDAC8 was mainly detected in the cytoplasm and co-localized with smooth muscle α-actin, where it is thought to play an important role in the contractile capacity of these cells [273].

The class IIa HDACs, HDAC4, HDAC5, HDAC7 and HDAC9, contain a highly conserved C-terminal catalytic domain comprising around 400 amino acids homologous to yeast HDA1 and an N-terminal domain unique to this sub-group of HDACs (Fig. 2). *Drosophila* and *C. elegans* each possess one copy of a gene encoding this sub-type of the HDAC family, and both contain motifs found in the N-terminal regions of the mammalian enzymes [33, 300]. Whilst class IIa HDACs often display distinct patterns of expression, they are also co-expressed in certain tissues and cell types, indicating that an element of redundancy in their biological functions may exist [66, 68, 93, 274].

The class IIb HDACs, HDAC6, HDAC10, are characterized by duplicated HDAC domains, although this duplication is partial in the case of HDAC10 as the C-terminal HDAC domain lacks the active pocket residues required for enzymatic activity (Fig. 2). The enzymatic activities of HDAC6 and HDAC10 are more resistant to the HDAC inhibitors trapoxin and sodium butyrate than those of class I and class IIa HDACs [71, 96]. HDAC6 is normally localized in the cytoplasm, but may undergo partial translocation to the nucleus after cell-cycle arrest [269]. HDAC10 is also primarily cytoplasmic, but shows significant nuclear staining in several cell lines [64, 96, 129, 258]. HDAC6 shows some degree of tissue-specific gene expression [93] whilst HDAC10 is widely expressed in adult human tissues and cultured mammalian cells [129, 258]. Another member of the HDAC family, HDAC11, was recently cloned [75] but little is known about the biological function of this enzyme, except that it is mainly localized to the nucleus, has a restricted pattern of expression and associates with HDAC6. HDAC11 cannot be classified as either class I or class II on the basis of catalytic domain homology, and it has been suggested that it constitutes a class IV HDAC [92].

2.1
The Biological Roles of Histone Deacetylases

Studies on histone deacetylases in model organisms such as *S. cerevisiae* [151] and the many interactions that have been established between HDACs and transcriptional regulators, cofactors, structural and other proteins in humans suggest a wide variety of biological roles [38, 46, 270]. One of the themes that has become clear in recent years is that HDACs cannot simply be regarded as histone-modifying enzymes, and their activities are implicated in the modification of a wide range of proteins, including a number of oncoproteins [112, 292].

The role of histone deacetylases in relation to normal myelopoiesis and the pathogenesis of APL is well documented [179, 256]. APL translocation-associated PLZF has also been shown to co-localize with HDAC4 in myelodysplastic MDS cells, and HDAC4 appeared to mediate its transcriptional repression [30]. HDAC4 can also be recruited, via interactions with 53BP1, to nuclear foci after double-strand DNA damage occurs, perhaps playing a role in control of cell-cycle checkpoints [128]. Additional example for the importance of HDACs in haematopoiesis is illustrated by their interactions with BCL6, another BTB/POZ family transcription factor hat plays an important role in lymphoid development [240] as well as in the pathogenesis of non-Hodgkin's lymphoma (NHL) [40, 137, 288]. BCL6 interacts with both class I and IIa HDACs, either directly or through co-repressor complexes. BCL6 recruits the HDAC1- and HDAC2-containing Sin3A repressor complex [42, 106, 114], and the N-terminal BTB/POZ domain can bind either to SMRT/NCoR [52, 53, 113, 282] or to BCoR, another co-repressor protein [114]. BCL6 also interacts directly with HDAC1 [42] and a conserved region in the N-terminal domain of class IIa HDACs [158]. Thus, both class I and IIa HDACs can be recruited to BCL6-regulated promoters by either direct interactions with BCL6 or indirect recruitment via co-repressors.

Class IIa HDACs are also important for thymic T cell development; they undergo negative selection through apoptosis if they receive a strong signal from major histocompatibility complex self-peptide via their antigen receptors. In response to calcium signalling, the apoptotic process is activated by the orphan steroid receptor Nur77 [293], expression of which is tightly controlled through two myocyte enhancer factor 2 (MEF2)-binding sites in the promoter [283]. HDAC7 is highly expressed in CD4/CD8 double-positive thymocytes, where it associates with MEF2-D and represses the *NUR77* gene until T cell activation occurs and the HDAC is re-localized to the cytoplasm [50].

Of the class IIb HDACs, only HDAC6 has been extensively characterized. HDAC6 is localized to the cytoplasm where its primary catalytic substrate appears to be α-tubulin, which it specifically deacetylates at Lys^{40} [111, 173]. Moreover, HDAC6 interacts and co-localizes with a member of the NAD^+-dependent class III HDAC family, SIRT2, which also deacetylates α-tubulin at Lys^{40} [191]. It is noteworthy that acetylation of α-tubulin is a marker of microtubule stability [206]. HDAC6 also associates with p97/VCP and phospholipase A2-activating protein, which are both involved in the control of ubiquitination [238]. The link with ubiquitination is reinforced by the fact that HDAC6 contains a C-terminal zinc finger motif [known as a polyubiquitin-associated zinc finger (PAZ) domain], which shares significant homology with several ubiquitin-specific proteases [238] and mediates binding of ubiquitin to HDAC6 [107, 238]. Interestingly, HDAC6 co-localizes and interacts with the dynein motor complex [111, 132], which transports aggregated, misfolded proteins to aggresomes [147]. These complexes degrade the protein aggregates, which are not dealt with effectively by the proteasome, and loss of

HDAC6 severely impairs aggresome formation [132]. These data indicate that HDAC6 also functions as a link between aggresomes and the active transport of ubiquitinated protein aggregates, playing a crucial role in the management of cellular stress.

Another important role for HDACs is in regulation of the cell cycle. E2F, which controls the G1/S phase transition by regulating specific checkpoint genes, functions as a repressor when bound by retinoblastoma protein (Rb) [63]. This effect is mediated mainly through HDAC recruitment by Rb [18, 167]. E2F/Rb control of the cell cycle is disrupted in virtually every human cancer and this often occurs through inactivation of the *RB1* gene [239], thus deregulating HDAC activity and favouring cell proliferation.

Several mouse models of HDAC function have been generated, which consist of *HDAC1*, *HDAC5* and *HDAC9* knock-outs, and a mouse expressing an HDAC5 mutant [29, 39, 154, 302]. The mice null for HDAC5 or HDAC9 did not show serious health problems, but when *HDAC5/HDAC9* double knockouts were generated, the embryos displayed multi-focal haemorrhages, and the few animals that survived to adulthood were severely growth retarded. These data support the notion that an element of redundancy may exist in the functions of class IIa HDACs. In contrast to loss of *HDAC5* or *HDAC9* alone, a knock-out of *HDAC1* was found to result in embryonic lethality before embryonic day (E)10.5 due to major proliferation defects and developmental retardation [154]. Also in contrast to the knock-out of *HDAC5*, expression of a mutated HDAC5 protein that cannot undergo nucleocytoplasmic transport (see next section) led to a significantly more severe phenotype [39]. Mice constitutively expressing the mutant were embryonic lethal and, in subsequent experiments, most adults conditionally expressing the mutant from the cardiac-specific α-myosin heavy chain promoter died within 1 month of doxycycline withdrawal.

2.2
Regulation of Histone Deacetylase Activities

Gene regulation arising from alternative splicing is recognized as an increasingly important mechanism in the creation of proteomic complexity [90], and recent data suggest that up to 74% of human multi-exon genes are alternatively spliced [123]. Previously, expression analyses indicated that both class I and II HDACs existed as single isoforms. However, an inspection of the nucleotide sequence database at the National Center for Biotechnology Information reveals that HDAC7 is alternatively spliced, and also various transcript variants have been reported for HDAC3, HDAC9 and HDAC10 [64, 91, 201]. The most extensively spliced histone deacetylase gene is *HDAC9*, which generates at least 24 different messenger RNA (mRNA) species through alternative splicing [201]. Some of these *HDAC9* transcript variants encode proteins with potentially distinct biological activities, for example the MITR (MEF2-interacting transcription repressor) isoform, which lacks the catalytic domain [246].

There is evidence that co-repressor availability plays an important part in regulating HDAC activity, as both class I and class IIa HDACs are enzymatically inactive as purified recombinant proteins generated by in vitro translation, or as glutathione S-transferase (GST) fusion proteins in *E. coli* [66, 67, 97, 159]. In vitro-translated HDAC3, however, becomes enzymatically active when bound to SMRT/NCoR [67, 97]. In this context, post-translational modification of HDACs by reversible phosphorylation is a vital mechanism of control. For example, HDAC1 and HDAC2 serve as substrates for various protein kinases and differential phosphorylation regulates complex-formation, subsequently modulating the level of deacetylase activity and substrate specificity [20, 74, 202, 250, 259]. Full activity of HDAC3 requires phosphorylation of Ser^{424}, a non-conserved residue among the class I HDACs [304]. By contrast, HDAC8 is negatively regulated by cyclic AMP-dependent protein kinase A (PKA)-mediated phosphorylation at Ser^{39} [157]. HDAC activity may also be modulated by sumoylation, with HDAC1 modified at Lys^{444} and Lys^{476} [36, 43], and HDAC4 at Lys^{559} [143]. HDAC6 and HDAC9 are also small ubiquitin-like modifier (SUMO)-modified, indicating that sumoylation may have an important role in the control of HDAC functions [143, 201].

The class IIa HDACs undergo nucleocytoplasmic shuttling in response to calcium signalling, a re-localization that removes these enzymes from their nuclear substrates [94, 130, 174, 275, 303]. This trafficking is dependent on the phosphorylation of conserved N-terminal serine residues in class IIa HDACs that are closely related to the consensus phosphorylation sites for Ca^{2+}/CaM-dependent protein kinases (CaMKs) [94, 130, 275] or protein kinase D (PKD) [195, 268], a downstream effector of protein kinase C (PKC) [268]. Phosphorylation by CaMK or PKD of class IIa HDACs promotes their association with 14-3-3 proteins, leading to cytoplasmic sequestration [94, 130, 174, 175, 268, 275] and suppression of their nuclear activities [163, 174]. Class IIa HDACs contain a conserved C-terminal chromosome region maintenance 1 (CRM1)-dependent nuclear export signal [175, 276] and also a N-terminal localization signal (NLS) [276], located in the same region as two of the CaMK/PKD phosphorylation sites. It is believed that the binding of 14-3-3 proteins could affect class IIa HDAC localization, at least in part, by masking the NLS and altering the balance of the competing effects of nuclear export and import signals.

An additional level of regulation of HDAC activity that has come to attention through recent research is the direct interaction of histone acetyltransferase (HAT) complexes with HDACs. HDAC1 co-immunoprecipitates with the nuclear HAT, PCAF (p300/CBP associated factor), and the two proteins co-localize in HeLa cells. Another HAT, GCN5 (global non-repressed 5) interacts with HDAC1 and HDAC2 and the Sin3A complex, and also with HDAC3 and NCoR [285]. Moreover, HDAC1 interacts with the C/H3 domain of p300 [242] and HDAC6 associates with the SUMO-modified CRD1 domain of this HAT, causing it to function as a transcriptional repressor. In this context, p300-mediated repression is relieved by histone deacetylase inhibition and short interfering RNA (siRNA)-mediated reduction of HDAC6 expression [84]. Consistent with the finding that HDACs can interact physically with transcriptional co-activators, they have also been implicated in gene activation [45, 131, 229]. Also, in mouse embryonic fibroblasts derived from NCoR-null embryos, RAR/RXR binding to DR+1 (separated by one base pair) retinoic acid response elements (RARE) was associated with gene repression rather than the anticipated activation as found with DR+5 RARE. The ligand-dependent activation of a DR+1-containing promoter was restored by addition of NCoR and, consistent with the known association between NCoR and HDAC3, specific depletion of HDAC3 activity via antibodies or dominant-negative forms abolished activation [120].

3
Histone Deacetylase Inhibitors

The discovery that HDACs are involved in cancer, together with the knowledge that the activities of these enzymes could be inhibited by small molecules has prompted a great deal of research with the goal of the discovery of new drugs. Structurally, a wide variety of HDAC inhibitors (HDACi) exist and can be

Table 1 Structural groups of HDAC inhibitors

Group	Classification	Examples
1	Hydroxamic acids	Trichostatin A (TSA), suberoylanilide hydroxamic acid (SAHA)
2	Short chain fatty acids	Butyrate, phenylbutyrate, valproic acid
3	Benzamides	MS-275, N-acetyldinaline
4	Cyclic peptides	Fungal metabolites such as trapoxin A, apicidin and depsipeptide
5	Cyclic hydroxamic-acid-containing peptide (CHAP)	Synthetic hybrids of hydroxamic acids and cyclic tetrapeptides

classified into groups as detailed in Table 1. The anti-tumoural activities of HDACi arise from their ability to specifically target cancer cells via modulation of cellular processes such as apoptosis, the cell cycle, and differentiation pathways that are deregulated in neoplastic cells.

3.1
Hydroxamic Acids

The general structure of these molecules consists of a polar hydroxamic acid site (used to chelate the cation at the bottom of the HDAC catalytic pocket), which is separated by a spacer arm from a hydrophobic moiety that acts as a cap for the catalytic tube of the deacetylase (Fig. 3). These compounds constitute the broadest set of HDACi, and most are very potent but reversible inhibitors of both class I and II (except HDAC6) HDACs, with an IC_{50} (inhibitory concentration 50%) in the low nanomolar to micromolar range in vitro. The most well-known member of this group of inhibitors is trichostatin A (TSA), which was originally developed as an anti-fungal agent [260,

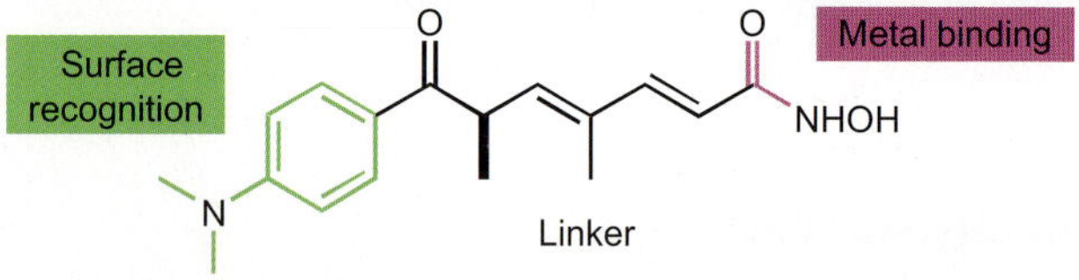

Fig. 3 Structural characteristics of hydroxamic acid-based HDACi. Based on crystallographic studies of hydroxamic acid-based HDACi [trichostatin A, (TSA) shown here] bound to the bacterial deacetylase HDLP and HDAC8, their general structural characteristics comprise a metal binding group, which targets the catalytic site, a linker region and surface recognition group. These structural characteristics can also be extended to other classes of HDACi

Fig. 4a–e Selected HDAC inhibitors. The chemical structures of various histone deacetylase inhibitors (HDACi) are shown as indicated. The *upper left panel* (**a**) contains examples of the hydroxamic acid-based HDACi trichostatin A (TSA), suberoylanilide hydroxamic acid (SAHA) and LAQ-824, with the hydroxamic acid moiety highlighted in *magenta*. **b** The structures of the short chain fatty acids phenylbutyrate and valproic acid with the carboxylic acid group coloured *red*. Also indicated is the structure of Pivanex, AN-9 (pivaloyloxymethyl butyrate) and its metabolites. **c** MS-275 and *N*-acetyldinaline (CI-994), with the benzamide moieties of these HDACi highlighted in *orange*. **d** The structure of FK-228 (depsipeptide), with the disulphide bridge that is reduced in vivo indicated in *green*. **e** The naturally occurring cyclic peptide trapoxin A, with the epoxide group shown in *blue*, and also the synthetic hybrid peptide CHAP31, with the hydroxamic acid moiety highlighted in *magenta*

290, 291]. Although TSA was a very potent HDACi, solubility problems and lack of specificity motivated the search for other inhibitors [266]. Moreover, TSA displayed no anti-tumour activity during in vivo studies of human melanoma xenografts in nude mice, most likely due to metabolic inactivation in the liver and kidney [212]. Many HDACi have, however, used the structural characteristics of TSA as a template, including closely related compounds such as suberoylanilide hydroxamic acid (SAHA) [221] and Scriptaid [249], and recently developed drugs such as LAQ-824 [6, 219] and PXD-101 [207], which are structurally more complex (Fig. 4a).

In the context of APL, the hydroxamic acid-based HDACi, TSA and SAHA, were able to induce apoptosis in NB4 cells harbouring the t(15;17) translocation and also an ATRA-resistant subclone, NB4 306 [4]. The degree of apoptosis was both time- and concentration-dependent, and apoptosis was markedly diminished in the presence of caspase inhibitors. A decrease in the level the anti-apoptotic regulator Daxx was also observed. Similar data were obtained by He et al. with TSA and SAHA in NB4 cells, and with SAHA in transgenic mice expressing PLZF-RARα and RARα-PLZF fusion proteins [102], which develop ATRA- and As_2O_3-resistant APL [100]. SAHA induced apoptosis in bone marrow cells collected from PLZF-RARα/RARα-PLZF mice and potentiated ATRA-induced differentiation. In vivo, SAHA treatment in combination with ATRA achieved complete remission in over 50% of the PLZF-RARα/RARα-PLZF mice, which lasted for up to 7 weeks and was accompanied by an increase in the levels of acetylated histone H4.

Despite the extensive range of hydroxamic acid-based HDACi, only SAHA has progressed to a phase II/III clinical trial setting. SAHA was originally evaluated in a phase I clinical trial using an intravenous preparation, and although treatment led to an increase in histone acetylation, the drug suffered from similar solubility and pharmacokinetic problems to TSA [136]. These problems led to the development of an orally administered version of SAHA, which has been used with successful results [77]. A phase II/III clinical trial of SAHA is currently underway for patients suffering from advanced cutaneous T cell lymphoma (Table 2). A great deal of expectation initially surrounded another hydroxamic acid-based HDACi, LAQ-824, which displayed very promising results in vitro [6, 28, 218, 223]. However, in a phase I clinical trial, intravenous administration caused patients to develop serious cardiac problems. Consequently, development the drug by Novartis has ceased and it has been replaced by a modified version, LBH-589, which was also initially administered intravenously [13, 65, 82]. An oral formulation of LBH-589 has now, however, been developed and is undergoing a phase I/II clinical trial [12] (Table 2).

3.2
Short Chain Fatty Acids

This category of HDAC inhibitors comprises, among others, butyrate [24, 236], valproic acid [89, 203] and phenylbutyrate [156] (Fig. 4b). Some studies have also investigated an in vivo metabolite of phenylbutyrate, phenylacetate [27, 87, 257]. Members of this class of HDACi are considerably less potent than

Table 2 Selected HDAC inhibitors that are currently undergoing clinical trials. (Unreferenced data were sourced from the website http://clinicaltrials.gov/ provided by the National Institutes of Health)

HDAC inhibitor	Disease	Associated therapy	Start date	Phase	Institution	Reference(s)
SAHA (oral)	Solid tumours, haematological malignancies		Feb-2000	Phase I	MSK, NCI	[135]
	Cutaneous TCL, MF, SS		Feb-2004	Phase II/III	Merk	
LBH-589 (oral)	Advanced haematological Malignancies			Phase I/II	Novartis	[12, 13, 65, 82]
MS-275	Lymphoma, solid tumours		Apr-2001	Phase I	NCI	[228]
	AML, CML, MDS	5-Azacytidine	Feb-2005	Phase I	SKCC	
	Metastatic or advanced solid tumours or lymphomas	13-*cis*-RA (isotretinoin)	Dec-2004	Phase I	SKCC	
CI-994 (*N*-Acetyldinaline)	MM, plasma cell neoplasia		May-2000	Phase II	H. Lee Moffitt, NCI	[185]
	NSCLC, pancreatic cancer	Gemcitabine	Oct-1999	Phase I/II	Parke-Davis	
	Advanced cancer	Capecitabine		Phase I	UChicago	[264]
	Advanced solid tumours	Carboplatin, paclitaxel (taxol)		Phase I	Pfizer	[198]
FK228 (Depsipeptide)	Cutaneous/peripheral TCL		Dec-2000	Phase II	NCI	[204, 205]
	Mesothelioma, NSCLC, SCC	Decitabine	May-2002	Phase I	NCI	[235]
	FL, SLL	Fludarabine, rituximab	Mar-2004	Phase I/II	UMG, NCI	
	Malignancies involving lungs, oesophagus, or pleura	Flavopiridol	Oct-2004	Phase I	NCI	
	AML, CLL		Sep-2001	Phase I	OSU, NCI	[19]
Pivanex, AN-9	NSCLC		Jan-1999	Phase I	Titan	[217]

Table 2 (continued)

HDAC inhibitor	Disease	Associated therapy	Start date	Phase	Institution	Reference(s)
(Butyrate prodrug)	NSCLC	Docetaxel	Sep-2003	Phase II	Titan	
	Malignant melanoma		Jan-2004	Phase I/II	Titan	
	CLL, SLL		May-2004	Phase II	Titan	
Phenylbutyrate (oral)	Refractory solid tumours			Phase I	SKCC	[81]
Phenylbutyrate (i.v.)	MDS, adult solid tumours, leukaemia, lymphoma	5-Azacytidine	May-2000	Phase I	SKCC, NCI	[226]
Phenylbutyrate (i.v.)	Adult AML, atypical CML, CMML, MDS	ATRA (tretinoin)	Sep-2000	Phase I	SKCC, NCI	
Phenylbutyrate (i.v.)	Colon, rectal cancer	Fluorouracil, indomethacin, interferon γ	Nov-1999	Phase I/II	Mount Sinai	
Valproic Acid	Advanced cancer			Phase I		[7]
	AML, MDS	Decitabine	Jan-2004	Phase I/II	MD Anderson	[78]
	Metastatic solid tumours	Epirubicin (topoisomerase II inhibitor)		Phase I		[182]
MGCD0103	Advanced solid tumours, NHL		Dec-2004	Phase I	MethylGene	[79, 126]

AML, acute myeloid leukaemia; ATRA, all-*trans* retinoic acid; CLL, chronic lymphocytic leukaemia; CML, chronic myeloid leukaemia; CMML, chronic myelomonocytic leukaemia; FL, follicular lymphoma; HDAC, histone deacetylase; MDS, myelodysplastic syndrome; MF, mycosis fungoides; MM, multiple myeloma; MSK, Memorial Sloan-Kettering Cancer Center; NCI, National Cancer Institute; NHL, non-Hodgkin's lymphoma; NSCLC, non-small cell lung cancer; OSU, Ohio State University; SCC, small cell carcinoma; SKCC, Sidney Kimmel Cancer Centre at John Hopkins University; SLL, small lymphocytic lymphoma; SS, sezary syndrome; TCL, T cell lymphoma; UMG, University of Maryland Greenebaum Cancer Center hydroxamic acids, with IC_{50} values occurring in vitro at millimolar concentrations and at very high doses in vivo.

The prodrug form of butyrate, pivaloyloxymethyl butyrate (known as Pivanex, AN-9) [8, 105], which must undergo chemical conversion by metabolic processes before becoming an active pharmacological agent (Fig. 4b), has been shown to display selective toxicity towards acute leukaemia and drug-resistant primary leukaemia and cancer cell lines, including HL60 AML (M2) cells [10]. The studies in NB4 cells discussed for hydroxamic acid HDACi also showed induction of apoptosis by butyrate [4], and apoptosis and differentiation by phenylbutyrate [102]. The results for phenylbutyrate mirrored previous data from studies carried out in ML-1 AML cells [55]. Recently, death receptor-dependent apoptosis in PML-RARα transgenic mice was demonstrated after treatment with valproic acid [117]. Induction of apoptosis was found to be p53-independent and dependent on tumour necrosis factor (TNF)-related apoptosis inducing ligand (TRAIL) and Fas signalling pathways. Moreover, leukaemic cells, but not haematopoietic progenitors, displayed an increase in the levels of TRAIL, DR5 FasL and Fas upon valproic acid treatment. Short chain fatty acids also display pleiotropic activity, effecting phosphorylation, methylation and cytoskeletal structure [150]. However, they are currently amongst the best-studied HDACi and, in America, the Food and Drug Administration has previously given clinical approval for valproic acid to be used in the treatment of epilepsy, and phenylbutyrate in patients with urea cycle disorders. Pivanex is currently in clinical trials [197, 217], as is phenylbutyrate [26, 81, 88] and valproic acid [7, 78, 182] (Table 2).

3.3
Benzamides

Benzamides have an IC_{50} in the micromolar range, and the two representatives of this class of HDACi that have attracted most attention are MS-275 (Fig. 4c) [251] and acetyldinaline (CI-994) [60, 162, 237]. The mechanism by which the benzamides exert their activities is not clearly understood, but it is has been suggested that the diaminophenyl group enters the catalytic site and chelates the Zn^{2+} cation. Recent research has shown MS-275 to inhibit the activity of HDAC1 more than HDAC3 and to a much greater degree than HDAC8 [108]. Moreover, in contrast to several other HDACi tested, use of MS-275 does not lead to a build-up of acetylated α-tubulin, most likely due to a lack of activity towards HDAC6 [85].

The effects of MS-275 have been examined in human histiocytic lymphoma U937 and acute myeloid leukaemia HL60 cells by Rosato et al., who found that micromolar concentrations induced differentiation (1 μM), or apoptosis (5 µM) [224]. Apoptosis was characterized by an increase in reactive oxygen species (ROS), a loss in mitochondrial membrane potential and cytosolic release of cytochrome *c* leading to activation of the caspase cascade. Degradation of anti-apoptotic proteins such as Bcl-2, Mcl-1 and XIAP, as well as BID (BH3 death domain agonist) cleavage was also reported. Apoptosis directed through the extrinsic pathway mediated by FasL was not found to play a significant role.

Recent research has shown that MS-275 (and also SAHA and valproic acid) can induce apoptosis in NB4, HL60 and U937 cells through up-regulation of TRAIL expression [184]. The major part of the work carried out for this study utilized MS-275, which was found to induce expression of p21^{WAF1} and TRAIL, and to a lesser degree DR4 and DR5, whilst down-regulating cyclin D2. AML and APL patient blast cells also responded to MS-275 treatment with TRAIL induction and apoptosis, whereas CD34^{+ve} progenitor cells were insensitive to the apoptogenic effects of this HDACi. Both MS-275 (phase I) [228] and CI-994 (phase II) [185, 198, 209, 264] are undergoing clinical trials (Table 2).

3.4
Cyclic Peptides

These irreversible inhibitors constitute the most structurally complex HDACi (Fig. 4) and have an IC$_{50}$ in the nanomolar range. The best-characterized examples are a fungal metabolite, apicidin [41], the microbial metabolites trapoxin A and B [119] and FK228 (also known as depsipeptide and FR901228) [263]. Trapoxin A and B HDACi are thought to trap HDACs through the reaction of the epoxide moiety with the zinc cation or an amino acid in the binding pocket. FK228, which is derived from *Chromobacterium violaceum*, is the only cyclic peptide undergoing clinical trials, where it is being investigated in both solid tumours and haematological malignancies [19, 172, 204, 205, 230, 235]. In a phase I/II clinical trail this HDACi has been shown to be effective in patients with refractory cutaneous (overall response rate of 50%) or peripheral T cell (partial response of 24%) lymphoma [204, 205] (Table 2). The mechanism by which FK228 inhibits HDACs is not known with certainty but it has been proposed that the disulphide bridge is reduced inside the cell and releases a free thiol analogue, redFK, as the active species. This is then able to fit inside the HDAC catalytic pocket and interact with the zinc cation, forming a covalent bond [72]. FK228 can therefore be thought of as a naturally occurring prodrug.

In the context of APL, nanomolar concentrations of FK228 were cytotoxic to and, in combination with ATRA, induced differentiation in NB4 cells [148]. Moreover, in vivo administration of ATRA and FK228 in combination synergistically inhibited the growth of established tumours of NB4 cells subcutaneously transplanted in NOD-SCID mice. FK228 was also found to restore transcription of silenced genes [e.g. interleukin (IL)-3] and induce cell differentiation in AML1/ETO-positive Kasumi cells and blasts from a patient with t(8;21) AML [145]. The activity of FK228 was enhanced by 5-aza-2′-deoxycytidine, a DNMT inhibitor, resulting in enhanced histone acetylation, IL-3 expression and cytotoxicity. Cyclic peptides have also been combined with hydroxamic acid groups, a class of HDACi referred to as cyclic hydroxamic-acid-containing peptide (CHAP) [71, 146], and this underlies the rationale behind the development of an HDAC6-specific hexapeptide hydroxamic acid inhibitor based on the α-tubulin sequence [125].

3.5
Molecular Mechanisms Underlying Biological Effects of HDACi

Although it is likely that not all biological effects of HDACi are a direct consequence of HDAC inhibition, effects of HDAC inhibition on gene expression are consistent with effects that a given HDACi exerts on a biological function of a specific cancer cell. There have been relatively few studies comparing global alterations to gene expression as a result of treatment with different HDACi [85, 180, 199]. The data indicated that structurally diverse HDACi significantly affect a relatively small number of genes—between 10% (>2-fold change in expression [85]) and 20% (>2-fold change in expression [199]). Similarly, effects of different inhibitors on patterns of gene expression suggest that certain loci are particularly susceptible to the effects of these agents. Nevertheless, small subsets of regulated genes exist, which are specific for a given inhibitor [199], and this may reflect an inhibitor and/or cell type-specific response.

The gene expression analyses confirm that many of the target genes for HDACi encode proteins involved in regulation of cell proliferation and apoptosis. Induction of tumour cell apoptosis by HDACi is usually associated with up-regulated expression of genes encoding proteins involved in the extrinsic death receptor-mediated apoptotic pathway such as DR5, Fas, FasL or TRAIL [86, 117, 153, 184]. With regard to the intrinsic (via disruption of the mitochondrial membrane) apoptotic pathway, genes encoding pro-apoptotic proteins Bak and Bax [252] are up-regulated, whilst the anti-apoptotic Bcl-2, Bcl-XL, Mcl-1 and XIAP [25, 57, 138, 224] are down-regulated. Cell-cycle control genes that are affected include $p21^{WAF1}$ [220], which is up-regulated, or loss of cyclin D1 expression [231]. This results in hypophosphorylation of Rb and G1 arrest, preventing S phase progression [161].

HDACi-induced differentiation has been demonstrated in a variety of malignancies, and PLZF-RARα-associated APL provides an excellent example of the efficacy of HDACi in this context. Unlike PML-RARα associated APL, which responds to treatment with pharmacological concentrations of ATRA as a result of ligand-induced conformational changes in the fusion protein and release of the co-repressor complex, PLZF-RARα recruits HDAC activity in an ATRA-insensitive manner. However, combined treatment of ATRA and HDACi leads to differentiation and apoptosis of PLZF-RARα-positive cells [98, 101, 144].

HDACi-induced apoptosis may also be influenced by events that do not rely on changes in expression of target genes. SAHA treatment is associated with cleavage and activation of the pro-apoptotic Bcl-2 family member BID and production of ROS, which induces mitochondrial damage, initiating the intrinsic apoptotic pathway [227]. MS-275 also elevated ROS levels [224], and this activity of these HDACi, which specifically affects cancer cells, appears to be, at least in part, due to differential induction of thioredoxin [265]. Thioredoxin acts as a scavenger of ROS, and the fact that it is induced in normal, but not transformed, cells helps to explain why normal cells are more resistant to HDACi-induced cell death. Recent research has indicated that another way in which HDACi (in this case depsipeptide) can facilitate apoptosis is through redistribution of TRAIL receptors to membrane lipid rafts, increasing sensitivity to TRAIL-induced apoptosis [267].

An effect of HDACi activities that, as yet, has not been extensively explored and could prove to be extremely important relates to modification of the acetylation status of non-histone proteins such as α-tubulin and transcription factors [292]. A good example of the potential importance of this aspect of HDACi function is the tumour-suppressor protein p53, for which acetylation is important for stability and the ability to activate transcription [9]. Deacetylation by either the class III deacetylase SIR2 [155] or HDAC1 [110, 165] leads to inhibition of p53 transcriptional activity and prevents apoptosis. Recently, p53 has been found to be specifically deacetylated and degraded via interactions with PML-RARα [116] and could be an important target, at least in some cancers, as it is necessary for TSA- and SAHA-mediated apoptosis [103]. Another important mechanism of action of HDACi is the modulation of genes involved in hypoxia-induced angiogenesis such as *VEGF* and *HIF-1α* [51, 176, 233, 234, 281, 301]. Finally, in analogy to the arsenic trioxide-induced degradation of PML-RARα [44], treatment of cells with valproic acid has been shown to cause the specific degradation of HDAC2 [149].

3.6
Combination Therapy

Whilst some HDACi are in clinical trials as monotherapy, most are now being tested in combination with other drugs such as DNA demethylating agents, retinoids or chemotherapy (Tables 2 and 3). Better understanding of the molecular mechanisms that underlie biological effects of various HDACi has facilitated a more rational design of combination therapies. The molecular basis for the use of HDACi in combination with ATRA was mentioned previously, and this concept is being extended to synthetic retinoids and drugs that elevate levels of cyclic AMP such as pentoxifylline, which also promote differentiation of APL cells by targeting activities of the fusion oncoprotein [127, 299]. The cross-talk between DNA methylation and histone modification has also encouraged combinatorial targeting of these processes in anti-cancer therapy [34, 59]. Another effect of HDACi, for example with MS-275 and SAHA, is to sensitize cells to chemotherapeutic agents [3, 166], and several clinical trials are ongoing based on this principle. There are a number of other innovative strategies employing the use of HDACi in combination with other therapies, and details of the various rationales underlying them are shown in Table 3.

4
Future Directions

It is clear that HDACi have a strong therapeutic potential, and this class of enzymes represents a bone fide target for anti-cancer drug development. However, there remains much to learn with respect to the specific substrates of individual family members, target genes that they may act upon and what their precise roles are as they function in concert with other chromatin modifiers to shape particular domains. In this regard, recent research has indicated that HDAC3 preferentially deacetylates histone H4 at position Lys^5, then Lys^8, Lys^{12} and Lys^{16} [99], which is in agreement with previous hypotheses on the mechanisms of H4 tail acetylation. Moreover, whilst the situation in humans is undoubtedly more complex, work in *S. cerevisiae* and more recently in *C. elegans* has indicated non-redundant roles for different HDACs in regulation of specific genes [222, 280].

A somewhat disappointing characteristic of the HDACi that have so far have been developed is overall lack of selectivity towards individual family members, although some inhibitors are less effective against certain HDACs. This may be explained in part by the finding that area surrounding the catalytic pocket of HDAC8 actually alters its conformation to accommodate

Table 3 Combinatorial therapies targeting cancer epigenetics

HDACi	Combination therapy	Scientific rationale	Reference(s)
SAHA, TSA, Pivanex	Chemotherapy	Pretreatment of cells with HDACi promoted chromatin decondensation, increasing the efficiency of several anti-cancer drugs targeting DNA. Pivanex down-regulated levels of NADPH- cytochrome P450 reductase and DT-diaphorase mRNA, sensitizing cells to doxorubicin treatment	[142, 188]
CBHA, FK228, MS-275, TSA	γ-Irradiation	HDACs have been implicated in double-stranded DNA repair. Combined HDACi and γ-irradiation treatment prolonged γ-H2AX foci expression and enhanced the radiosensitivity of cells and xenografts.	[22, 23, 140, 305]
NaB, SAHA, tubacin	Bortezomib (26S proteasome inhibitor)	HDACi induce NF-κB DNA binding. Combined treatment using bortezomib with HDACi NaB and SAHA resulted in increased ROS generation and diminished NF-κB activation. HDAC6 is required for aggresome-mediated degradation of ubiquitinated proteins. Combined treatment with bortezomib and tubacin inhibits both pathways, leading to accumulation of ubiquitinated proteins followed by cell stress and cytotoxicity	[2, 48, 49, 104, 200, 295, 296]
Tubacin	Lonafarnib (farnesyl transferase inhibitor), paclitaxel, taxol (microtubule-stabilizer)	Microtubule stabilization and acetylation, and suppression of microtubule dynamics is enhanced by tubacin inhibition of HDAC6, leading to mitotic arrest and cell death	[170]
LBH-589, NaB, SAHA	17-AAG (HSP90 inhibitor)	In Bcr-Abl+ve (including STI-571 resistant) AML cells and those with activating mutation of Flt-3, the hsp90 inhibitor 17-AAG prevents their association with the chaperone, resulting in polyubiquitination and proteasomal degradation. Combined treatment with HDACi greatly enhances apoptosis	[80, 214, 216]
NaB, SAHA, TSA	Perifosine, D-21266 (alkyl-lysophospholipid)	Alkyl-lysophospholipids selectively target tumour cell membranes. Combined treatment of HDACi with perifosine synergistically induced mitochondrial dysfunction, increased ROS generation and caspase activation, leading to apoptosis and decreased cell growth	[215]

Table 3 (continued)

HDACi	Combination therapy	Scientific rationale	Reference(s)
Apicidin, FK228, phenyl-butyrate	STI-571, imatinib, Gleevec (tyrosine kinase inhibitor)	Combined treatment of STI-571 with HDACi enhances apoptosis in Bcr-Abl+ve AML cells and causes apoptosis in STI-571-resistant cells	[141, 189, 190, 294]
SAHA	CI-1033 (pan-ErbB tyrosine kinase inhibitor)	Combination therapy decreased EGFR and AKT signalling and increased caspase activity	[31]
FK228, NaB, SAHA, TSA	TRAIL	HDACi potentiate apoptosis induced death receptor ligation	[115, 245]
FK228, NaB, SAHA	Flavopiridol (CDK inhibitor)	HDACi induce NF-κB DNA binding. This is abrogated by flavopiridol, enhancing apoptosis. Flavopiridol also enhances apoptosis by down-regulating anti-apoptotic proteins (e.g. XIAP) and p21^{WAF1} (preventing cell cycle arrest)	[3, 76, 186, 187, 225]
Apicidin, NaB, SAHA	Topo II inhibitors	HDACi up-regulate topo II expression, increasing sensitivity to topo II inhibitors. Pre-treatment with SAHA promoted chromatin decondensation also potentiating DNA damage by topo II inhibitors	[152, 169, 177, 193]
LAQ-824	PTK-787/ZK-222584 (VEGFR tyrosine kinase inhibitor)	VEGF-induced angiogenesis is impaired through inhibition of VEGF signalling by PTK-787/ZK-222584 and down-regulation of angiogenesis-related genes such as HIF-1α and VEGF by LAQ-824	[211]
FK228, NaB, SAHA, TSA	TRAIL, TNFα	Activation of the extrinsic, receptor-mediated apoptotic pathway by HDACi sensitizes cells to treatment with death receptor ligands	[115, 245, 267]
FK228	Bcl-2 antisense oligonucleotide (G3139)	Anti-apoptotic Bcl-2 blocks HDACi activity. Combined treatment with Bcl-2 antisense oligonucleotide and HDACi enhanced apoptosis and cytotoxicity	[56]

Table 3 (continued)

HDACi	Combination therapy	Scientific rationale	Reference(s)
FK228, phenylbutyrate, NaB, SAHA, scriptaid, TSA, VPA	5-Azacytidine, decitabine	Combined treatment with DNMT inhibitors and HDACi overcomes promoter hypermethylation-associated gene silencing, and synergistically inhibit growth and induce apoptosis	[14, 17, 21, 73, 134, 145, 181, 210, 241, 247, 279, 286]
MS-275, NaB, SAHA	Fludarabine, fluorouracil	Nucleoside analogues cause cytotoxicity due to incorporation into DNA and RNA. This effect is enhanced by combined use with HDACi	[1, 166, 193]
CBHA, FK228, MS-275, NaB, phenylbutyrate, SAHA, TSA, VPA	13-*cis*-RA, ATRA, As$_2$O$_3$	RARα fusion oncoproteins aberrantly recruit HDAC-containing repressor complexes and silence expression of target genes. Combined treatment with retinoids and HDACi reactivate repressed genes. The PML-RARα oncoprotein may also be specifically degraded as a result of As$_2$O$_3$ treatment	[4, 35, 37, 47, 98, 101, 122, 144, 148, 178, 181, 277, 278]

ATRA, all-*trans*-retinoic acid; *decitabine*, 5-aza-2′-deoxycytidine; *HDACi*, HDAC inhibitor(s); *IL-2*, interleukin-2; *NaB*, sodium butyrate; *NADPH*, nicotinamide adenine dinucleotide phosphate, reduced; *RA*, retinoic acid; *topo*, topoisomerase structurally different HDACi [243]. This malleability, if it extends to other family members, may also account for the ability of these enzymes to deacetylate diverse target proteins. Newly published data, however, show that an HDAC6-specific inhibitor, tubacin, may have therapeutic potential in multiple myeloma through targeting of its aggresome function [104]. Targeting the α-tubulin acetylation activity of HDAC6 with tubacin in combination with lonafarnib (a farnesyl transferase inhibitor) and paclitaxel also proved effective in non-small cell lung cancer cell lines [170]. Moreover, class I specific HDACi [194], and also an inhibitor that inhibits HDAC4 but not HDAC1 [168] have been recently described. The class IIa specific inhibitor did not, however, induce apoptosis or granulocytic differentiation in U937 cells in comparison with SAHA [168]. Finally, MethylGene (Montreal, Canada) has recently published two abstracts detailing the development of a novel and allegedly specific HDACi, MGCD0103; however, the details of the basic research have not been revealed [79, 126].

The rational use of HDACi currently in clinical trials with other agents has great potential to target and enhance the activity of these drugs towards a particular malignancy. An exciting line of investigation currently being explored that has potential for use in combination therapy with HDACi utilizes peptides that block specific oncoprotein–co-repressor interactions [208, 213]. Peptides targeting the interface between PML-RARα and NCoR/SMRT restored ATRA sensitivity to differentiation resistant NB4 cells [213]. Similarly, peptides disrupting interaction between NCoR and BCL6 induce apoptosis of diffuse large B cell lymphoma cell lines [208]. In the future, this principle could readily be extended to HDACs themselves as the domains of interaction with partner proteins are mapped, potentially revealing more specific targets for development of small molecular drugs. Another option is to follow the example of valproic acid, and further investigation of compounds that promote selective degradation rather than those that inhibit directly could also yield improved selectivity. Other potential targets are the enzymes responsible for the modulation of HDAC activities such as kinases or phosphatases [74].

Clearly we are now well into the era of rational design of anti-cancer therapeutics, and a number of target-based therapies that reach the clinic is rapidly growing [299]. As the biological activities of individual HDACs are elucidated and novel, perhaps more specific, HDACi are developed, the potential for a highly effective use of these agents in combination therapies that are specifically tailored to different cancer types draws ever closer.

Acknowledgements The authors would like to acknowledge support from the Leukaemia Research Fund of Great Britain, the Samuel Waxman Cancer Research Foundation, the Key Kendall Leukaemia Fund and National Cancer Institute.

References

1. Acharya MR, Figg WD (2004) Histone deacetylase inhibitor enhances the antileukemic activity of an established nucleoside analogue. Cancer Biol Ther 3:719–720
2. Adachi M, Zhang Y, Zhao X, Minami T, Kawamura R, Hinoda Y, Imai K (2004) Synergistic effect of histone deacetylase inhibitors FK228 and m-carboxycinnamic acid bis-hydroxamide with proteasome inhibitors PSI and PS-341 against gastrointestinal adenocarcinoma cells. Clin Cancer Res 10:3853–3862
3. Almenara J, Rosato R, Grant S (2002) Synergistic induction of mitochondrial damage and apoptosis in human leukemia cells by flavopiridol and the histone deacetylase inhibitor suberoylanilide hydroxamic acid (SAHA). Leukemia 16:1331–1343
4. Amin HM, Saeed S, Alkan S (2001) Histone deacetylase inhibitors induce caspase-dependent apoptosis and downregulation of daxx in acute promyelocytic leukaemia with t(15;17). Br J Haematol 115:287–297
5. Antequera F, Bird A (1993) Number of CpG islands and genes in human and mouse. Proc Natl Acad Sci U S A 90:11995–11999
6. Atadja P, Hsu M, Kwon P, Trogani N, Bhalla K, Remiszewski S (2004) Molecular and cellular basis for the anti-proliferative effects of the HDAC inhibitor LAQ824. Novartis Found Symp 259:249–66; discussion 266–268, 285–288
7. Atmaca A, Maurer A, Heinzel T, Gottlicher M, Neumann A, Al-Batran SE, Martin E, Bartsch I, Knuth A, Jaeger E (2004) A dose-escalating phase I study with valproic acid (VPA) in patients (pts) with advanced cancer. J Clin Oncol 23:Abstr 3169
8. Aviram A, Zimrah Y, Shaklai M, Nudelman A, Rephaeli A (1994) Comparison between the effect of butyric acid and its prodrug pivaloyloxymethylbutyrate on histones hyperacetylation in an HL-60 leukemic cell line. Int J Cancer 56:906–909
9. Barlev NA, Liu L, Chehab NH, Mansfield K, Harris KG, Halazonetis TD, Berger SL (2001) Acetylation of p53 activates transcription through recruitment of coactivators/histone acetyltransferases. Mol Cell 8:1243–1254
10. Batova A, Shao LE, Diccianni MB, Yu AL, Tanaka T, Rephaeli A, Nudelman A, Yu J (2002) The histone deacetylase inhibitor AN-9 has selective toxicity to acute leukemia and drug-resistant primary leukemia and cancer cell lines. Blood 100:3319–3324
11. Baylin S, Bestor TH (2002) Altered methylation patterns in cancer cell genomes: cause or consequence? Cancer Cell 1:299–305
12. Beck J, Fischer T, George D, Huber C, Calvo E, Atadja P, Peng B, Kwong C, Sharma S, Patnaik A (2005) Phase I pharmacokinetic (PK) and pharmacodynamic (PD) study of ORAL LBH589B: a novel histone deacetylase (HDAC) inhibitor. J Clin Oncol 24:Abstr 3148
13. Beck J, Fischer T, Rowinsky E, Huber C, Mita M, Atadja P, Peng B, Kwong C, Dugan M, Patnaik A (2004) Phase I pharmacokinetic and pharmacodynamic study of LBH-589A: a novel histone deacetylase inhibitor. J Clin Oncol 23:Abstr 3025
14. Belinsky SA, Klinge DM, Stidley CA, Issa JP, Herman JG, March TH, Baylin SB (2003) Inhibition of DNA methylation and histone deacetylation prevents murine lung cancer. Cancer Res 63:7089–7093

15. Bestor TH (2000) The DNA methyltransferases of mammals. Hum Mol Genet 9:2395–2402
16. Bird A (2002) DNA methylation patterns and epigenetic memory. Genes Dev 16:6–21
17. Boivin AJ, Momparler LF, Hurtubise A, Momparler RL (2002) Antineoplastic action of 5-aza-2′-deoxycytidine and phenylbutyrate on human lung carcinoma cells. Anticancer Drugs 13:869–874
18. Brehm A, Miska EA, McCance DJ, Reid JL, Bannister AJ, Kouzarides T (1998) Retinoblastoma protein recruits histone deacetylase to repress transcription. Nature 391:597–601
19. Byrd JC, Marcucci G, Parthun MR, Xiao JJ, Klisovic RB, Moran M, Lin TS, Liu S, Sklenar AR, Davis ME, Lucas DM, Fischer B, Shank R, Tejaswi SL, Binkley P, Wright J, Chan KK, Grever MR (2005) A phase 1 and pharmacodynamic study of depsipeptide (FK228) in chronic lymphocytic leukemia and acute myeloid leukemia. Blood 105:959–967
20. Cai R, Kwon P, Yan-Neale Y, Sambuccetti L, Fischer D, Cohen D (2001) Mammalian histone deacetylase 1 protein is posttranslationally modified by phosphorylation. Biochem Biophys Res Commun 283:445–453
21. Cameron EE, Bachman KE, Myohanen S, Herman JG, Baylin SB (1999) Synergy of demethylation and histone deacetylase inhibition in the re-expression of genes silenced in cancer. Nat Genet 21:103–107
22. Camphausen K, Burgan W, Cerra M, Oswald KA, Trepel JB, Lee MJ, Tofilon PJ (2004) Enhanced radiation-induced cell killing and prolongation of gammaH2AX foci expression by the histone deacetylase inhibitor MS-275. Cancer Res 64:316–321
23. Camphausen K, Scott T, Sproull M, Tofilon PJ (2004) Enhancement of xenograft tumor radiosensitivity by the histone deacetylase inhibitor MS-275 and correlation with histone hyperacetylation. Clin Cancer Res 10:6066–6071
24. Candido EP, Reeves R, Davie JR (1978) Sodium butyrate inhibits histone deacetylation in cultured cells. Cell 14:105–113
25. Cao XX, Mohuiddin I, Ece F, McConkey DJ, Smythe WR (2001) Histone deacetylase inhibitor downregulation of bcl-xl gene expression leads to apoptotic cell death in mesothelioma. Am J Respir Cell Mol Biol 25:562–568
26. Carducci MA, Gilbert J, Bowling MK, Noe D, Eisenberger MA, Sinibaldi V, Zabelina Y, Chen TL, Grochow LB, Donehower RC (2001) A Phase I clinical and pharmacological evaluation of sodium phenylbutyrate on an 120-h infusion schedule. Clin Cancer Res 7:3047–3055
27. Carducci MA, Nelson JB, Chan-Tack KM, Ayyagari SR, Sweatt WH, Campbell PA, Nelson WG, Simons JW (1996) Phenylbutyrate induces apoptosis in human prostate cancer and is more potent than phenylacetate. Clin Cancer Res 2:379–387
28. Catley L, Weisberg E, Tai YT, Atadja P, Remiszewski S, Hideshima T, Mitsiades N, Shringarpure R, LeBlanc R, Chauhan D, Munshi NC, Schlossman R, Richardson P, Griffin J, Anderson KC (2003) NVP-LAQ824 is a potent novel histone deacetylase inhibitor with significant activity against multiple myeloma. Blood 102:2615–2622
29. Chang S, McKinsey TA, Zhang CL, Richardson JA, Hill JA, Olson EN (2004) Histone deacetylases 5 and 9 govern responsiveness of the heart to a subset of stress signals and play redundant roles in heart development. Mol Cell Biol 24:8467–8476

30. Chauchereau A, Mathieu M, de Saintignon J, Ferreira R, Pritchard LL, Mishal Z, Dejean A, Harel-Bellan A (2004) HDAC4 mediates transcriptional repression by the acute promyelocytic leukaemia-associated protein PLZF. Oncogene 23:8777–8784
31. Chinnaiyan P, Varambally S, Tomlins S, Huang S, Chinnaiyan A, Harari P (2004) Enhancing the anti-tumor activity of ErbB blockade with histone deacetylase (HDAC) inhibition. J Clin Oncol 23:Abstr 3029
32. Choi JH, Kwon HJ, Yoon BI, Kim JH, Han SU, Joo HJ, Kim DY (2001) Expression profile of histone deacetylase 1 in gastric cancer tissues. Jpn J Cancer Res 92:1300–1304
33. Choi KY, Ji YJ, Jee C, Kim do H, Ahnn J (2002) Characterization of CeHDA-7, a class II histone deacetylase interacting with MEF-2 in Caenorhabditis elegans. Biochem Biophys Res Commun 293:1295–1300
34. Claus R, Lubbert M (2003) Epigenetic targets in hematopoietic malignancies. Oncogene 22:6489–6496
35. Coffey DC, Kutko MC, Glick RD, Butler LM, Heller G, Rifkind RA, Marks PA, Richon VM, La Quaglia MP (2001) The histone deacetylase inhibitor, CBHA, inhibits growth of human neuroblastoma xenografts in vivo, alone and synergistically with all-trans retinoic acid. Cancer Res 61:3591–3594
36. Colombo R, Boggio R, Seiser C, Draetta GF, Chiocca S (2002) The adenovirus protein Gam1 interferes with sumoylation of histone deacetylase 1. EMBO Rep 3:1062–1068
37. Cote S, Rosenauer A, Bianchini A, Seiter K, Vandewiele J, Nervi C, Miller WH Jr (2002) Response to histone deacetylase inhibition of novel PML/RARalpha mutants detected in retinoic acid-resistant APL cells. Blood 100:2586–2596
38. Cress WD, Seto E (2000) Histone deacetylases, transcriptional control, and cancer. J Cell Physiol 184:1–16
39. Czubryt MP, McAnally J, Fishman GI, Olson EN (2003) Regulation of peroxisome proliferator-activated receptor gamma coactivator 1 alpha (PGC-1 alpha) and mitochondrial function by MEF2 and HDAC5. Proc Natl Acad Sci U S A 100:1711–1716
40. Dalla-Favera R, Migliazza A, Chang CC, Niu H, Pasqualucci L, Butler M, Shen Q, Cattoretti G (1999) Molecular pathogenesis of B cell malignancy: the role of BCL-6. Curr Top Microbiol Immunol 246:257–263; discussion 263–265
41. Darkin-Rattray SJ, Gurnett AM, Myers RW, Dulski PM, Crumley TM, Allocco JJ, Cannova C, Meinke PT, Colletti SL, Bednarek MA, Singh SB, Goetz MA, Dombrowski AW, Polishook JD, Schmatz DM (1996) Apicidin: a novel antiprotozoal agent that inhibits parasite histone deacetylase. Proc Natl Acad Sci U S A 93:13143–13147
42. David G, Alland L, Hong SH, Wong CW, DePinho RA, Dejean A (1998) Histone deacetylase associated with mSin3A mediates repression by the acute promyelocytic leukemia-associated PLZF protein. Oncogene 16:2549–2556
43. David G, Neptune MA, DePinho RA (2002) SUMO-1 modification of histone deacetylase 1 (HDAC1) modulates its biological activities. J Biol Chem 17:17
44. Davison K, Mann KK, Miller WH Jr (2002) Arsenic trioxide: mechanisms of action. Semin Hematol 39:3–7

45. De Nadal E, Zapater M, Alepuz PM, Sumoy L, Mas G, Posas F (2004) The MAPK Hog1 recruits Rpd3 histone deacetylase to activate osmoresponsive genes. Nature 427:370–374
46. De Ruijter AJ, Van Gennip AH, Caron HN, Kemp S, Van Kuilenburg AB (2003) Histone deacetylases (HDACs): characterization of the classical HDAC family. Biochem J 370:737–749
47. Demary K, Wong L, Spanjaard RA (2001) Effects of retinoic acid and sodium butyrate on gene expression, histone acetylation and inhibition of proliferation of melanoma cells. Cancer Lett 163:103–107
48. Denlinger CE, Keller MD, Mayo MW, Broad RM, Jones DR (2004) Combined proteasome and histone deacetylase inhibition in non-small cell lung cancer. J Thorac Cardiovasc Surg 127:1078–1086
49. Denlinger CE, Rundall BK, Jones DR (2004) Proteasome inhibition sensitizes non-small cell lung cancer to histone deacetylase inhibitor-induced apoptosis through the generation of reactive oxygen species. J Thorac Cardiovasc Surg 128:740–748
50. Dequiedt F, Kasler H, Fischle W, Kiermer V, Weinstein M, Herndier BG, Verdin E (2003) HDAC7, a thymus-specific class II histone deacetylase, regulates Nur77 transcription and TCR-mediated apoptosis. Immunity 18:687–698
51. Deroanne CF, Bonjean K, Servotte S, Devy L, Colige A, Clausse N, Blacher S, Verdin E, Foidart JM, Nusgens BV, Castronovo V (2002) Histone deacetylases inhibitors as anti-angiogenic agents altering vascular endothelial growth factor signaling. Oncogene 21:427–436
52. Dhordain P, Albagli O, Lin RJ, Ansieau S, Quief S, Leutz A, Kerckaert JP, Evans RM, Leprince D (1997) Corepressor SMRT binds the BTB/POZ repressing domain of the LAZ3/BCL6 oncoprotein. Proc Natl Acad Sci U S A 94:10762–10767
53. Dhordain P, Lin RJ, Quief S, Lantoine D, Kerckaert JP, Evans RM, Albagli O (1998) The LAZ3(BCL-6) oncoprotein recruits a SMRT/mSIN3A/histone deacetylase containing complex to mediate transcriptional repression. Nucleic Acids Res 26:4645–4651
54. Di Croce L, Raker VA, Corsaro M, Fazi F, Fanelli M, Faretta M, Fuks F, Lo Coco F, Kouzarides T, Nervi C, Minucci S, Pelicci PG (2002) Methyltransferase recruitment and DNA hypermethylation of target promoters by an oncogenic transcription factor. Science 295:1079–1082
55. DiGiuseppe JA, Weng LJ, Yu KH, Fu S, Kastan MB, Samid D, Gore SD (1999) Phenylbutyrate-induced G1 arrest and apoptosis in myeloid leukemia cells: structure-function analysis. Leukemia 13:1243–1253
56. Doi S, Soda H, Oka M, Tsurutani J, Kitazaki T, Nakamura Y, Fukuda M, Yamada Y, Kamihira S, Kohno S (2004) The histone deacetylase inhibitor FR901228 induces caspase-dependent apoptosis via the mitochondrial pathway in small cell lung cancer cells. Mol Cancer Ther 3:1397–1402
57. Duan H, Heckman CA, Boxer LM (2005) Histone deacetylase inhibitors down-regulate bcl-2 expression and induce apoptosis in t(14;18) lymphomas. Mol Cell Biol 25:1608–1619
58. Eberharter A, Becker PB (2002) Histone acetylation: a switch between repressive and permissive chromatin. Second in review series on chromatin dynamics. EMBO Rep 3:224–229

59. Egger G, Liang G, Aparicio A, Jones PA (2004) Epigenetics in human disease and prospects for epigenetic therapy. Nature 429:457–463
60. el-Beltagi HM, Martens AC, Lelieveld P, Haroun EA, Hagenbeek A (1993) Acetyldinaline: a new oral cytostatic drug with impressive differential activity against leukemic cells and normal stem cells—preclinical studies in a relevant rat model for human acute myelocytic leukemia. Cancer Res 53:3008–3014
61. el-Deiry WS, Nelkin BD, Celano P, Yen RW, Falco JP, Hamilton SR, Baylin SB (1991) High expression of the DNA methyltransferase gene characterizes human neoplastic cells and progression stages of colon cancer. Proc Natl Acad Sci U S A 88:3470–3474
62. Feinberg AP, Tycko B (2004) The history of cancer epigenetics. Nat Rev Cancer 4:143–153
63. Ferreira R, Naguibneva I, Pritchard LL, Ait-Si-Ali S, Harel-Bellan A (2001) The Rb/chromatin connection and epigenetic control: opinion. Oncogene 20:3128–3133
64. Fischer DD, Cai R, Bhatia U, Asselbergs FA, Song C, Terry R, Trogani N, Widmer R, Atadja P, Cohen D (2002) Isolation and characterization of a novel class II histone deacetylase, HDAC10. J Biol Chem 277:6656–6666
65. Fischer T, Patnaik A, Bhalla K, Beck J, Morganroth J, Laird GH, Sharma S, Scott JW, Dugan M, Giles F (2005) Results of cardiac monitoring during phase I trials of a novel histone deacetylase (HDAC) inhibitor LBH589 in patients with advanced solid tumors and hematologic malignancies. J Clin Oncol 24:Abstr 3106
66. Fischle W, Dequiedt F, Fillion M, Hendzel MJ, Voelter W, Verdin E (2001) Human HDAC7 histone deacetylase activity is associated with HDAC3 in vivo. J Biol Chem 276:35826–35835
67. Fischle W, Dequiedt F, Hendzel MJ, Guenther MG, Lazar MA, Voelter W, Verdin E (2002) Enzymatic activity associated with class II HDACs is dependent on a multiprotein complex containing HDAC3 and SMRT/N-CoR. Mol Cell 9:45–57
68. Fischle W, Emiliani S, Hendzel MJ, Nagase T, Nomura N, Voelter W, Verdin E (1999) A new family of human histone deacetylases related to Saccharomyces cerevisiae HDA1p. J Biol Chem 274:11713–11720
69. Fischle W, Wang Y, Allis CD (2003) Histone and chromatin cross-talk. Curr Opin Cell Biol 15:172–183
70. Fuks F, Burgers WA, Brehm A, Hughes-Davies L, Kouzarides T (2000) DNA methyltransferase Dnmt1 associates with histone deacetylase activity. Nat Genet 24:88–91
71. Furumai R, Komatsu Y, Nishino N, Khochbin S, Yoshida M, Horinouchi S (2001) Potent histone deacetylase inhibitors built from trichostatin A and cyclic tetrapeptide antibiotics including trapoxin. Proc Natl Acad Sci U S A 98:87–92
72. Furumai R, Matsuyama A, Kobashi N, Lee KH, Nishiyama M, Nakajima H, Tanaka A, Komatsu Y, Nishino N, Yoshida M, Horinouchi S (2002) FK228 (depsipeptide) as a natural prodrug that inhibits class I histone deacetylases. Cancer Res 62:4916–4921
73. Gagnon J, Shaker S, Primeau M, Hurtubise A, Momparler RL (2003) Interaction of 5-aza-2′-deoxycytidine and depsipeptide on antineoplastic activity and activation of 14-3-3sigma, E-cadherin and tissue inhibitor of metalloproteinase 3 expression in human breast carcinoma cells. Anticancer Drugs 14:193–202

74. Galasinski SC, Resing KA, Goodrich JA, Ahn NG (2002) Phosphatase inhibition leads to histone deacetylases 1 and 2 phosphorylation and disruption of corepressor interactions. J Biol Chem 277:19618–19626
75. Gao L, Cueto MA, Asselbergs F, Atadja P (2002) Cloning and functional characterization of HDAC11, a novel member of the human histone deacetylase family. J Biol Chem 277:25748–25755
76. Gao N, Dai Y, Rahmani M, Dent P, Grant S (2004) Contribution of disruption of the nuclear factor-kappaB pathway to induction of apoptosis in human leukemia cells by histone deacetylase inhibitors and flavopiridol. Mol Pharmacol 66:956–963
77. Garcia-Manero G, Cannalli AA, Wierda W, Cortes J, O'Brien S, Cupo A, Secrist JP, Davis J, Faderl S, Giles F, Chiao JH, Richon V, Issa JP (2003) Phase I study of oral suberoylanilide hydroxamic acid (SAHA) in patients (pts) with advanced leukemias or myelodysplastic syndromes (MDS). Blood 102:254b
78. Garcia-Manero G, Kantarjian H, Sanchez-Gonzalez B, Verstovsek S, Ravandi F, Ryttling M, Cortes J, Yang H, Fiorentino J, Rosner G, Issa JP (2005) Results of a phase I/II study of the combination of 5-aza-2-deoxycytidine and valproic acid in patients with acute myeloid leukemia and myelodysplastic syndrome. J Clin Oncol 24:Abstr 6544
79. Gelmon K, Tolcher A, Carducci M, Reid GK, Li Z, Kalita A, Callejas V, Longstreth J, Besterman JM, Siu LL (2005) Phase I trials of the oral histone deacetylase (HDAC) inhibitor MGCD0103 given either daily or 3x weekly for 14 days every 3 weeks in patients (pts) with advanced solid tumors. J Clin Oncol 24:Abstr 3147
80. George P, Bali P, Annavarapu S, Scuto A, Fiskus W, Guo F, Sigua C, Sondarva G, Moscinski L, Atadja P, Bhalla K (2005) Combination of the histone deacetylase inhibitor LBH589 and the hsp90 inhibitor 17-AAG is highly active against human CML-BC cells and AML cells with activating mutation of FLT-3. Blood 105:1768–1776
81. Gilbert J, Baker SD, Bowling MK, Grochow L, Figg WD, Zabelina Y, Donehower RC, Carducci MA (2001) A phase I dose escalation and bioavailability study of oral sodium phenylbutyrate in patients with refractory solid tumor malignancies. Clin Cancer Res 7:2292–2300
82. Giles F, Fischer T, Cortes J, Beck J, Ravandi F, Garcia-Manero G, Kantarjian H, Peng B, Rae P, Laird G, Sharma S, Dugan M, Albitar M, Bhalla K (2004) A phaseI/II study of intravenous LBH589, a novel histone deacetylase (HDAC) inhibitor, in patients with advanced hematalogic malignances. Blood 104:499a
83. Duplicated reference deleted in proof
84. Girdwood D, Bumpass D, Vaughan OA, Thain A, Anderson LA, Snowden AW, Garcia-Wilson E, Perkins ND, Hay RT (2003) P300 transcriptional repression is mediated by SUMO modification. Mol Cell 11:1043–1054
85. Glaser KB, Staver MJ, Waring JF, Stender J, Ulrich RG, Davidsen SK (2003) Gene expression profiling of multiple histone deacetylase (HDAC) inhibitors: defining a common gene set produced by HDAC inhibition in T24 and MDA carcinoma cell lines. Mol Cancer Ther 2:151–163
86. Glick RD, Swendeman SL, Coffey DC, Rifkind RA, Marks PA, Richon VM, La Quaglia MP (1999) Hybrid polar histone deacetylase inhibitor induces apoptosis and CD95/CD95 ligand expression in human neuroblastoma. Cancer Res 59:4392–4399

87. Gore SD, Samid D, Weng LJ (1997) Impact of the putative differentiating agents sodium phenylbutyrate and sodium phenylacetate on proliferation, differentiation, and apoptosis of primary neoplastic myeloid cells. Clin Cancer Res 3:1755–1762
88. Gore SD, Weng LJ, Figg WD, Zhai S, Donehower RC, Dover G, Grever MR, Griffin C, Grochow LB, Hawkins A, Burks K, Zabelena Y, Miller CB (2002) Impact of prolonged infusions of the putative differentiating agent sodium phenylbutyrate on myelodysplastic syndromes and acute myeloid leukemia. Clin Cancer Res 8:963–970
89. Gottlicher M, Minucci S, Zhu P, Kramer OH, Schimpf A, Giavara S, Sleeman JP, Lo Coco F, Nervi C, Pelicci PG, Heinzel T (2001) Valproic acid defines a novel class of HDAC inhibitors inducing differentiation of transformed cells. EMBO J 20:6969–6978
90. Graveley BR (2001) Alternative splicing: increasing diversity in the proteomic world. Trends Genet 17:100–107
91. Gray SG, Iglesias AH, Teh BT, Dangond F (2003) Modulation of splicing events in histone deacetylase 3 by various extracellular and signal transduction pathways. Gene Expr 11:13–21
92. Gregoretti IV, Lee YM, Goodson HV (2004) Molecular evolution of the histone deacetylase family: functional implications of phylogenetic analysis. J Mol Biol 338:17–31
93. Grozinger CM, Hassig CA, Schreiber SL (1999) Three proteins define a class of human histone deacetylases related to yeast Hda1p. Proc Natl Acad Sci U S A 96:4868–4873
94. Grozinger CM, Schreiber SL (2000) Regulation of histone deacetylase 4 and 5 and transcriptional activity by 14-3-3-dependent cellular localization. Proc Natl Acad Sci U S A 97:7835–7840
95. Grunstein M (1997) Histone acetylation in chromatin structure and transcription. Nature 389:349–352
96. Guardiola AR, Yao TP (2002) Molecular cloning and characterization of a novel histone deacetylase HDAC10. J Biol Chem 277:3350–3356
97. Guenther MG, Barak O, Lazar MA (2001) The SMRT and N-CoR corepressors are activating cofactors for histone deacetylase 3. Mol Cell Biol 21:6091–6101
98. Guidez F, Ivins S, Zhu J, Soderstrom M, Waxman S, Zelent A (1998) Reduced retinoic acid-sensitivities of nuclear receptor corepressor binding to PML- and PLZF-RARalpha underlie molecular pathogenesis and treatment of acute promyelocytic leukemia. Blood 91:2634–2642
99. Hartman HB, Yu J, Alenghat T, Ishizuka T, Lazar MA (2005) The histone-binding code of nuclear receptor co-repressors matches the substrate specificity of histone deacetylase 3. EMBO Rep 6:445–451
100. He L, Bhaumik M, Tribioli C, Rego EM, Ivins S, Zelent A, Pandolfi PP (2000) Two critical hits for promyelocytic leukemia. Mol Cell 6:1131–1141
101. He LZ, Guidez F, Tribioli C, Peruzzi D, Ruthardt M, Zelent A, Pandolfi PP (1998) Distinct interactions of PML-RARalpha and PLZF-RARalpha with co-repressors determine differential responses to RA in APL. Nat Genet 18:126–135

102. He LZ, Tolentino T, Grayson P, Zhong S, Warrell RP Jr, Rifkind RA, Marks PA, Richon VM, Pandolfi PP (2001) Histone deacetylase inhibitors induce remission in transgenic models of therapy-resistant acute promyelocytic leukemia. J Clin Invest 108:1321–1330
103. Henderson C, Mizzau M, Paroni G, Maestro R, Schneider C, Brancolini C (2003) Role of caspases, Bid, and p53 in the apoptotic response triggered by histone deacetylase inhibitors trichostatin-A (TSA) and suberoylanilide hydroxamic acid (SAHA). J Biol Chem 278:12579–12589
104. Hideshima T, Bradner JE, Wong J, Chauhan D, Richardson P, Schreiber SL, Anderson KC (2005) Small-molecule inhibition of proteasome and aggresome function induces synergistic antitumor activity in multiple myeloma. Proc Natl Acad Sci U S A 102:8567–8572
105. Hobdy E, Murren J (2004) AN-9 (Titan). Curr Opin Investig Drugs 5:628–634
106. Hong SH, David G, Wong CW, Dejean A, Privalsky ML (1997) SMRT corepressor interacts with PLZF and with the PML-retinoic acid receptor alpha (RARalpha) and PLZF-RARalpha oncoproteins associated with acute promyelocytic leukemia. Proc Natl Acad Sci U S A 94:9028–9033
107. Hook SS, Orian A, Cowley SM, Eisenman RN (2002) Histone deacetylase 6 binds polyubiquitin through its zinc finger (PAZ domain) and copurifies with deubiquitinating enzymes. Proc Natl Acad Sci U S A 99:13425–13430
108. Hu E, Dul E, Sung CM, Chen Z, Kirkpatrick R, Zhang GF, Johanson K, Liu R, Lago A, Hofmann G, Macarron R, de los Frailes M, Perez P, Krawiec J, Winkler J, Jaye M (2003) Identification of novel isoform-selective inhibitors within class I histone deacetylases. J Pharmacol Exp Ther 307:720–728
109. Huang ME, Ye YC, Chen SR, Zhao JC, Gu LJ, Cai JR, Zhao L, Xie JX, Shen ZX, Wang ZY (1987) All-trans retinoic acid with or without low dose cytosine arabinoside in acute promyelocytic leukemia. Report of 6 cases. Chin Med J (Engl) 100:949–953
110. Huang Y, Tan M, Gosink M, Wang KK, Sun Y (2002) Histone deacetylase 5 is not a p53 target gene, but its overexpression inhibits tumor cell growth and induces apoptosis. Cancer Res 62:2913–2922
111. Hubbert C, Guardiola A, Shao R, Kawaguchi Y, Ito A, Nixon A, Yoshida M, Wang XF, Yao TP (2002) HDAC6 is a microtubule-associated deacetylase. Nature 417:455–458
112. Huo X, Zhang J (2005) Important roles of reversible acetylation in the function of hematopoietic transcription factors. J Cell Mol Med 9:103–112
113. Huynh KD, Bardwell VJ (1998) The BCL-6 POZ domain and other POZ domains interact with the co-repressors N-CoR and SMRT. Oncogene 17:2473–2484
114. Huynh KD, Fischle W, Verdin E, Bardwell VJ (2000) BCoR, a novel corepressor involved in BCL-6 repression. Genes Dev 14:1810–1823
115. Inoue S, MacFarlane M, Harper N, Wheat LM, Dyer MJ, Cohen GM (2004) Histone deacetylase inhibitors potentiate TNF-related apoptosis-inducing ligand (TRAIL)-induced apoptosis in lymphoid malignancies. Cell Death Differ 11 Suppl 2:S193–206
116. Insinga A, Monestiroli S, Ronzoni S, Carbone R, Pearson M, Pruneri G, Viale G, Appella E, Pelicci P, Minucci S (2004) Impairment of p53 acetylation, stability and function by an oncogenic transcription factor. EMBO J 23:1144–1154

117. Insinga A, Monestiroli S, Ronzoni S, Gelmetti V, Marchesi F, Viale A, Altucci L, Nervi C, Minucci S, Pelicci PG (2005) Inhibitors of histone deacetylases induce tumor-selective apoptosis through activation of the death receptor pathway. Nat Med 11:71–76
118. Issa JP (2004) CpG island methylator phenotype in cancer. Nat Rev Cancer 4:988–993
119. Itazaki H, Nagashima K, Sugita K, Yoshida H, Kawamura Y, Yasuda Y, Matsumoto K, Ishii K, Uotani N, Nakai H, et al (1990) Isolation and structural elucidation of new cyclotetrapeptides, trapoxins A and B, having detransformation activities as antitumor agents. J Antibiot (Tokyo) 43:1524–1532
120. Jepsen K, Hermanson O, Onami TM, Gleiberman AS, Lunyak V, McEvilly RJ, Kurokawa R, Kumar V, Liu F, Seto E, Hedrick SM, Mandel G, Glass CK, Rose DW, Rosenfeld MG (2000) Combinatorial roles of the nuclear receptor corepressor in transcription and development. Cell 102:753–763
121. Jepsen K, Rosenfeld MG (2002) Biological roles and mechanistic actions of co-repressor complexes. J Cell Sci 115:689–698
122. Jing Y, Xia L, Waxman S (2002) Targeted removal of PML-RARalpha protein is required prior to inhibition of histone deacetylase for overcoming all-trans retinoic acid differentiation resistance in acute promyelocytic leukemia. Blood 100:1008–1013
123. Johnson JM, Castle J, Garrett-Engele P, Kan Z, Loerch PM, Armour CD, Santos R, Schadt EE, Stoughton R, Shoemaker DD (2003) Genome-wide survey of human alternative pre-mRNA splicing with exon junction microarrays. Science 302:2141–2144
124. Jones PL, Veenstra GJ, Wade PA, Vermaak D, Kass SU, Landsberger N, Strouboulis J, Wolffe AP (1998) Methylated DNA and MeCP2 recruit histone deacetylase to repress transcription. Nat Genet 19:187–191
125. Jose B, Okamura S, Kato T, Nishino N, Sumida Y, Yoshida M (2004) Toward an HDAC6 inhibitor: synthesis and conformational analysis of cyclic hexapeptide hydroxamic acid designed from alpha-tubulin sequence. Bioorg Med Chem 12:1351–1356
126. Kalita A, Maroun C, Bonfils C, Gelmon K, Siu LL, Tolcher A, Carducci M, Besterman JM, Reid GK, Li Z (2005) Pharmacodynamic effect of MGCD0103, an oral isotype-selective histone deacetylase (HDAC) inhibitor, on HDAC enzyme inhibition and histone acetylation induction in phase I clinical trials in patients (pts) with advanced solid tumors or non-Hodgkin's lymphoma (NHL). J Clin Oncol 24:Abstr 9631
127. Kamashev D, Vitoux D, De The H (2004) PML-RARA-RXR oligomers mediate retinoid and rexinoid/cAMP cross-talk in acute promyelocytic leukemia cell differentiation. J Exp Med 199:1163–1174
128. Kao GD, McKenna WG, Guenther MG, Muschel RJ, Lazar MA, Yen TJ (2003) Histone deacetylase 4 interacts with 53BP1 to mediate the DNA damage response. J Cell Biol 160:1017–1027
129. Kao HY, Lee CH, Komarov A, Han CC, Evans RM (2002) Isolation and characterization of mammalian HDAC10, a novel histone deacetylase. J Biol Chem 277:187–193

130. Kao HY, Verdel A, Tsai CC, Simon C, Juguilon H, Khochbin S (2001) Mechanism for nucleocytoplasmic shuttling of histone deacetylase 7. J Biol Chem 276:47496–47507
131. Kato H, Tamamizu-Kato S, Shibasaki F (2004) Histone deacetylase 7 associates with hypoxia-inducible factor 1alpha and increases transcriptional activity. J Biol Chem 279:41966–41974
132. Kawaguchi Y, Kovacs JJ, McLaurin A, Vance JM, Ito A, Yao TP (2003) The deacetylase HDAC6 regulates aggresome formation and cell viability in response to misfolded protein stress. Cell 115:727–738
133. Kawai H, Li H, Avraham S, Jiang S, Avraham HK (2003) Overexpression of histone deacetylase HDAC1 modulates breast cancer progression by negative regulation of estrogen receptor alpha. Int J Cancer 107:353–358
134. Keen JC, Yan L, Mack KM, Pettit C, Smith D, Sharma D, Davidson NE (2003) A novel histone deacetylase inhibitor, scriptaid, enhances expression of functional estrogen receptor alpha (ER) in ER negative human breast cancer cells in combination with 5-aza 2'-deoxycytidine. Breast Cancer Res Treat 81:177–186
135. Kelly WK, O'Connor OA, Krug LM, Chiao JH, Heaney M, Curley T, Macgregore-Cortelli B, Tong W, Secrist JP, Schwartz L, Richardson S, Chu E, Olgac S, Marks PA, Scher H, Richon VM (2005) Phase I study of an oral histone deacetylase inhibitor, suberoylanilide hydroxamic Acid, in patients with advanced cancer. J Clin Oncol 23:3923–3931
136. Kelly WK, Richon VM, O'Connor O, Curley T, MacGregor-Curtelli B, Tong W, Klang M, Schwartz L, Richardson S, Rosa E, Drobnjak M, Cordon-Cordo C, Chiao JH, Rifkind R, Marks PA, Scher H (2003) Phase I clinical trial of histone deacetylase inhibitor: suberoylanilide hydroxamic acid administered intravenously. Clin Cancer Res 9:3578–3588
137. Kerckaert JP, Deweindt C, Tilly H, Quief S, Lecocq G, Bastard C (1993) LAZ3, a novel zinc-finger encoding gene, is disrupted by recurring chromosome 3q27 translocations in human lymphomas. Nat Genet 5:66–70
138. Khan SB, Maududi T, Barton K, Ayers J, Alkan S (2004) Analysis of histone deacetylase inhibitor, depsipeptide (FR901228), effect on multiple myeloma. Br J Haematol 125:156–161
139. Khorasanizadeh S (2004) The nucleosome: from genomic organization to genomic regulation. Cell 116:259–272
140. Kim JH, Shin JH, Kim IH (2004) Susceptibility and radiosensitization of human glioblastoma cells to trichostatin A, a histone deacetylase inhibitor. Int J Radiat Oncol Biol Phys 59:1174–1180
141. Kim JS, Jeung HK, Cheong JW, Maeng H, Lee ST, Hahn JS, Ko YW, Min YH (2004) Apicidin potentiates the imatinib-induced apoptosis of Bcr-Abl-positive human leukaemia cells by enhancing the activation of mitochondria-dependent caspase cascades. Br J Haematol 124:166–178
142. Kim MS, Blake M, Baek JH, Kohlhagen G, Pommier Y, Carrier F (2003) Inhibition of histone deacetylase increases cytotoxicity to anticancer drugs targeting DNA. Cancer Res 63:7291–7300
143. Kirsh O, Seeler JS, Pichler A, Gast A, Muller S, Miska E, Mathieu M, Harel-Bellan A, Kouzarides T, Melchior F, Dejean A (2002) The SUMO E3 ligase RanBP2 promotes modification of the HDAC4 deacetylase. EMBO J 21:2682–2691

144. Kitamura K, Hoshi S, Koike M, Kiyoi H, Saito H, Naoe T (2000) Histone deacetylase inhibitor but not arsenic trioxide differentiates acute promyelocytic leukaemia cells with t(11;17) in combination with all-trans retinoic acid. Br J Haematol 108:696–702
145. Klisovic MI, Maghraby EA, Parthun MR, Guimond M, Sklenar AR, Whitman SP, Chan KK, Murphy T, Anon J, Archer KJ, Rush LJ, Plass C, Grever MR, Byrd JC, Marcucci G (2003) Depsipeptide (FR 901228) promotes histone acetylation, gene transcription, apoptosis and its activity is enhanced by DNA methyltransferase inhibitors in AML1/ETO-positive leukemic cells. Leukemia 17:350–358
146. Komatsu Y, Tomizaki KY, Tsukamoto M, Kato T, Nishino N, Sato S, Yamori T, Tsuruo T, Furumai R, Yoshida M, Horinouchi S, Hayashi H (2001) Cyclic hydroxamic-acid-containing peptide 31, a potent synthetic histone deacetylase inhibitor with antitumor activity. Cancer Res 61:4459–4466
147. Kopito RR (2000) Aggresomes, inclusion bodies and protein aggregation. Trends Cell Biol 10:524–530
148. Kosugi H, Ito M, Yamamoto Y, Towatari M, Ueda R, Saito H, Naoe T (2001) In vivo effects of a histone deacetylase inhibitor, FK228, on human acute promyelocytic leukemia in NOD/Shi-scid/scid mice. Jpn J Cancer Res 92:529–536
149. Kramer OH, Zhu P, Ostendorff HP, Golebiewski M, Tiefenbach J, Peters MA, Brill B, Groner B, Bach I, Heinzel T, Gottlicher M (2003) The histone deacetylase inhibitor valproic acid selectively induces proteasomal degradation of HDAC2. EMBO J 22:3411–3420
150. Kruh J (1982) Effects of sodium butyrate, a new pharmacological agent, on cells in culture. Mol Cell Biochem 42:65–82
151. Kurdistani SK, Grunstein M (2003) Histone acetylation and deacetylation in yeast. Nat Rev Mol Cell Biol 4:276–284
152. Kurz EU, Wilson SE, Leader KB, Sampey BP, Allan WP, Yalowich JC, Kroll DJ (2001) The histone deacetylase inhibitor sodium butyrate induces DNA topoisomerase II alpha expression and confers hypersensitivity to etoposide in human leukemic cell lines. Mol Cancer Ther 1:121–131
153. Kwon SH, Ahn SH, Kim YK, Bae GU, Yoon JW, Hong S, Lee HY, Lee YW, Lee HW, Han JW (2002) Apicidin, a histone deacetylase inhibitor, induces apoptosis and Fas/Fas ligand expression in human acute promyelocytic leukemia cells. J Biol Chem 277:2073–2080
154. Lagger G, O'Carroll D, Rembold M, Khier H, Tischler J, Weitzer G, Schuettengruber B, Hauser C, Brunmeir R, Jenuwein T, Seiser C (2002) Essential function of histone deacetylase 1 in proliferation control and CDK inhibitor repression. EMBO J 21:2672–2681
155. Langley E, Pearson M, Faretta M, Bauer UM, Frye RA, Minucci S, Pelicci PG, Kouzarides T (2002) Human SIR2 deacetylates p53 and antagonizes PML/p53-induced cellular senescence. EMBO J 21:2383–2396
156. Lea MA, Tulsyan N (1995) Discordant effects of butyrate analogues on erythroleukemia cell proliferation, differentiation and histone deacetylase. Anticancer Res 15:879–883
157. Lee H, Rezai-Zadeh N, Seto E (2004) Negative regulation of histone deacetylase 8 activity by cyclic AMP-dependent protein kinase A. Mol Cell Biol 24:765–773

158. Lemercier C, Brocard MP, Puvion-Dutilleul F, Kao HY, Albagli O, Khochbin S (2002) Class II histone deacetylases are directly recruited by BCL6 transcriptional repressor. J Biol Chem 277:22045–22052
159. Li J, Staver MJ, Curtin ML, Holms JH, Frey RR, Edalji R, Smith R, Michaelides MR, Davidsen SK, Glaser KB (2004) Expression and functional characterization of recombinant human HDAC1 and HDAC3. Life Sci 74:2693–2705
160. Licht JD (2001) AML1 and the AML1-ETO fusion protein in the pathogenesis of t(8;21) AML. Oncogene 20:5660–5679
161. Lipinski MM, Jacks T (1999) The retinoblastoma gene family in differentiation and development. Oncogene 18:7873–7882
162. LoRusso PM, Demchik L, Foster B, Knight J, Bissery MC, Polin LM, Leopold WR 3rd, Corbett TH (1996) Preclinical antitumor activity of CI-994. Invest New Drugs 14:349–356
163. Lu J, McKinsey TA, Zhang CL, Olson EN (2000) Regulation of skeletal myogenesis by association of the MEF2 transcription factor with class II histone deacetylases. Mol Cell 6:233–244
164. Lund AH, van Lohuizen M (2004) Epigenetics and cancer. Genes Dev 18:2315–2335
165. Luo J, Su F, Chen D, Shiloh A, Gu W (2000) Deacetylation of p53 modulates its effect on cell growth and apoptosis. Nature 408:377–381
166. Maggio SC, Rosato RR, Kramer LB, Dai Y, Rahmani M, Paik DS, Czarnik AC, Payne SG, Spiegel S, Grant S (2004) The histone deacetylase inhibitor MS-275 interacts synergistically with fludarabine to induce apoptosis in human leukemia cells. Cancer Res 64:2590–2600
167. Magnaghi-Jaulin L, Groisman R, Naguibneva I, Robin P, Lorain S, Le Villain JP, Troalen F, Trouche D, Harel-Bellan A (1998) Retinoblastoma protein represses transcription by recruiting a histone deacetylase. Nature 391:601–605
168. Mai A, Massa S, Pezzi R, Simeoni S, Rotili D, Nebbioso A, Scognamiglio A, Altucci L, Loidl P, Brosch G (2005) Class II (IIa)-selective histone deacetylase inhibitors. 1. Synthesis and biological evaluation of novel (aryloxopropenyl)pyrrolyl hydroxyamides. J Med Chem 48:3344–3353
169. Marchion DC, Bicaku E, Daud AI, Richon V, Sullivan DM, Munster PN (2004) Sequence-specific potentiation of topoisomerase II inhibitors by the histone deacetylase inhibitor suberoylanilide hydroxamic acid. J Cell Biochem 92:223–237
170. Marcus AI, Zhou J, O'Brate A, Hamel E, Wong J, Nivens M, El-Naggar A, Yao TP, Khuri FR, Giannakakou P (2005) The synergistic combination of the farnesyl transferase inhibitor lonafarnib and paclitaxel enhances tubulin acetylation and requires a functional tubulin deacetylase. Cancer Res 65:3883–3893
171. Margueron R, Trojer P, Reinberg D (2005) The key to development: interpreting the histone code? Curr Opin Genet Dev 15:163–176
172. Marshall JL, Rizvi N, Kauh J, Dahut W, Figuera M, Kang MH, Figg WD, Wainer I, Chaissang C, Li MZ, Hawkins MJ (2002) A phase I trial of depsipeptide (FR901228) in patients with advanced cancer. J Exp Ther Oncol 2:325–332
173. Matsuyama A, Shimazu T, Sumida Y, Saito A, Yoshimatsu Y, Seigneurin-Berny D, Osada H, Komatsu Y, Nishino N, Khochbin S, Horinouchi S, Yoshida M (2002) In vivo destabilization of dynamic microtubules by HDAC6-mediated deacetylation. EMBO J 21:6820–6831

174. McKinsey TA, Zhang CL, Olson EN (2000) Activation of the myocyte enhancer factor-2 transcription factor by calcium/calmodulin-dependent protein kinase-stimulated binding of 14-3-3 to histone deacetylase 5. Proc Natl Acad Sci U S A 97:14400–14405
175. McKinsey TA, Zhang CL, Olson EN (2001) Identification of a signal-responsive nuclear export sequence in class II histone deacetylases. Mol Cell Biol 21:6312–6321
176. Mie Lee Y, Kim SH, Kim HS, Jin Son M, Nakajima H, Jeong Kwon H, Kim KW (2003) Inhibition of hypoxia-induced angiogenesis by FK228, a specific histone deacetylase inhibitor, via suppression of HIF-1alpha activity. Biochem Biophys Res Commun 300:241–246
177. Mikhailov A, Shinohara M, Rieder CL (2004) Topoisomerase II and histone deacetylase inhibitors delay the G2/M transition by triggering the p38 MAPK checkpoint pathway. J Cell Biol 166:517–526
178. Minucci S, Horn V, Bhattacharyya N, Russanova V, Ogryzko VV, Gabriele L, Howard BH, Ozato K (1997) A histone deacetylase inhibitor potentiates retinoid receptor action in embryonal carcinoma cells. Proc Natl Acad Sci U S A 94:11295–11300
179. Mistry AR, Pedersen EW, Solomon E, Grimwade D (2003) The molecular pathogenesis of acute promyelocytic leukaemia: implications for the clinical management of the disease. Blood Rev 17:71–97
180. Mitsiades CS, Mitsiades NS, McMullan CJ, Poulaki V, Shringarpure R, Hideshima T, Akiyama M, Chauhan D, Munshi N, Gu X, Bailey C, Joseph M, Libermann TA, Richon VM, Marks PA, Anderson KC (2004) Transcriptional signature of histone deacetylase inhibition in multiple myeloma: biological and clinical implications. Proc Natl Acad Sci U S A 101:540–545
181. Mongan NP, Gudas LJ (2005) Valproic acid, in combination with all-trans retinoic acid and 5-aza-2'-deoxycytidine, restores expression of silenced RARbeta2 in breast cancer cells. Mol Cancer Ther 4:477–486
182. Munster PN, Marchion DC, Bicaku E, Sullivan P, Beam C, Mahany J, Lush R, Sullivan DM, Daud A (2005) Phase I trial of the histone deacetylase inhibitor, valproic acid and the topoisomerase II inhibitor, epirubicin: a clinical and translational study. J Clin Oncol 24:Abstr 3084
183. Nan X, Ng HH, Johnson CA, Laherty CD, Turner BM, Eisenman RN, Bird A (1998) Transcriptional repression by the methyl-CpG-binding protein MeCP2 involves a histone deacetylase complex. Nature 393:386–389
184. Nebbioso A, Clarke N, Voltz E, Germain E, Ambrosino C, Bontempo P, Alvarez R, Schiavone EM, Ferrara F, Bresciani F, Weisz A, de Lera AR, Gronemeyer H, Altucci L (2005) Tumor-selective action of HDAC inhibitors involves TRAIL induction in acute myeloid leukemia cells. Nat Med 11:77–84
185. Nemunaitis JJ, Orr D, Eager R, Cunningham CC, Williams A, Mennel R, Grove W, Olson S (2003) Phase I study of oral CI-994 in combination with gemcitabine in treatment of patients with advanced cancer. Cancer J 9:58–66
186. Nguyen DM, Schrump WD, Chen GA, Tsai W, Nguyen P, Trepel JB, Schrump DS (2004) Abrogation of p21 expression by flavopiridol enhances depsipeptide-mediated apoptosis in malignant pleural mesothelioma cells. Clin Cancer Res 10:1813–1825

187. Nguyen DM, Schrump WD, Tsai WS, Chen A, Stewart JHt, Steiner F, Schrump DS (2003) Enhancement of depsipeptide-mediated apoptosis of lung or esophageal cancer cells by flavopiridol: activation of the mitochondria-dependent death-signaling pathway. J Thorac Cardiovasc Surg 125:1132–1142
188. Niitsu N, Kasukabe T, Yokoyama A, Okabe-Kado J, Yamamoto-Yamaguchi Y, Umeda M, Honma Y (2000) Anticancer derivative of butyric acid (Pivaly-loxymethyl butyrate) specifically potentiates the cytotoxicity of doxorubicin and daunorubicin through the suppression of microsomal glycosidic activity. Mol Pharmacol 58:27–36
189. Nimmanapalli R, Fuino L, Bali P, Gasparetto M, Glozak M, Tao J, Moscinski L, Smith C, Wu J, Jove R, Atadja P, Bhalla K (2003) Histone deacetylase inhibitor LAQ824 both lowers expression and promotes proteasomal degradation of Bcr-Abl and induces apoptosis of imatinib mesylate-sensitive or -refractory chronic myelogenous leukemia-blast crisis cells. Cancer Res 63:5126–5135
190. Nimmanapalli R, Fuino L, Stobaugh C, Richon V, Bhalla K (2003) Cotreatment with the histone deacetylase inhibitor suberoylanilide hydroxamic acid (SAHA) enhances imatinib-induced apoptosis of Bcr-Abl-positive human acute leukemia cells. Blood 101:3236–3239
191. North BJ, Marshall BL, Borra MT, Denu JM, Verdin E (2003) The human Sir2 ortholog, SIRT2, is an NAD+-dependent tubulin deacetylase. Mol Cell 11:437–444
192. North BJ, Verdin E (2004) Sirtuins: Sir2-related NAD-dependent protein deacetylases. Genome Biol 5:224
193. Ocker M, Alajati A, Ganslmayer M, Zopf S, Luders M, Neureiter D, Hahn EG, Schuppan D, Herold C (2005) The histone-deacetylase inhibitor SAHA potentiates proapoptotic effects of 5-fluorouracil and irinotecan in hepatoma cells. J Cancer Res Clin Oncol 131:385–394
194. Park JH, Jung Y, Kim TY, Kim SG, Jong HS, Lee JW, Kim DK, Lee JS, Kim NK, Bang YJ (2004) Class I histone deacetylase-selective novel synthetic inhibitors potently inhibit human tumor proliferation. Clin Cancer Res 10:5271–5281
195. Parra M, Kasler H, McKinsey TA, Olson EN, Verdin E (2005) Protein kinase D1 phosphorylates HDAC7 and induces its nuclear export after T-cell receptor activation. J Biol Chem 280:13762–13770
196. Pasqualucci L, Bereschenko O, Niu H, Klein U, Basso K, Guglielmino R, Cattoretti G, Dalla-Favera R (2003) Molecular pathogenesis of non-Hodgkin's lymphoma: the role of Bcl-6. Leuk Lymphoma 44 Suppl 3:S5–12
197. Patnaik A, Rowinsky EK, Villalona MA, Hammond LA, Britten CD, Siu LL, Goetz A, Felton SA, Burton S, Valone FH, Eckhardt SG (2002) A phase I study of pivaloyloxymethyl butyrate, a prodrug of the differentiating agent butyric acid, in patients with advanced solid malignancies. Clin Cancer Res 8:2142–2148
198. Pauer LR, Olivares J, Cunningham C, Williams A, Grove W, Kraker A, Olson S, Nemunaitis J (2004) Phase I study of oral CI-994 in combination with carboplatin and paclitaxel in the treatment of patients with advanced solid tumors. Cancer Invest 22:886–896

199. Peart MJ, Smyth GK, van Laar RK, Bowtell DD, Richon VM, Marks PA, Holloway AJ, Johnstone RW (2005) Identification and functional significance of genes regulated by structurally different histone deacetylase inhibitors. Proc Natl Acad Sci U S A 102:3697–3702
200. Pei XY, Dai Y, Grant S (2004) Synergistic induction of oxidative injury and apoptosis in human multiple myeloma cells by the proteasome inhibitor bortezomib and histone deacetylase inhibitors. Clin Cancer Res 10:3839–3852
201. Petrie K, Guidez F, Howell L, Healy L, Waxman S, Greaves M, Zelent A (2003) The histone deacetylase 9 gene encodes multiple protein isoforms. J Biol Chem 278:16059–16072
202. Pflum MK, Tong JK, Lane WS, Schreiber SL (2001) Histone deacetylase 1 phosphorylation promotes enzymatic activity and complex formation. J Biol Chem 276:47733–47741
203. Phiel CJ, Zhang F, Huang EY, Guenther MG, Lazar MA, Klein PS (2001) Histone deacetylase is a direct target of valproic acid, a potent anticonvulsant, mood stabilizer, and teratogen. J Biol Chem 276:36734–36741
204. Piekarz R, Frye R, Turner B, Wright J, Leonard J, Allen S, Bates S (2004) Update on the phase II trial and correlative studies of depsipeptide in patients with cutaneous T-cell lymphoma and relapsed peripheral T-cell lymphoma. J Clin Oncol 23:Abstr 3028
205. Piekarz RL, Robey R, Sandor V, Bakke S, Wilson WH, Dahmoush L, Kingma DM, Turner ML, Altemus R, Bates SE (2001) Inhibitor of histone deacetylation, depsipeptide (FR901228), in the treatment of peripheral and cutaneous T-cell lymphoma: a case report. Blood 98:2865–2868
206. Piperno G, LeDizet M, Chang XJ (1987) Microtubules containing acetylated alpha-tubulin in mammalian cells in culture. J Cell Biol 104:289–302
207. Plumb JA, Finn PW, Williams RJ, Bandara MJ, Romero MR, Watkins CJ, La Thangue NB, Brown R (2003) Pharmacodynamic response and inhibition of growth of human tumor xenografts by the novel histone deacetylase inhibitor PXD101. Mol Cancer Ther 2:721–728
208. Polo JM, Dell'Oso T, Ranuncolo SM, Cerchietti L, Beck D, Da Silva GF, Prive GG, Licht JD, Melnick A (2004) Specific peptide interference reveals BCL6 transcriptional and oncogenic mechanisms in B-cell lymphoma cells. Nat Med 10:1329–1335
209. Prakash S, Foster BJ, Meyer M, Wozniak A, Heilbrun LK, Flaherty L, Zalupski M, Radulovic L, Valdivieso M, LoRusso PM (2001) Chronic oral administration of CI-994: a phase 1 study. Invest New Drugs 19:1–11
210. Primeau M, Gagnon J, Momparler RL (2003) Synergistic antineoplastic action of DNA methylation inhibitor 5-AZA-2′-deoxycytidine and histone deacetylase inhibitor depsipeptide on human breast carcinoma cells. Int J Cancer 103:177–184
211. Qian DZ, Wang X, Kachhap SK, Kato Y, Wei Y, Zhang L, Atadja P, Pili R (2004) The histone deacetylase inhibitor NVP-LAQ824 inhibits angiogenesis and has a greater antitumor effect in combination with the vascular endothelial growth factor receptor tyrosine kinase inhibitor PTK787/ZK222584. Cancer Res 64:6626–6634

212. Qiu L, Kelso MJ, Hansen C, West ML, Fairlie DP, Parsons PG (1999) Anti-tumour activity in vitro and in vivo of selective differentiating agents containing hydroxamate. Br J Cancer 80:1252–1258
213. Racanicchi S, Maccherani C, Liberatore C, Billi M, Gelmetti V, Panigada M, Rizzo G, Nervi C, Grignani F (2005) Targeting fusion protein/corepressor contact restores differentiation response in leukemia cells. EMBO J 24:1232–1242
214. Rahmani M, Reese E, Dai Y, Bauer C, Kramer LB, Huang M, Jove R, Dent P, Grant S (2005) Cotreatment with suberanoylanilide hydroxamic acid and 17-allylamino 17-demethoxygeldanamycin synergistically induces apoptosis in Bcr-Abl+ Cells sensitive and resistant to STI571 (imatinib mesylate) in association with down-regulation of Bcr-Abl, abrogation of signal transducer and activator of transcription 5 activity, and Bax conformational change. Mol Pharmacol 67:1166–1176
215. Rahmani M, Reese E, Dai Y, Bauer C, Payne SG, Dent P, Spiegel S, Grant S (2005) Coadministration of histone deacetylase inhibitors and perifosine synergistically induces apoptosis in human leukemia cells through Akt and ERK1/2 inactivation and the generation of ceramide and reactive oxygen species. Cancer Res 65:2422–2432
216. Rahmani M, Yu C, Dai Y, Reese E, Ahmed W, Dent P, Grant S (2003) Coadministration of the heat shock protein 90 antagonist 17-allylamino-17-demethoxygeldanamycin with suberoylanilide hydroxamic acid or sodium butyrate synergistically induces apoptosis in human leukemia cells. Cancer Res 63:8420–8427
217. Reid T, Valone F, Lipera W, Irwin D, Paroly W, Natale R, Sreedharan S, Keer H, Lum B, Scappaticci F, Bhatnagar A (2004) Phase II trial of the histone deacetylase inhibitor pivaloyloxymethyl butyrate (Pivanex, AN-9) in advanced non-small cell lung cancer. Lung Cancer 45:381–386
218. Remiszewski SW (2003) The discovery of NVP-LAQ824: from concept to clinic. Curr Med Chem 10:2393–2402
219. Remiszewski SW, Sambucetti LC, Bair KW, Bontempo J, Cesarz D, Chandramouli N, Chen R, Cheung M, Cornell-Kennon S, Dean K, Diamantidis G, France D, Green MA, Howell KL, Kashi R, Kwon P, Lassota P, Martin MS, Mou Y, Perez LB, Sharma S, Smith T, Sorensen E, Taplin F, Trogani N, Versace R, Walker H, Weltchek-Engler S, Wood A, Wu A, Atadja P (2003) N-Hydroxy-3-phenyl-2-propenamides as novel inhibitors of human histone deacetylase with in vivo antitumor activity: discovery of (2E)-N-hydroxy-3-[4-[[(2-hydroxyethyl)[2-(1H-indol-3-yl)ethyl]amino]methyl]phenyl]-2-propenamide (NVP-LAQ824). J Med Chem 46:4609–4624
220. Richon VM, Sandhoff TW, Rifkind RA, Marks PA (2000) Histone deacetylase inhibitor selectively induces p21WAF1 expression and gene-associated histone acetylation. Proc Natl Acad Sci U S A 97:10014–10019
221. Richon VM, Webb Y, Merger R, Sheppard T, Jursic B, Ngo L, Civoli F, Breslow R, Rifkind RA, Marks PA (1996) Second generation hybrid polar compounds are potent inducers of transformed cell differentiation. Proc Natl Acad Sci U S A 93:5705–5708
222. Robyr D, Suka Y, Xenarios I, Kurdistani SK, Wang A, Suka N, Grunstein M (2002) Microarray deacetylation maps determine genome-wide functions for yeast histone deacetylases. Cell 109:437–446

223. Romanski A, Bacic B, Bug G, Pfeifer H, Gul H, Remiszewski S, Hoelzer D, Atadja P, Ruthardt M, Ottmann OG (2004) Use of a novel histone deacetylase inhibitor to induce apoptosis in cell lines of acute lymphoblastic leukemia. Haematologica 89:419–426
224. Rosato RR, Almenara JA, Grant S (2003) The histone deacetylase inhibitor MS-275 promotes differentiation or apoptosis in human leukemia cells through a process regulated by generation of reactive oxygen species and induction of p21CIP1/WAF1 1. Cancer Res 63:3637–3645
225. Rosato RR, Almenara JA, Yu C, Grant S (2004) Evidence of a functional role for p21WAF1/CIP1 down-regulation in synergistic antileukemic interactions between the histone deacetylase inhibitor sodium butyrate and flavopiridol. Mol Pharmacol 65:571–581
226. Rudek MA, Zhao M, He P, Hartke C, Gilbert J, Gore SD, Carducci MA, Baker SD (2005) Pharmacokinetics of 5-azacitidine administered with phenylbutyrate in patients with refractory solid tumors or hematologic malignancies. J Clin Oncol 23:3906–3911
227. Ruefli AA, Ausserlechner MJ, Bernhard D, Sutton VR, Tainton KM, Kofler R, Smyth MJ, Johnstone RW (2001) The histone deacetylase inhibitor and chemotherapeutic agent suberoylanilide hydroxamic acid (SAHA) induces a cell-death pathway characterized by cleavage of Bid and production of reactive oxygen species. Proc Natl Acad Sci U S A 98:10833–10838
228. Ryan QC, Headlee D, Acharya M, Sparreboom A, Trepel JB, Ye J, Figg WD, Hwang K, Chung EJ, Murgo A, Melillo G, Elsayed Y, Monga M, Kalnitskiy M, Zwiebel J, Sausville EA (2005) Phase I and pharmacokinetic study of MS-275, a histone deacetylase inhibitor, in patients with advanced and refractory solid tumors or lymphoma. J Clin Oncol 23:3912–3922
229. Sakamoto S, Potla R, Larner AC (2004) Histone deacetylase activity is required to recruit RNA polymerase II to the promoters of selected interferon stimulated early response genes. J Biol Chem 279:40362–40367
230. Sandor V, Bakke S, Robey RW, Kang MH, Blagosklonny MV, Bender J, Brooks R, Piekarz RL, Tucker E, Figg WD, Chan KK, Goldspiel B, Fojo AT, Balcerzak SP, Bates SE (2002) Phase I trial of the histone deacetylase inhibitor, depsipeptide (FR901228, NSC 630176), in patients with refractory neoplasms. Clin Cancer Res 8:718–728
231. Sandor V, Senderowicz A, Mertins S, Sackett D, Sausville E, Blagosklonny MV, Bates SE (2000) P21-dependent g(1)arrest with downregulation of cyclin D1 and upregulation of cyclin E by the histone deacetylase inhibitor FR901228. Br J Cancer 83:817–825
232. Sanz MA, Martin G, Gonzalez M, Leon A, Rayon C, Rivas C, Colomer D, Amutio E, Capote FJ, Milone GA, De La Serna J, Roman J, Barragan E, Bergua J, Escoda L, Parody R, Negri S, Calasanz MJ, Bolufer P (2004) Risk-adapted treatment of acute promyelocytic leukemia with all-trans-retinoic acid and anthracycline monochemotherapy: a multicenter study by the PETHEMA group. Blood 103:1237–1243

233. Sasakawa Y, Naoe Y, Noto T, Inoue T, Sasakawa T, Matsuo M, Manda T, Mutoh S (2003) Antitumor efficacy of FK228, a novel histone deacetylase inhibitor, depends on the effect on expression of angiogenesis factors. Biochem Pharmacol 66:897–906
234. Sawa H, Murakami H, Ohshima Y, Murakami M, Yamazaki I, Tamura Y, Mima T, Satone A, Ide W, Hashimoto I, Kamada H (2002) Histone deacetylase inhibitors such as sodium butyrate and trichostatin A inhibit vascular endothelial growth factor (VEGF) secretion from human glioblastoma cells. Brain Tumor Pathol 19:77–81
235. Schrump DS, Nguyen DM, Kunst TE, Hancox A, Figg WD, Steinberg SM, Pishchik V, Becerra Y (2002) Phase I study of sequential deoxyazacytidine/depsipeptide infusion in patients with malignancies involving lungs or pleura. Clin Lung Cancer 4:186–192
236. Sealy L, Chalkley R (1978) The effect of sodium butyrate on histone modification. Cell 14:115–121
237. Seelig MH, Berger MR (1996) Efficacy of dinaline and its methyl and acetyl derivatives against colorectal cancer in vivo and in vitro. Eur J Cancer 32A:1968–1976
238. Seigneurin-Berny D, Verdel A, Curtet S, Lemercier C, Garin J, Rousseaux S, Khochbin S (2001) Identification of components of the murine histone deacetylase 6 complex: link between acetylation and ubiquitination signaling pathways. Mol Cell Biol 21:8035–8044
239. Sellers WR, Kaelin WG Jr (1997) Role of the retinoblastoma protein in the pathogenesis of human cancer. J Clin Oncol 15:3301–3312
240. Shaffer AL, Yu X, He Y, Boldrick J, Chan EP, Staudt LM (2000) BCL-6 represses genes that function in lymphocyte differentiation, inflammation, and cell cycle control. Immunity 13:199–212
241. Shaker S, Bernstein M, Momparler LF, Momparler RL (2003) Preclinical evaluation of antineoplastic activity of inhibitors of DNA methylation (5-aza-2'-deoxycytidine) and histone deacetylation (trichostatin A, depsipeptide) in combination against myeloid leukemic cells. Leuk Res 27:437–444
242. Simone C, Stiegler P, Forcales SV, Bagella L, De Luca A, Sartorelli V, Giordano A, Puri PL (2004) Deacetylase recruitment by the C/H3 domain of the acetyltransferase p300. Oncogene 23:2177–2187
243. Somoza JR, Skene RJ, Katz BA, Mol C, Ho JD, Jennings AJ, Luong C, Arvai A, Buggy JJ, Chi E, Tang J, Sang BC, Verner E, Wynands R, Leahy EM, Dougan DR, Snell G, Navre M, Knuth MW, Swanson RV, McRee DE, Tari LW (2004) Structural snapshots of human HDAC8 provide insights into the class I histone deacetylases. Structure (Camb) 12:1325–1334
244. Song J, Noh JH, Lee JH, Eun JW, Ahn YM, Kim SY, Lee SH, Park WS, Yoo NJ, Lee JY, Nam SW (2005) Increased expression of histone deacetylase 2 is found in human gastric cancer. Apmis 113:264–268
245. Sonnemann J, Gange J, Kumar KS, Muller C, Bader P, Beck JF (2005) Histone deacetylase inhibitors interact synergistically with tumor necrosis factor-related apoptosis-inducing ligand (TRAIL) to induce apoptosis in carcinoma cell lines. Invest New Drugs 23:99–109

246. Sparrow DB, Miska EA, Langley E, Reynaud-Deonauth S, Kotecha S, Towers N, Spohr G, Kouzarides T, Mohun TJ (1999) MEF-2 function is modified by a novel co-repressor, MITR. EMBO J 18:5085–5098
247. Steiner FA, Hong JA, Fischette MR, Beer DG, Guo ZS, Chen GA, Weiser TS, Kassis ES, Nguyen DM, Lee S, Trepel JB, Schrump DS (2005) Sequential 5-aza 2'-deoxycytidine/depsipeptide FK228 treatment induces tissue factor pathway inhibitor 2 (TFPI-2) expression in cancer cells. Oncogene 24:2386–2397
248. Strahl BD, Allis CD (2000) The language of covalent histone modifications. Nature 403:41–45
249. Su GH, Sohn TA, Ryu B, Kern SE (2000) A novel histone deacetylase inhibitor identified by high-throughput transcriptional screening of a compound library. Cancer Res 60:3137–3142
250. Sun JM, Chen HY, Moniwa M, Litchfield DW, Seto E, Davie JR (2002) The transcriptional repressor Sp3 is associated with CK2-phosphorylated histone deacetylase 2. J Biol Chem 277:35783–35786
251. Suzuki T, Ando T, Tsuchiya K, Fukazawa N, Saito A, Mariko Y, Yamashita T, Nakanishi O (1999) Synthesis and histone deacetylase inhibitory activity of new benzamide derivatives. J Med Chem 42:3001–3003
252. Suzuki T, Yokozaki H, Kuniyasu H, Hayashi K, Naka K, Ono S, Ishikawa T, Tahara E, Yasui W (2000) Effect of trichostatin A on cell growth and expression of cell cycle- and apoptosis-related molecules in human gastric and oral carcinoma cell lines. Int J Cancer 88:992–997
253. Szyf M, Pakneshan P, Rabbani SA (2004) DNA demethylation and cancer: therapeutic implications. Cancer Lett 211:133–143
254. Tallman MS, Andersen JW, Schiffer CA, Appelbaum FR, Feusner JH, Woods WG, Ogden A, Weinstein H, Shepherd L, Willman C, Bloomfield CD, Rowe JM, Wiernik PH (2002) All-trans retinoic acid in acute promyelocytic leukemia: long-term outcome and prognostic factor analysis from the North American Intergroup protocol. Blood 100:4298–4302
255. Taunton J, Hassig CA, Schreiber SL (1996) A mammalian histone deacetylase related to the yeast transcriptional regulator Rpd3p. Science 272:408–411
256. Tenen DG, Hromas R, Licht JD, Zhang DE (1997) Transcription factors, normal myeloid development, and leukemia. Blood 90:489–519
257. Thibault A, Cooper MR, Figg WD, Venzon DJ, Sartor AO, Tompkins AC, Weinberger MS, Headlee DJ, McCall NA, Samid D, et al (1994) A phase I and pharmacokinetic study of intravenous phenylacetate in patients with cancer. Cancer Res 54:1690–1694
258. Tong JJ, Liu J, Bertos NR, Yang XJ (2002) Identification of HDAC10, a novel class II human histone deacetylase containing a leucine-rich domain. Nucleic Acids Res 30:1114–1123
259. Tsai SC, Seto E (2002) Regulation of histone deacetylase 2 by protein kinase CK2. J Biol Chem 277:31826–31833
260. Tsuji N, Kobayashi M, Nagashima K, Wakisaka Y, Koizumi K (1976) A new antifungal antibiotic, trichostatin. J Antibiot (Tokyo) 29:1–6
261. Turner BM (2000) Histone acetylation and an epigenetic code. Bioessays 22:836–845
262. Turner BM (2002) Cellular memory and the histone code. Cell 111:285–291

263. Ueda H, Nakajima H, Hori Y, Goto T, Okuhara M (1994) Action of FR901228, a novel antitumor bicyclic depsipeptide produced by Chromobacterium violaceum no. 968, on Ha-ras transformed NIH3T3 cells. Biosci Biotechnol Biochem 58:1579–1583
264. Undevia SD, Kindler HL, Janisch L, Olson SC, Schilsky RL, Vogelzang NJ, Kimmel KA, Macek TA, Ratain MJ (2004) A phase I study of the oral combination of CI-994, a putative histone deacetylase inhibitor, and capecitabine. Ann Oncol 15:1705–1711
265. Ungerstedt JS, Sowa Y, Xu WS, Shao Y, Dokmanovic M, Perez G, Ngo L, Holmgren A, Jiang X, Marks PA (2005) Role of thioredoxin in the response of normal and transformed cells to histone deacetylase inhibitors. Proc Natl Acad Sci U S A 102:673–678
266. Vanhaecke T, Papeleu P, Elaut G, Rogiers V (2004) Trichostatin A-like hydroxamate histone deacetylase inhibitors as therapeutic agents: toxicological point of view. Curr Med Chem 11:1629–1643
267. Vanoosten RL, Moore JM, Ludwig AT, Griffith TS (2005) Depsipeptide (FR901228) enhances the cytotoxic activity of TRAIL by redistributing TRAIL receptor to membrane lipid rafts. Mol Ther 11:542–552
268. Vega RB, Harrison BC, Meadows E, Roberts CR, Papst PJ, Olson EN, McKinsey TA (2004) Protein kinases C and D mediate agonist-dependent cardiac hypertrophy through nuclear export of histone deacetylase 5. Mol Cell Biol 24:8374–8385
269. Verdel A, Curtet S, Brocard MP, Rousseaux S, Lemercier C, Yoshida M, Khochbin S (2000) Active maintenance of mHDA2/mHDAC6 histone-deacetylase in the cytoplasm. Curr Biol 10:747–749
270. Verdin E, Dequiedt F, Kasler HG (2003) Class II histone deacetylases: versatile regulators. Trends Genet 19:286–293
271. Vidal M, Gaber RF (1991) RPD3 encodes a second factor required to achieve maximum positive and negative transcriptional states in Saccharomyces cerevisiae. Mol Cell Biol 11:6317–6327
272. Waltregny D, De Leval L, Glenisson W, Ly Tran S, North BJ, Bellahcene A, Weidle U, Verdin E, Castronovo V (2004) Expression of histone deacetylase 8, a class I histone deacetylase, is restricted to cells showing smooth muscle differentiation in normal human tissues. Am J Pathol 165:553–564
273. Waltregny D, Glenisson W, Tran SL, North BJ, Verdin E, Colige A, Castronovo V (2005) Histone deacetylase HDAC8 associates with smooth muscle alpha-actin and is essential for smooth muscle cell contractility. FASEB J 19:966–968
274. Wang AH, Bertos NR, Vezmar M, Pelletier N, Crosato M, Heng HH, Th'ng J, Han J, Yang XJ (1999) HDAC4, a human histone deacetylase related to yeast HDA1, is a transcriptional corepressor. Mol Cell Biol 19:7816–7827
275. Wang AH, Kruhlak MJ, Wu J, Bertos NR, Vezmar M, Posner BI, Bazett-Jones DP, Yang XJ (2000) Regulation of histone deacetylase 4 by binding of 14-3-3 proteins. Mol Cell Biol 20:6904–6912
276. Wang AH, Yang XJ (2001) Histone deacetylase 4 possesses intrinsic nuclear import and export signals. Mol Cell Biol 21:5992–6005

277. Wang XF, Qian DZ, Ren M, Kato Y, Wei Y, Zhang L, Fansler Z, Clark D, Nakanishi O, Pili R (2005) Epigenetic modulation of retinoic acid receptor beta2 by the histone deacetylase inhibitor MS-275 in human renal cell carcinoma. Clin Cancer Res 11:3535–3542
278. Warrell RP Jr, He LZ, Richon V, Calleja E, Pandolfi PP (1998) Therapeutic targeting of transcription in acute promyelocytic leukemia by use of an inhibitor of histone deacetylase. J Natl Cancer Inst 90:1621–1625
279. Weiser TS, Guo ZS, Ohnmacht GA, Parkhurst ML, Tong-On P, Marincola FM, Fischette MR, Yu X, Chen GA, Hong JA, Stewart JH, Nguyen DM, Rosenberg SA, Schrump DS (2001) Sequential 5-aza-2′-deoxycytidine-depsipeptide FR901228 treatment induces apoptosis preferentially in cancer cells and facilitates their recognition by cytolytic T lymphocytes specific for NY-ESO-1. J Immunother 24:151–161
280. Whetstine JR, Ceron J, Ladd B, Dufourcq P, Reinke V, Shi Y (2005) Regulation of tissue-specific and extracellular matrix-related genes by a class I histone deacetylase. Mol Cell 18:483–490
281. Williams RJ (2001) Trichostatin A, an inhibitor of histone deacetylase, inhibits hypoxia-induced angiogenesis. Expert Opin Investig Drugs 10:1571–1573
282. Wong CW, Privalsky ML (1998) Components of the SMRT corepressor complex exhibit distinctive interactions with the POZ domain oncoproteins PLZF, PLZF-RARalpha, and BCL-6. J Biol Chem 273:27695–27702
283. Woronicz JD, Lina A, Calnan BJ, Szychowski S, Cheng L, Winoto A (1995) Regulation of the Nur77 orphan steroid receptor in activation-induced apoptosis. Mol Cell Biol 15:6364–6376
284. Wu J, Grunstein M (2000) 25 years after the nucleosome model: chromatin modifications. Trends Biochem Sci 25:619–623
285. Yamagoe S, Kanno T, Kanno Y, Sasaki S, Siegel RM, Lenardo MJ, Humphrey G, Wang Y, Nakatani Y, Howard BH, Ozato K (2003) Interaction of histone acetylases and deacetylases in vivo. Mol Cell Biol 23:1025–1033
286. Yang H, Hoshino K, Sanchez-Gonzalez B, Kantarjian H, Garcia-Manero G (2005) Antileukemia activity of the combination of 5-aza-2′-deoxycytidine with valproic acid. Leuk Res 29:739–748
287. Yang WM, Tsai SC, Wen YD, Fejer G, Seto E (2002) Functional domains of histone deacetylase-3. J Biol Chem 277:9447–9454
288. Ye BH, Lista F, Lo Coco F, Knowles DM, Offit K, Chaganti RS, Dalla-Favera R (1993) Alterations of a zinc finger-encoding gene, BCL-6, in diffuse large-cell lymphoma. Science 262:747–750
289. Yoder JA, Walsh CP, Bestor TH (1997) Cytosine methylation and the ecology of intragenomic parasites. Trends Genet 13:335–340
290. Yoshida M, Horinouchi S, Beppu T (1995) Trichostatin A and trapoxin: novel chemical probes for the role of histone acetylation in chromatin structure and function. Bioessays 17:423–430
291. Yoshida M, Kijima M, Akita M, Beppu T (1990) Potent and specific inhibition of mammalian histone deacetylase both in vivo and in vitro by trichostatin A. J Biol Chem 265:17174–17179
292. Yoshida M, Shimazu T, Matsuyama A (2003) Protein deacetylases: enzymes with functional diversity as novel therapeutic targets. Prog Cell Cycle Res 5:269–278

293. Youn HD, Sun L, Prywes R, Liu JO (1999) Apoptosis of T cells mediated by Ca2+-induced release of the transcription factor MEF2. Science 286:790–793
294. Yu C, Rahmani M, Almenara J, Subler M, Krystal G, Conrad D, Varticovski L, Dent P, Grant S (2003) Histone deacetylase inhibitors promote STI571-mediated apoptosis in STI571-sensitive and -resistant Bcr/Abl+ human myeloid leukemia cells. Cancer Res 63:2118–2126
295. Yu C, Rahmani M, Conrad D, Subler M, Dent P, Grant S (2003) The proteasome inhibitor bortezomib interacts synergistically with histone deacetylase inhibitors to induce apoptosis in Bcr/Abl+ cells sensitive and resistant to STI571. Blood 102:3765–3774
296. Yu C, Rahmani M, Dent P, Grant S (2004) The hierarchical relationship between MAPK signaling and ROS generation in human leukemia cells undergoing apoptosis in response to the proteasome inhibitor Bortezomib. Exp Cell Res 295:555–566
297. Zelent A, Greaves M, Enver T (2004) Role of the TEL-AML1 fusion gene in the molecular pathogenesis of childhood acute lymphoblastic leukaemia. Oncogene 23:4275–4283
298. Zelent A, Guidez F, Melnick A, Waxman S, Licht JD (2001) Translocations of the RARalpha gene in acute promyelocytic leukemia. Oncogene 20:7186–7203
299. Zelent A, Petrie K, Chen Z, Lotan R, Lubbert M, Tallman MS, Ohno R, Degos L, Waxman S (2005) Molecular target-based treatment of human cancer: summary of the 10th international conference on differentiation therapy. Cancer Res 65:1–7
300. Zeremski M, Stricker JR, Fischer D, Zusman SB, Cohen D (2003) Histone deacetylase dHDAC4 is involved in segmentation of the Drosophila embryo and is regulated by gap and pair-rule genes. Genesis 35:31–38
301. Zgouras D, Becker U, Loitsch S, Stein J (2004) Modulation of angiogenesis-related protein synthesis by valproic acid. Biochem Biophys Res Commun 316:693–697
302. Zhang CL, McKinsey TA, Chang S, Antos CL, Hill JA, Olson EN (2002) Class II histone deacetylases act as signal-responsive repressors of cardiac hypertrophy. Cell 110:479–488
303. Zhang CL, McKinsey TA, Olson EN (2001) The transcriptional corepressor MITR is a signal-responsive inhibitor of myogenesis. Proc Natl Acad Sci U S A 98:7354–7359
304. Zhang X, Ozawa Y, Lee H, Wen YD, Tan TH, Wadzinski BE, Seto E (2005) Histone deacetylase 3 (HDAC3) activity is regulated by interaction with protein serine/threonine phosphatase 4. Genes Dev 19:827–839
305. Zhang Y, Adachi M, Zhao X, Kawamura R, Imai K (2004) Histone deacetylase inhibitors FK228, N-(2-aminophenyl)-4-[N-(pyridin-3-yl-methoxycarbonyl)amino-methyl]benzamide and m-carboxycinnamic acid bis-hydroxamide augment radiation-induced cell death in gastrointestinal adenocarcinoma cells. Int J Cancer 110:301–308

Monoclonal Antibody Therapy of APL

P. G. Maslak (✉) · J. G. Jurcic · D. A. Scheinberg

Memorial Sloan-Kettering Cancer Center and Weill Medical College
of Cornell University, New York, NY 10021, USA
maslakp@mskcc.org

1	Introduction	205
2	Background	206
3	Therapies	209
4	Conclusion	214
	References	215

Abstract Acute promyelocytic leukemia (APL) is a rare subtype of acute myeloid leukemia (AML) for which a number of targeted therapies have been developed. The "targets" have included both genotypic and phenotypic features of the disease. The application of monoclonal antibodies (MAbs) to this disease to date have been limited to a relatively small number of studies where this therapy has been used to supplement effective approaches to the disease. The preliminary results have been promising, and further development of this modality as an effective adjunct to existing treatment regimens will most certainly occur in the near future.

1
Introduction

Acute myelogenous leukemia (AML) is a disorder of malignant hematopoiesis that has remained difficult to cure. Although the disease itself is relatively rare, AML remains an important entity nonetheless because it serves as a model for a fundamental understanding of cancer and provides a "testing ground" for newer therapeutic strategies including agents that target the underlying biology of the disease. Acute promyelocytic leukemia (APL), a subtype of AML, is the prototypical example of this continuum from scientific understanding to clinical management. Although the initial drug-based approaches were based on empiricism, the information gained as the disease has become more intensely studied in the laboratory has allowed the clinical model to be refined, resulting in a clinical management approach to the disease that is radically different from the standard of care employed 15 years ago. The same cannot be said for the other diseases classified as AML.

2
Background

APL is a disease where the genotype determines the phenotype, which in turn, is recognized as a clinical syndrome. Over 95% of cases of APL are characterized by a balanced translocation between chromosomes 15 and 17 [1, 2]. The breakpoints for the translocation usually occur at the q22 loci on chromosome 15 and at q21 on chromosome 17. When detected by conventional karyotyping, the 15;17 translocation is definitive evidence of the diagnosis of APL. More recently, the availability of specific chromosomal probes has facilitated the application of fluorescence in situ hybridization (FISH) to detect the characteristic translocation and provide rapid confirmatory testing.

The molecular consequences of t(15;17) are not only of fundamental importance in the process of leukemogenesis (see below) but also provides a distinct marker for establishing the diagnosis and monitoring the response to therapy [3–6]. The (15;17) translocation results in a fusion of a portion of the gene for the retinoic acid receptor-α (RARα) on chromosome 17 to part of the promyelocytic leukemia (PML) gene on chromosome 15. The break within the RAR gene invariably occurs in the second intron of the gene. The point of rearrangement in PML, however, can occur at one of two major breakpoints, and such variability may then result in three isoforms of the transcript. Breakpoints with PML intron 3 (bcr3) yield a shorter messenger RNA (mRNA) transcript than breakpoints within intron 6 (bcr1), which result in the "long form" of the transcript [7]. Breakpoints within intron 6 of PML can also occur at a second site (bcr2) and result in a transcript of variable length. The breakpoint site has been reported by some investigators to have prognostic implications, as those newly diagnosed patients who have been found to have the short form of the transcript have a shorter disease-free period and lower rates of overall survival [8, 9].

Other investigators have disputed the prognostic significance of this finding as an independent variable but instead have correlated the isoform with other disease-related variables (such as leukocytosis) known to have prognostic significance [10].

The PML-RARα fusion transcript does, however, have profound implications for cellular metabolism, and experimental models for malignant transformation have been developed [11–15]. The most basic hypothesis states that APL results from transcriptional dysregulation of myeloid differentiation effected by the PML-RARα gene product. Under normal physiologic conditions in a myeloid progenitor, RARα is thought to play an important role in differentiation based on the ability to recruit various nuclear corepressors like SMRT/N-CoR and mSin3. The transcription corepressors can then bind various histone deacetylases' "closing" chromatin conformation, resulting in transcriptional repression of downstream target genes responsible for the process of differentiation. Under normal physiologic conditions, retinoic acid (RA) binding causes a dissociation of the corepressor complex, recruits transcriptional activators, and "opens" the structure of the chromatin, allowing transcription of the target genes responsible for myeloid maturation. The PML-RARα complex acts differently by virtue of its increased affinity for the corepressor complex. Physiologic doses of RA ($<10^{-8}$ M) are unable to effect dissociation of the complex, resulting in continued transcriptional repression and maturation arrest. The administration of all-*trans* retinoic acid (ATRA) results in the supraphysiologic levels required to dislodge the corepressor complex and restore the normal physiologic response of the wildtype receptor.

Although the vast majority of APL cases encountered in clinical practice are found to have t(15;17), chromosomal—and hence, molecular—variants have been shown to exist. Although rare as clinical entities, these variants have provided experimental data that in turn have refined the APL model of leukemogenesis. On a cytogenetic level, the most common variants involve translocations between chromosome 17 and either chromosome 5 or 11 [16–20]. On a molecular level, these variants retain the same break within the RARα intron but differ in the partner gene located on the alternate chromosome(s). The change in the wildtype RARα results in a change of function. The most notable among the molecular variants is the fusion of the RAR gene with the promyelocytic leukemia zinc finger gene (PLZF-RARα) which results from t(11;17) (q23q21). This entity is resistant to the effects of ATRA and also renders this form of APL relatively resistant to standard chemotherapy [21].

Using reverse transcriptase polymerase chain reaction (RT-PCR) to detect the PML-RARα fusion product has become a standard tool in the clinical management of APL [22–24]. Since the t(15;17) and the PML-RARα fusion product are genetic changes specific for APL, their detection can be used to confirm the diagnosis. The assay is widely available and has a relatively rapid turnaround time. In addition to acting as a confirmatory test at diagnosis, the detection of PML-RARα can be used to monitor response and test for minimal residual disease in the face of morphologically documented remission [9, 22–26]. This ability to detect minimal residual disease via a molecular marker is in sharp contrast to most other forms of AML, in which response may solely be assessed by conventional microscopy. Therefore, in APL, the concept of remission can be redefined to include more stringent molecular criteria. In many cases, molecular relapse can be detected prior to the reemergence of the leukemia cells in the blood or the bone marrow. Such information can be used to optimize therapy, as several groups have reported a potential benefit to treating disease in molecular relapse prior to the advent of the full clinical syndrome. Effective treatment regimens upon their completion render the RT-PCR assay for PML-RARα negative. The conversion of a negative result to a positive finding that is reproducible on two sequential assays is predictive of clinical relapse and, given the data cited above, will often trigger therapeutic intervention. These findings have led to the standard recommendation for clinical management that patients with APL be serially monitored with RT-PCR for PML-RARα every 3 months during the first 2 years after remission is achieved when the risk of relapse is the greatest [9]. In addition, this ability to follow a molecular assay to monitor minimal residual disease makes APL the ideal disease to test the application of monoclonal antibody therapy, a modality that may work best in the setting of a decreased disease burden.

While the molecular genetics of this disorder has received much attention in recent years, the majority of cases of APL are diagnosed through conventional microscopy and immunophenotyping. Most cases of APL are of the hypergranular variety [27]. The cytoplasm contains large granules that often obscure the nuclear cytoplasmic border. This is in sharp contrast to normal promyelocytes where the separation between the normal cellular components is maintained. In addition, the abnormal promyelocytes may have a folded, reniform nucleus. Some cells contain multiple Auer rods and have been labeled faggot ("bundle of sticks") cells. Morphologic microgranular variants have been described, but virtually all of these subtypes have been found to have t(15;17) or PML/RARα on cytogenetic or molecular testing [28, 29]. More recently, a morphologic appearance of the PLZF/RAR variant has been reported to share some morphologic features of a myelodysplastic syndrome in addition to APL characteristics [30]. Given the rarity of this entity, however, this generally does not pose a significant problem for the clinician who could still rely on DNA-based testing to identify this subtype.

Although immunophenotyping is not diagnostic of this disorder, APL does have an immunophenotypic profile that is consistent with the disease [31, 32]. Generally, the two most important cell surface markers are CD33 and HLA-DR. CD33 is a myeloid differentiation marker that arises as cells pass from the blast to promyelocyte stage. Therefore, the presence of this marker is consistent with the observation that these cells have undertaken a limited degree of differentiation. It has taken on new significance with the emergence of monoclonal antibodies that target this antigen and the findings that these drugs can be used as therapeutic agents (see below). In contrast to most other subtypes of AML, HLA-DR is absent from APL cells. In addition, the presence of such cross lineage markers as CD2, CD56, and CD68 has been reported [33]. In some series these immunophenotypes have been correlated with either clinical outcomes or other biologic features.

3
Therapies

The key to the clinical management of APL is the ability to successfully recognize the disorder and institute specific therapy. This concept has evolved through the years as therapeutic agents targeted to the specific biology of the disease have become available to the clinician. Prior to the advent of these agents, recognition was still important but only because it characterized the degree of supportive care the patient would require in order to survive induction therapy.

Since the 1970s, the mainstay of AML induction therapy has been the combination of an anthracycline and cytosine arabinoside (Ara-C). The application of such therapy to APL was generally, however, associated with a higher induction mortality than the other forms of AML [34, 35]. This could primarily be attributed to an exacerbation of the underlying DIC (disseminated intravascular coagulopathy), which occurs with lysis of the leukemic promyelocytes. The effect of cytotoxic therapy is particularly pronounced in patients who present with high peripheral white blood cell counts. In either case, the application of stringent monitoring of coagulation parameters, as well as the early application of aggressive blood product support, eventually decreased the peri-induction mortality to around 10% [36].

The standard paradigm for AML therapy that eventually developed called for one induction course followed by at least two courses of dose-attenuated postremission (consolidation) therapy. As the data matured, it became apparent that outcomes for APL using this approach as standard therapy were superior to those seen in other AML subtypes [34, 35]. Therefore, if an individual patient could survive the induction period, the chance of survival was superior, and APL began to be considered a "good risk" form of AML. In addition, the outcomes seen with standard chemotherapy-based postremission regimens were comparable to survival reported with bone marrow transplantation (BMT), causing most experts to reserve BMT for relapsed patients.

The emergence of high-dose Ara-C as the preferred postremission therapy prompted a further divergence in treatment approach between APL and the other AML subtypes. While the use of high-dose Ara-C appeared to benefit groups of young patients with AML, particularly those with t(8;21) or inv 16, the effect on APL was relatively minimal, In fact, retrospective analysis revealed that it was the dose intensity of the anthracycline instead of Ara-C that assumed primary importance in the treatment of this disorder [37, 38]. Therefore, regimens that exploited this strategy were adopted as the standard in place of the high-dose Ara-C-based regimens.

The introduction of ATRA changed the management of APL even further and ushered in a new era of effective, targeted therapy of oncologic therapeutics. Unlike imatinib, which arose out of a painstakingly planned drug development program, the introduction of ATRA as a clinical agent was the result of empiricism born of a necessity to develop an effective therapy in the face of relatively limited clinical resources. The success from the initial Chinese trials rapidly gave rise to a number of other nonrandomized trials that also reported high complete remission (CR) rates. It soon became evident from these studies that the clinical response to ATRA was correlated with the presence of the 15;17 translocation or PML/RARα as assessed by conventional karyotyping or RT-PCR [39–43]. Two other important observations were made as ATRA progressed to phase II studies. The first was that up to 50% of patients developed "RA or differentiation syndrome" [44]. This was an adult respiratory distress syndrome (ARDS)-like reaction characterized by pulmonary infiltrates, fever, weight gain, and serositis that could be rapidly fatal if left unrecognized and untreated. Many of the initial fatalities on the ATRA resulted from RA syndrome. As more experience with the syndrome was acquired, the practice of vigilant monitoring with the early institution of high-dose dexamethasone resulted in a significant decrease in the mortality and morbidity of this toxicity. The other important observation was that remissions obtained solely with ATRA were brief in duration [45, 46]. Therefore, the continued administration of ATRA as postremission therapy was inadequate to maintain remission and effect cure. Subsequently, both single-arm and randomized studies revealed that combining ATRA with standard induction chemotherapy and following this induction therapy with several cycles of anthracycline-based regimens resulted in remissions that were not only durable but superior to those achieved with chemotherapy alone [46–49].

The model for ATRA-based upfront therapy of APL was further modified by the results of a large European study that addressed the issue of scheduling ATRA/chemotherapy [50]. In this trial, 413 untreated APL patients were prospectively randomized between concurrent ATRA plus daunorubicin/Ara-C and sequential ATRA followed by the identical chemotherapy. Patients who achieved CR then received 1–2 additional course of chemotherapy (one course if age >65 years) and were then randomized to receive either 2 years of maintenance therapy consisting of ATRA alone, methotrexate plus 6-mercaptopurine

(6-MP), ATRA plus methotrexate and 6-MP, or no maintenance (observation alone). The proportion of patients achieving CR (92%) did not differ among the two different induction regimens. The clinical benefit appeared to result from a reduction in the risk of relapse, which at 2 years was 6% in the concurrent cohort and 16% in the sequential group ($p = 0.04$). Patients who received some form of maintenance therapy had superior overall survival to those who received no maintenance therapy. In addition, another potential benefit from the concurrent ATRA/chemotherapy group was a greater than 50% reduction in the incidence of RA syndrome.

These data were, therefore, instrumental in shaping the current standard of care for APL therapy. Combined modality therapy is employed as induction followed by at least two courses of anthracycline-based regimens as postremission therapy. This therapy, in turn, is followed by 2 years of ATRA +/− chemotherapy administered on an intermittent schedule. Recently, some groups have reported similar outcomes by omitting the maintenance phase, but the regimens used generally employed more dose-intensive chemotherapy than is standard practice [51]. These results await further validation by other investigators.

The difficulty with the modern approach to therapy is that it is not without toxicity. The initial excitement regarding ATRA was prompted by the idea that it was a targeted therapy specific to the APL cells. The superior results obtained by adding chemotherapy to ATRA shifted the approach from a strictly targeted modality to one which included some of the toxicity associated with cytotoxic therapy. Such toxicities have received renewed interest, as reports of secondary myelodysplastic syndrome in up to 6% of patients have surfaced and have prompted investigators to seek alternatives to chemotherapy-based strategies [52].

Monoclonal antibodies (MAbs) may represent a relatively nontoxic approach to supplementing the already effective therapy of APL. With the commercial availability of such agents as rituximab and alemtuzumab, MAbs are becoming an increasingly important therapeutic modality for cancer as a whole. Leukemia is a disease well suited to these agents because of the accessibility of the malignant cells in the blood, bone marrow, and other hematopoietic organs. In addition, the well-described immunophenotypes of the various disorders provide distinct antigenic targets.

Most of the studies for the antibody therapy of AML have used CD33 as the target antigen. CD33 is a cell-surface glycoprotein found on the majority of myeloid leukemias and committed myelomonocytic progenitors, but not on mature granulocytes, hematopoietic stem cells, or nonhematopoietic tissues [53]. Early studies showed that traced-labeled ^{131}I-M195, a murine MAb that targets CD33, rapidly targets leukemia cells in patients [54]. Furthermore, the clinical activity of this immunoconjugate was demonstrated in a small cohort of patients with relapsed APL [55]. Therapy with M195, however, was limited by a lack of intrinsic antileukemic activity and by the formation of human anti-mouse antibodies, which alters its pharmacokinetics. Humanized M195 (HuM195) was then constructed by grafting the complementarity-determining regions of murine M195 into a human IgG1 framework and backbone. HuM195 can mediate leukemia cell killing in vitro by antibody-dependent cell-mediated cytotoxicity and can fix human complement [56]. An initial phase I study with HuM195 demonstrated leukemia cell targeting and pharmacology that was similar to murine M195. No significant immunogenicity was seen, allowing the construct to be developed as an agent for human disease [57].

The observation that high doses of murine M195 eliminated HL60 cells in an athymic nude mouse model provided the rationale for a strategy employing supersaturating doses of HuM195 [58]. Ten patients with relapsed or refractory myeloid leukemia were treated with two courses of HuM195 (12–36 mg/m^2 daily for 4 days) 2 weeks apart [59]. One patient with refractory AML, presenting with less than 10% bone marrow blasts, achieved a CR lasting over 5 years. A 6% response rate was confirmed in a larger, multicenter phase II study. All responses occurred in patients who had less than 30% blasts at presentation, illustrating the concept that this therapy is most effective when the leukemia burden is minimal [60].

Because of the activity seen in patients with lower blast counts, the role of HuM195 in cytoreduced disease was examined in a randomized phase III trial [61]. Patients with relapsed or refractory AML received mitoxantrone, etoposide, and cytarabine alone or with HuM195. No difference in adverse events or treatment-related mortality between the two groups was seen. The overall response rate [CR+CRp (CR with incomplete platelet recovery)] was 36% in the HuM195 group ($n = 94$) compared to 28% in the control group ($n = 97$), although this difference was not statistically significant ($p = 0.28$).

APL presents the perfect venue for a study of the utility of HuM195 in the treatment of minimal residual disease because, as discussed above, an effective induction strategy already exists for this disorder and a theme of many current investigations is modification of postremission therapy to minimize the exposure to standard chemotherapy and ameliorate toxicity. Serial monitoring of bone marrow by RT-PCR for PML/RARα provided a surrogate marker to assess the effect of postremission therapy. After attaining clinical remission with ATRA, 31 patients with newly diagnosed APL were treated with HuM195 followed by three cycles of idarubicin and cytarabine as consolidation and six monthly courses of HuM195 as maintenance [62]. Half of the 24 patients evaluable for conversion of positive RT-PCR assays became negative after HuM195 without additional therapy. The 5-year disease-free survival was 93%, compared with 73% among patients receiving ATRA induction followed by consolidation chemotherapy without HuM195 in earlier studies.

Further modification of postremission therapy of APL was investigated by administering HuM195 followed by arsenic trioxide in 15 patients with newly diagnosed APL using a risk-adapted approach based on RT-PCR monitoring of residual disease [63]. Patients in molecular remission (MR) after arsenic trioxide received one course of idarubicin as consolidation. Up to three cycles of idarubicin could be administered, however, depending upon the time at which MR was achieved. Of the patients with a positive RT-PCR assay after induction, 4 of 7 became negative after HuM195, and all patients achieved MR after arsenic trioxide. All patients are in clinical remission with a median follow-up duration of 25 months, although one molecular relapse was seen. This patient achieved MR following treatment with arsenic trioxide and then proceeded to allogeneic stem cell transplantation and is currently alive without evidence of disease with approximately a 23-month follow-up. These preliminary results suggests that the use of HuM195 and other newer agents, such as arsenic trioxide, may reduce the number of standard chemotherapy courses required for long-term remission in APL.

Another targeted MAb-based therapy that has received much attention in AML is the drug gemtuzumab ozogamicin (GO). GO consists of a recombinant humanized anti-CD33 MAb conjugated to calicheamicin, a potent antitumor antibiotic. Within the acidic environment of lysosomes after internalization, calicheamicin dissociates from the antibody and migrates to the nucleus, where it causes double-stranded DNA breaks. In a phase I trial, 8 of 40 patients with relapsed or refractory AML treated with escalating doses of GO had reductions in marrow blasts to below 5%, and CRs were seen in 3 patients [64]. Subsequently, 142 patients with AML in first relapse were treated with two doses of GO (9 mg/m^2) 2 weeks apart in three phase II trials. Patients with secondary AML or prior MDS were excluded. Of the patients, 23 (16%) achieved a CR, and 19 (13%) had a CRp [65]. Grade 3 or 4 hyperbilirubinemia developed in 23% of patients, and elevated serum transaminases were seen in 17%. Hepatic venoocclusive disease (VOD) occurred in 4% of patients. When used as a single-agent for newly diagnosed AML in older patients, complete response rates of approximately 25% have been reported [66].

Other clinical studies have reported higher rates of VOD associated with GO. Among patients who received GO in first relapse and then underwent stem cell transplantation, 17% developed VOD [67]. Another study noted that 11 of 23 patients (48%) treated with GO after stem cell transplantation developed liver injury similar to classical VOD, termed sinusoidal obstruction syndrome [68]. In a series of 119 patients treated with GO at the MD Anderson Cancer Center, 14 (12%) developed VOD in the absence of stem cell transplantation. The majority of these patients, however, received GO in combination with other agents, including investigational drugs, or at more frequent intervals than originally described [69]. Hence, it would appear that despite the "targeted" nature of the drug, some unique toxicities are associated with its use.

GO has been used specifically in APL in a number of settings. In vitro, GO has been found to be effective against ATRA or arsenic trioxide-resistant cell lines that lack expression of the multidrug-resistant p-glycoprotein [70]. The MD Anderson group administered GO in combination with ATRA in 19 patients with untreated APL. A CR rate of 84% was reported, which was comparable to more traditional ATRA-based regimens used in APL [71]. Of the patients tested for PML/RARα following completion of the induction therapy, all were RT-PCR negative ($n = 12$), although 3 required the addition of idarubicin during the initial phase of treatment. The study also called for eight courses of GO to be administered as the sole form of postremission therapy. A preliminary report of these results yielded no relapses with relatively short follow-up. Lo-Coco et al. reported the experience using GO as monotherapy in 16 patients with molecular relapse of APL [72]. The GO was administered at a dose of 6 mg/m^2 for 2 doses and, for those patients achieving a new MR, an additional dose was administered for consolidation therapy. Overall, 81% of the patients responded to therapy. Of the responders, 50% achieved a sustained molecular remission for a median of 15 months (range 7–31 months), prompting the authors to conclude that this therapy was effective against minimal residual disease and, like the MD Anderson trial discussed above, set the stage for future studies exploring GO use in the postremission setting.

4
Conclusion

APL is a rare disease for which a number of targeted therapies have been developed. The targets have included both genotypic and phenotypic features of the disease. The application of MAbs to this disease to date has been rather limited. The preliminary results, however, have been promising, and the further development of this modality as an effective adjunct to existing treatment regimens will most certainly occur in the near future.

References

1. Rowley J, Golomb HM, Dougherty C (1997) 15/17 trans-location, a consistent chromosomal change in acute promyelocytic leukemia. Lancet 1:549–550
2. Larsen RA, Kondo K, Vardiman JW, et al (1984) Evidence for a 15;17 translocation in every patient with acute promyelocytic leukemia. Am J Med 76:827–841
3. de Thë H, Chomienne C, Lanotte M, et al (1990) The t(15;17) translocation of acute promyelocytic leukemia fuses the retinoic acid receptor alpha gene to a novel transcribed locus. Nature 347:558–561
4. Kakizuka A, Miller WH, Umesono K, et al (1991) Chromosomal translocation t(15;17) in human acute promyelocytic leukemia fuses RARa with a novel putative transcription factor, PLL. Cell 66:663
5. de Thë H, Lavau C, Marchio A, et al (1991) The PML/RARa fusion mRNA generated by the t(15;17) translocation in acute promyelocytic leukemia encodes a functionally altered RAR. Cell 66:675
6. Melnick A, Licht JD (1999) Deconstructing a disease: RARα, its fusion partners, and their roles in the pathogenesis of acute promyelocytic leukemia. Blood 93:3167–3215
7. Pandolfi PP, Alcalay M, Fagioli M, et al (1992) Genomic variability and alternative splicing generate multiple PML-RARα transcripts that encode aberrant PML proteins and PML/RARα isoforms in acute promyelocytic leukemia. EMBO J 11:1397–1407
8. Vahdat L, Maslak P, Miller WH, et al (1994) Early mortality and retinoic acid syndrome in acute promyelocytic leukemia: impact of leucocytosis, low-dose chemotherapy, PML/RARα isoform, and CD13 expression in patients treated with all-trans retinoic acid. Blood 84:3843–3849
9. Jurcic JG, Nimer SD, Scheinberg D, et al (2001) Prognostic significance of minimal residual disease detection and PML/RAR-α isoform type: long-term follow-up in acute promyelocytic leukemia. Blood 98:2651–2656
10. Gallagher RE, Willman CL, Slack JL, et al (1997) Association of PML/RARα fusion mRNA type with pre-treatment characteristics but not treatment outcome in acute promyelocytic leukemia: an intergroup molecular study. Blood 90:1656–1663
11. Hong SH, David G, Wong CW, et al (1997) SMRT corepressor interacts with PLZF and with the PML-retinoic acid receptor α (RARα) and PLZF-RARα oncoproteins associated with acute promyelocytic leukemia. Proc Natl Acad Sci USA 94:9028–9033
12. Guidez F, Ivins S, Zhu J, et al (1998) Reduced retinoic acid-sensitivities of nuclear receptor corepressor binding to PML- and PLZF-RARalpha underlie molecular pathogenesis and treatment of acute promyelocytic leukemia. Blood 91:2634–2642
13. Heinzel T, Lavinski R, Mullen T, et al (1997) A complex containing N-CoR, mSin3 and histone deacetylase, mediates transcriptional repression. Nature 387:43–48
14. Lin RJ, Nagy L, Inoue S, et al (1998) Role of histone deacetylase complex in acute promyelocytic leukaemia. Nature 391:811–814
15. Uteley RT, Ikeda K, Grant PA, et al (1998) Transcriptional activators direct histone acetyltransferase complexed to nucleosomes. Nature 30:498–502

16. Chen Z, Brand NJ, Chen A, et al (1993) Fusion between a novel Kruppel-like zinc finger gene and the retinoic acid receptor-α locus due to a variant t(11;17) translocation association with acute promyelocytic leukaemia. EMBO J 12:1161–1167
17. Licht JD, Chomienne C, Goy A, et al (1995) Clinical and molecular characterization of a rare syndrome of acute promyelocytic leukemia associated with trans-location (11;17). Blood 85:1083–1094
18. Redner RL, Chen JD, Rush EA, et al (2000) The t(5;17) acute promyelocytic leukemia fusion protein NPM-RAR interacts with co-repressor and co-activator proteins and exhibits both positive and negative transcriptional properties. Blood 95:2683–2690
19. Wells RA, Catzavelos C, Kamel-Reid S (1997) Fusion of retinoic acid receptor α to NUMA, the nuclear mitotic apparatus protein, by a variant translocation in acute promyelocytic leukaemia. Nat Genet 17:109–113
20. Arnould C, Phillippe C, Bourdon V, et al (1999) The signal transducer and activator of transcription STAT5b gene is a new partner of retinoic acid receptor alpha in acute promyelocytic-like leukaemia. Hum Mol Genet 8:1741–1749
21. He LZ, Guidez F, Tribioli C, et al (1998) Distinct interactions of PML-RARalpha and PLZF-RARalpha with co-repressors determine differential responses to RA in APL. Nat Genet 18:126–135
22. Miller WH Jr, Kakizuka A, Frankel SR, et al (1992) Reverse transcription polymerase chain reaction for the re-arranged retinoic acid receptor α clarifies diagnosis and detects minimal residual disease in acute promyelocytic leukemia. Proc Natl Acad Sci USA 89:2694–2698
23. Lo Coco F, Diverio D, Pandolfi PP, et al (1992) Molecular evaluation of residual disease as a predictor of relapse in acute promyelocytic leukemia. Lancet 340:1437–1438
24. Miller WH Jr, Levine K, De Blasio A, et al (1993) Detection of minimal residual disease in acute promyelocytic leukemia by a reverse transcription polymerase chain reaction. Blood 82:1689–1694
25. Grimwade D, Howe K, Langabeer S, et al (1996) Minimal residual disease detection in acute promyelocytic leukemia by reverse-transcriptase PCR: evaluation of PML-RARα and RARα-PML assessment in patients who ultimately relapse. Leukemia 10:61–66
26. Diverio D, Rossi V, Avvisati G, et al (1998) Early detection of relapse by prospective reverse transcriptase-polymerase chain reaction analysis of the PML/RARα fusion gene in patients with acute promyelocytic leukemia enrolled in the GIMEMA-AIEOP multicenter "AIDA" trial. Blood 92:784–789
27. Bennett JM, Catovsky D, Daniel MT, et al (1976) Proposal for the classification of the acute leukaemias (FAB Cooperative Group). Br J Haematol 33:451–458
28. Golomb HM, Rowley JD, Vardiman JW, et al (1980) Microgranular acute promyelocytic leukaemia: a distinct clinical, ultrastructural, and cytogenetic entity. Blood 55:253–259
29. Bennett JM, Catovsky D, Daniel MT, et al (1980) A variant form of hypergranular promyelocytic leukemia (M3). Br J Haematol 44:169–170

30. Sainty D, Liso V, Cantu-Rajnoldi A, et al (2000) A new morphological classification system for acute promyelocytic distinguishes cases with underlying PLZF-RARα rearrangements. Blood 96:1287–1296
31. Das Gupta A, Sapre RS, Shah AS, et al (1989) Cytochemical and immunophenotypic heterogeneity in acute promyelocytic leukemia. Acta Haematol 81:5–9
32. Paietta E, Andersen J, Gallagher R, et al (1994) The immunophenotype of acute promyelocytic leukemia (APL): an ECOG. Leukemia 8:1108–1112
33. Erbert WN, Asbahr H, Rule SA, et al (1994) Unique immunophenotype of acute promyelocytic leukaemia as defined by CD9 and CD68 antibodies. Br J Haematol 88:101–104
34. Cunningham I, Gee TS, Reich LM, et al (1989) Acute promyelocytic leukemia: treatment results during a decade at Memorial Hospital. Blood 73:1116–1122
35. Kantarjian H, Keating MJ, Walters RS, et al (1986) Acute promyelocytic leukemia: MD Anderson Hospital experience. Am J Med 80:789–797
36. Di Bona E, Avvisati G, Castaman G, et al (2000) Early haemorrhagic morbidity and mortality during remission induction with or without all-trans retinoic acid in acute promyelocytic leukemia. Br J Haematol 108:689–695
37. Head D, Kopecky KJ, Weick J, et al (1995) Effect of aggressive daunomycin therapy on survival in acute promyelocytic leukemia. Blood 86:1717–1728
38. Estey E, Thall PF, Pierce S, et al (1997) Treatment of newly diagnosed acute promyelocytic leukemia without cytarabine. J Clin Oncol 15:483–490
39. Huang ME, Ye YC, Chen SR, et al (1988) Use of all-trans retinoic acid in treatment of acute promyelocytic leukemia. Blood 72:567–572
40. Warrell RP Jr, Frankel SR, Miller WH Jr, et al (1991) Differentiation therapy of acute promyelocytic leukemia with tretinoin (all-trans-retinoid acid). N Engl J Med 324:1385–1393
41. Huang ME, Ye YC, Chen SR, et al (1987) All-trans retinoic acid with or without low dose cytosine arabinoside in acute promyelocytic leukemia-Report of 6 cases. Chin Med J 100:949–953
42. Fenaux P, Le Dely MC, Castaigne S, et al (1993) Effect of all-trans retinoic acid in newly diagnosed acute promyelocytic leukemia: results of a multicenter randomized trial. Blood 82:3241–3249
43. Lo Coco F, Avvisati G, Diverio D, et al (1991) Molecular evaluation of response to all-trans retinoic acid therapy in patients with acute promyelocytic leukemia. Blood 77:1657–1661
44. Frankel SR, Eardley A, Lauwers G, Weiss M, Warrell RP Jr (1992) The "retinoic acid syndrome" in acute promyelocytic leukemia. Ann Intern Med 117:292–296
45. Frankel SR, Eardley A, Heller G, et al (1994) All-trans retinoic acid for acute promyelocytic leukemia: results of the New York study. Ann Intern Med 120:278–286
46. Warrell RP Jr, Maslak P, Eardley A, et al (1994) Treatment of acute promyelocytic leukemia with all-trans retinoic acid: an update of the New York experience. Leukemia 8:929–933
47. Castaigne S, Chomienne C, Daniel MT, et al (1990) All-trans retinoic acid as a differentiating therapy for acute promyelocytic leukemias. I. Clinical Results. Blood 76:1704–1713

48. Avvisati G (1998) AIDA Protocol: the Italian way of treating APL (Abrstr). Br J Haematol 102:593a
49. Tallman MS, Andersen JW, Schiffer CA, et al (1997) All-trans retinoic acid in acute promyelocytic leukemia. N Engl J Med 337:1021–1028
50. Fenaux P, Chastang C, Chevret S, et al (1999) A randomized comparison of all trans-retinoic acid (ATRA) followed by chemotherapy and ATRA plus chemotherapy and the role of maintenance therapy in newly diagnosed acute promyelocytic leukemia. The European APL Group. Blood 94:1192–1200
51. Avvisati G, Petti MC, Lo Coco F, et al (2003) AIDA: the Italian way of treating acute promyelocytic leukemia (APL), final act (Abstr). Blood 102:487
52. Lobe I, Rigal-Huget FR, Vekoff A, et al (2003) Myelodysplastic syndrome after acute promyelocytic leukemia: the European APL group experience. Leukemia 17:1600–1604
53. Andrews RG, Takahashi M, Segal GM, et al (1986) The L4F3 antigen is expressed by unipotent colony-forming cells but not by their precursors. Blood 68:1030–1035
54. Scheinberg DA, Lovett D, Divgi CR, et al (1991) A phase I trial of monoclonal antibody M195 in acute myelogenous leukemia: specific bone marrow targeting and internalization of radionuclide. J Clin Oncol 9:478–490
55. Jurcic JG, Caron PC, Miller WH Jr, et al (1995) Sequential targeted therapy for relapsed acute promyelocytic leukemia with all-trans retinoic acid and anti-CD33 monoclonal antibody M195. Leukemia 9:244–248
56. Caron PC, Co MS, Bull MK, et al (1992) Biological and immunological features of humanized M195 (anti-CD33) monoclonal antibodies. Cancer Res 52:6761–6767
57. Caron PC, Jurcic JG, Scott AM, et al (1994) A phase 1B trial of humanized monoclonal antibody M195 (anti-CD33) in myeloid leukemia: specific targeting without immunogenicity. Blood 83:1760–1768
58. Xu Y, Scheinberg DA (1995) Elimination of human leukemia by monoclonal antibodies in an athymic nude mouse leukemia model. Clin Cancer Res 1:1179–1187
59. Caron PC, Dumont L, Scheinberg DA (1998) Supersaturating infusional humanized anti-CD33 monoclonal antibody HuM195 in myelogenous leukemia. Clin Cancer Res 4:1421–1428
60. Feldman E, Kalaycio M, Weiner G, et al (2003) Treatment of relapsed or refractory acute myeloid leukemia with humanized anti-CD33 monoclonal antibody HuM195. Leukemia 17:314–318
61. Feldman E, Stone RM, Brandwein J, et al (2002) Phase III randomized trial of an anti-CD33 monoclonal antibody (HuM195) in combination with chemotherapy compared to chemotherapy alone in adults with refractory or first-relapse acute myeloid leukemia (AML) (Abstr). Proc Am Soc Clin Oncol 21:261a
62. Jurcic JG, DeBlasio T, Dumont L, Yao TJ, Scheinberg DA (2000) Molecular remission induction with retinoic acid and anti-CD33 monoclonal antibody HuM195 in acute promyelocytic leukemia. Clin Cancer Res 6:372–380
63. Mulford DA, Maslak PG, Weiss MA, Scheinberg DA, Jurcic JG (2003) Reducing standard postremission chemotherapy in acute promyelocytic leukemia (APL) with risk-adapted therapy (Abrstr). Blood 102:619a–620a

64. Sievers EL, Appelbaum FR, Spielberger RT, et al (1999) Selective ablation of acute myeloid leukemia using antibody-targeted chemotherapy: a phase I study of an anti-CD33 calicheamicin immunoconjugate. Blood 93:3678–3684
65. Sievers EL, Larson RA, Staudtmauer EA, et al (2001) Efficacy and safety of gemtuzumab ozogamicin in patients with CD33-positive acute myeloid leukemia in first relapse. J Clin Oncol 19:3244–3254
66. Amadori S, Suciu S, Willemze R, Mandelli F, Selleslag D, Stauder R, Ho A, Denzlinger C, Leone G, Fabris P, Muus P, Vignetti M, Hagemeijer A, Beeldens F, Anak O, De Witte T; EORTC leukemia group; GIMEMA leukemia group (2004) Sequential administration of gemtuzumab ozogamcin and convential chemotherapy as first line therapy in elderly patients with acute myeloid leukemia: a phase II study (AML-15) of the EORTC and GIMEMA leukemia groups. Haematologica 89:950–956
67. Sievers E, Larson R, Estey E, et al (2002) Final report of prolonged disease-free survival in patients with acute myeloid leukemia in first relapse treated with gemtuzumab ozogamicin followed by hematpoietic stem cell transplantation (Abstr). Blood 100:89a
68. Rajvanshi P, Schulman H, Sievers E, et al (2002) Hepatic sinusoidal obstruction after gemtuzumab ozogamicin (Mylotarg) therapy. Blood 99:10–14
69. Giles FJ, Kantarjian HM, Kornblau SM, et al (2001) Mylotarg (gemtuzumab ozogamicin) therapy is associated with hepatic venoocclusive disease in patients who have not received stem cell transplantation. Cancer 92:406–413
70. Takeshita A, Shinjo K, Naito K, et al (2005) Efficacy of gemtuzumab ozogamicin on ATRA- and arsenic resistant acute promyelocytic leukemia (APL) cells. Leukemia 19:1306–1311
71. Estey E, Giles FJ, Beran M, et al (2002) Experience with gemtuzumab ozogamycin ("myelotarg") and all-trans retinoic acid in untreated acute promyelocytic leukemia. Blood 99:4222–4224
72. Lo-Coco F, Cimino G, Breccia M, et al (2004) Gemtuzumab ozogamicin (Myelotarg) as a single agent for molecularly relapsed acute promyelocytic leukemia. Blood 104:1995–1999

Targeting APL Fusion Proteins by Peptide Interference

A. Melnick

Department of Developmental and Molecular Biology and Medical Oncology, Albert Einstein College of Medicine, 1300 Morris Park Ave, Bronx, NY 10461, USA
amelnick@aecom.yu.edu

1	Introduction	222
2	Designing Therapeutic Peptides	224
2.1	Protein Transduction Domains	224
2.2	PTD Mechanism of Action	226
2.3	Working with PTDs	227
2.4	PTDs for Cancer Therapy	228
2.5	Could PTD Peptides Be Administered to Human Subjects?	228
3	Identifying Molecular Targets for Therapeutic Peptides	230
3.1	Transcription Factors as Therapeutic Targets	230
4	What Would the Clinical Applications of Peptide Interference Be in APL?	235
4.1	Peptide Interference for Frontline Therapy of APL	236
4.2	Peptides Interference for Retinoid Resistant APL	236
4.3	Peptides Interference for Retinoid Refractory APL	237
	References	238

Abstract A significant barrier to experimental therapeutics is the ability to identify and specifically target oncogenic proteins involved in the molecular pathogenesis of disease. In acute promyelocytic leukemia (APL), aberrant transcription factors and their associated machinery play a central role in mediating the malignant phenotype. The mechanism of action of APL chimeric fusion proteins involves their ability to either self-associate or interact with different partner proteins. Thus, targeting protein–protein interactions could have a significant impact in blocking the activity of APL oncoproteins. As therapeutic targets, the interface between interacting proteins may not always be amenable to highly specific small molecule blockade. In contrast, peptides are well-suited to this purpose and can be reliably delivered when fused to cell-permeable peptide domains. Therapeutic peptides can be designed to directly target APL fusion proteins, their downstream effectors, or other potentially synergistic oncogenic mechanisms of importance in APL blasts. In addition to serving as potential therapeutic agents, such reagents could serve as powerful reagents to dissect the molecular pathogenesis of APL.

1
Introduction

The study of the molecular basis and targeted therapeutics of acute promyelocytic leukemia (APL) is a remarkable success story and a paradigm for the specific biological targeting of cancer. Although now largely curable, advances continue to be made in APL molecular pathogenesis that will hopefully culminate in a nonchemotherapeutic cure for the disease. Many biological activities have been assigned to the APL fusion proteins, central among which is aberrant transcriptional repression by the respective retinoic acid receptor α (RARα) fusion proteins. Transcription-therapy targeting of APL oncoproteins by all-*trans* retinoic acid (ATRA) is highly effective, yet chemotherapy is still required for a cure (Tallman 2004). Induction or consolidation (or both) with arsenic trioxide might allow a further reduction in exposure to cytotoxic drugs (Shen et al. 2004). However, it is likely that additional therapeutic targets will need to be identified in both primary and relapsed or refractory APL that can be attacked with novel drugs to achieve long-term disease-free survival through specific molecular targeting.

One method to rapidly validate targets and generate novel APL drugs is using peptide-based drugs to disrupt critical protein–protein interactions that are required for the activity of APL oncogenes and their associated downstream pathways. Advances in cellular penetration techniques allow even relatively large peptides to be targeted to cell nuclei to disrupt transcriptional control mechanisms and other processes (Joliot and Prochiantz 2004; Wadia and Dowdy 2005). A significant advantage of such an approach is the relative ease with which peptides can be generated and tested compared to the expense and time required for screening small molecule libraries. Given the tremendous spectrum of actions described, for example, to the promyelocytic leukemia (PML)/RARα protein, specific peptide targeting of these functions could facilitate identification of which of these represent true therapeutic opportunities. From the scientific perspective, these peptides are ideal reagents for loss-of-function studies. Peptide drugs have the advantage over genetic studies such as RNA interference (RNAi) or gene knockouts in that precise time courses and dose-response curves can be generated so that direct effects can more readily be discriminated (Table 1). The goals of this manuscript are to discuss the use of cell-permeable peptides to deliver peptides that could interfere with oncogenic protein–protein interactions, to discuss selection of molecular targets for peptide interference, and to consider whether such agents might have therapeutic applications. A complete review of the molecular mechanism of action of APL fusion proteins is not intended, as this is offered elsewhere in this volume. Therefore, only a few examples of APL fusion

Table 1 Comparison of methods to block oncogenic pathways in APL

	Viral expression of peptides/RNAi	PTD—peptides	Small molecules	Knockouts
Cell types that can be targeted	Varies according to cell type	All cells are susceptible	All cells are susceptible	All cells are susceptible
Efficiency	Varies from cell to cell	Virtually 100%	Virtually 100%	100%
Expression levels	Vary from cell to cell	Dose dependent—same in all cells	Dose dependent—same in all cells	N/A
Genetic effects	Insertional mutations, inadvertent non-specific RNAi downregulation	None	None	Limited to targeted locus
Reproducibility	Variable according to cell system, excellent within a particular system	Always excellent	Always excellent	May be strain-dependent
Time to full effect	Hours to days	Minutes	Minutes	Days to months
Efficacy in vivo	Variable	Excellent	Excellent	Excellent
Cross BBB	Variable	Yes	Variable	N/A
Drawbacks	All the above	Synthetic peptides are expensive	Requires expensive screening methods	Limited to laboratory mice or cell lines. Extensive set up for each model system

N/A, not applicable

protein mechanisms are offered as examples or proof of principle, with the hope that this will trigger consideration of the many other molecular pathways discussed in the accompanying reviews as potential targets for peptide interference.

2
Designing Therapeutic Peptides

Therapeutic peptides can be designed that target cell surface molecules such as growth factor receptors and cell adhesion molecules, or that penetrate cells and target the nuclear or cytoplasmic compartments. Practically all of the therapeutic peptides in use today fall into the first category. The plasma membrane was traditionally regarded as a limiting factor for transport of molecules greater than 500 Da in size (i.e., the size of roughly three to four amino acids) (Wadia and Dowdy 2005). The interior of the cell was reserved to chemical compounds beneath this size cut-off. Small molecules are well suited to block discrete motifs such as enzymatic pockets, but may not be as well suited to interfere with more complex or more extensive protein interaction interfaces. Delivery of peptides to the interior of the cell would allow complex oncogenic protein–protein interactions to be disrupted.

2.1
Protein Transduction Domains

Fortunately, the size barrier to cell penetration can be overcome by fusing peptides or proteins to one of several protein transduction domains (PTDs). Most PTDs consist of variable chains of positively charged and hydrophobic residues usually between 5 and 20 amino acids long (Joliot and Prochiantz 2004). Examples of commonly used PTDs include natural domains such as the pTAT motif derived from the human immunodeficiency virus (HIV) TAT protein, and the penetratin motif derived from the *Drosophila* antennapedia protein, and artificially derived PTDs such as Arg9, a chain of nine arginine residues (Joliot and Prochiantz 2004; see Table 2 for comparison of PTDs). An emerging body of literature indicates that protein transduction may be a physiological property of cellular proteins such as growth factors and transcription factors (Belting et al. 2005). Thus, growth factors in addition to actions on the cell surface may penetrate cells, localize to the nuclei, and exert transcriptional or other effects (Olsnes et al. 2003). Homeoprotein transcription factors released from cells were recently proposed to form morphogenetic gradients by penetrating cells and regulating gene expression (Prochiantz and Joliot 2003).

PTDs have been used to successfully carry many different cargos and penetrate cells with virtually 100% efficiency comparable to small molecules (Nagahara et al. 1998). PTDs have the advantage over viral delivery systems in that all cell types can be transduced, there is no cell-cycle dependency, transduced proteins are maximally functional within minutes (not hours or days), and protein levels can be rigorously controlled and reproduced, and are equal

Table 2 Partial list of protein transduction domains

PTD type	Chemistry	Sequence	Reference(s)
TAT	Basic	YGRKKRRQRRR	Frankel and Pabo 1988; Green and Loewenstein 1988
Penetratin (Antp)	Basic/amphiphilic	RQIKIWFQNRRMKWKK	Derossi et al. 1994
Poly-arginine	Basic	$(R)_{7-11}$	Futaki et al. 2001
VP22	Basic/amphiphilic	DAATATRGRSAASRPTQRPRAPARSASRPRRPVQ	Elliott and O'Hare 1997
Transportan	Mixed	GWTLNSAGYLLGKINLKALAALAKKIL	Pooga et al. 1998
MAP	Basic/amphiphilic	KLALKLALKALKAALKLA	Oehlke et al. 1998
MTS	Hydrophobic	AAVALLPAVLLALLP	Lin et al. 1995
PEP-1	Mixed	KETWWETWWTEWSQPKKKRKV	Morris et al. 2001

TAT, penetratin, and poly-arginine are the most commonly used. Several of the many other cell penetrating domains along with their chemical structures are listed

from cell to cell (Barka et al. 2000). Moreover, cellular penetration is readily achieved both in vitro and in vivo (Wadia and Dowdy 2005). For example, the pTAT motif transported lacZ into all tissues and even crossed the blood–brain barrier after intraperitoneal administration into mice (Schwarze et al. 1999). Furthermore, cationic PTDs such as pTAT localize to cell nuclei, suggesting that these basic motifs may act as nuclear localization signals (NLS) (Vives et al. 1997; Wadia and Dowdy 2005). This property is particularly desirable to target transcription factors such as PML/RAR. For other PTDs, an NLS can be added to peptide constructs, with the only disadvantage being that this adds to the length of the peptide (Joliot and Prochiantz 2004). Alternatively, PTDs that normally migrate to the nucleus can be modified to target their cargo to the cytoplasm (Joliot and Prochiantz 2004). It is important to underline the complexity inherent in comparing and contrasting the often conflicting studies of PTD mechanisms of action as well as studies where the cell-penetrating activity of the different PTDs are tested head to head. The great diversity of chemical structures, cargos, epitope tags, labels, cell types, and experimental methods (etc.) make it difficult to generate an overall consensus mechanism, or to choose a "winner" among the several PTD motifs. It is possible that the best PTD for a specific cargo might need to be selected empirically. In our hands, the TAT motif has worked with very high efficiency, but may not be the best for other cargos. Other issues such as cargo linkage, length, composition, and position may also profoundly affect activity (Brooks et al. 2005).

2.2
PTD Mechanism of Action

Initial reports that protein transduction by PTDs was energy independent and could occur even at 4 C now seem most likely to be incorrect for most PTDs, attributed to phenomena such as fixation artifacts (Richard et al. 2003). Although individual PTDs might penetrate through different mechanisms (Joliot and Prochiantz 2004), much of the current data indicate that the cationic PTDs such as pTAT and penetratin undergo internalization via endocytosis (Console et al. 2003; Fischer et al. 2004; Letoha et al. 2005; Potocky et al. 2003; Wadia et al. 2004). It appears that positively charged PTDs are attracted to cells by negatively charged polymeric surface molecules such as proteoglycans and associate with lipid rafts (Console et al. 2003; Fittipaldi et al. 2003; Letoha et al. 2005; Tyagi et al. 2001; Wadia et al. 2004). In the case of TAT/cargo fusion constructs, lipid raft binding triggers dynamin-independent macropinocytosis, whereby membrane ruffles engulf TAT/cargo-coated lipid rafts (Wadia et al. 2004). The fact that all cells perform macropinocytosis explains the universality of PTD cellular penetration regardless of cell type. The resulting PTD-laden endosomes then undergo reduction of their pH (Wadia et al. 2004). Acidification of endosomes, possibly together with inherent macropinosome leakiness and the membrane destabilizing effects of PTD/lipid raft complexes results in escape of PTDs into the cytoplasm (Fischer et al. 2004; Potocky et al. 2003; Wadia et al. 2004). Released PTD is then amenable to nuclear transport via the importin system. The remaining bulk of PTDs are probably degraded within the endosomes or expelled by endosome recycling. It is possible that some cell types incorporate certain TAT-cargo fusions or unconjugated TAT via clathrin or caveolin-dependent endocytosis as well (Ferrari et al. 2003; Fittipaldi et al. 2003; Richard et al. 2005). Consistent with the macropinocytosis route (in which endosomal acidification occurs), it was recently shown that TAT-mediated delivery of cargo could be enhanced by adding TAT fused to the influenza virus fusogenic HA2 motif, that destabilizes endosomal membranes at low pH (Wadia et al. 2004). Combining pTAT-HA2 with a standard pTAT-cargo fusion enhanced the biological activity of the cargo peptide due to enhanced release of peptides from endosomes (Wadia et al. 2004). In our hands, the HA2 fusogenic motif is equally effective when included within the pTAT-cargo construct in *cis* (L. Cerchietti and A. Melnick, unpublished data), and thus should be considered by investigators performing peptide transduction for inclusion in their constructs.

2.3
Working with PTDs

Many targeting efforts begin by generating PTD fusion plasmids and expressing the recombinant peptide in appropriate strains of *Escherichia coli*. Most PTD constructs form inclusion bodies that require solubilization for subsequent purification steps. Purification is typically achieved by affinity chromatography of (HIS)6 or glutathione-*S*-transferase (GST)-tagged constructs (Wade et al. 1999) followed by a final purification step to remove additional impurities. It is critical to recognize that design flaws in the peptide constructs may significantly impair their functionality. For example, we found that addition of a FLAG epitope to the C-terminus of one our pTAT constructs considerably reduced its activity (J. Polo and A. Melnick, unpublished data). We hypothesized that the negatively charged FLAG motif was binding to the positively charged pTAT motif and impeding its function. Deleting this FLAG epitope eliminated the problem. TAT proteins can also be generated from mammalian cells, as cell lines have been generated that express and secret pTAT fusions proteins that can then be harvested or the conditioned media directly used to deliver peptides to other cells (Barka et al. 2004).

After exposure of cells to PTDs, the peptides localize mainly to the cell membrane or endosomes while only a small percentage enters the cytoplasm and nucleus. Lysis or fixation of cells causes surface and endosome-located peptide to rush into cells, giving the false impression that the most peptide is localized within the cells (Richard et al. 2003). Repeated washing of cells is insufficient to strip off peptide attached to the cell surface, so methods such as trypsin digestion are required to avoid this pitfall (Richard et al. 2003). Another way to overcome these artifacts is to perform live cell imaging, or functional assays in living cells. A functional experiment showing definitive proof of nuclear localization of a pTAT fusion in living cells revealed that a TAT-cre recombinase peptide could excise a floxed stop cassette from an integrated reporter construct and trigger expression of green fluorescent protein (GFP) (Wadia et al. 2004).

Chemical synthesis offers an alternative to recombinant peptide production. Many PTD sequences are difficult to synthesize and so particular attention must be paid to HPLC and mass spectroscopy readouts. Synthesis should be performed in a facility with experience in producing such peptides. Synthesis of long peptides might require that different components of the peptide be synthesized separately for subsequent chemical linkage. Chemical synthesis also offers the opportunity to generate therapeutic peptides consisting of D-amino acids in retro-inverso configuration to avoid degradation by cellular proteases (Snyder et al. 2004). For example, in a recent study where p53 C-terminal activating peptide was used to kill cancer cells, the retro-inverso version of the peptide was more potent and required less frequent dosing than the L-amino acid counterpart (Snowden et al. 2003).

2.4
PTDs for Cancer Therapy

Peptide transduction by the pTAT and other transduction domains is a promising method to deliver therapeutic agents for cancer and other diseases. A number of oncogenes and tumor suppressors that function as transcription factors, cell cycle regulators, signal transduction mediators, or apoptotic machinery have been targeted (see Table 3). For example, we recently designed a therapeutic PTD construct containing a 20-amino-acid peptide that blocks the ability of the N-terminal BTB/POZ (bric á brac tramtrack broad complex/pox virus zinc finger) domain of the BCL6 (B cell lymphoma 6) transcriptional repressor to recruit the SMRT, N-CoR, and BCoR corepressors (silencing-mediator for retinoid/thyroid hormone receptors, nuclear receptor corepressor, BCL6 corepressor) (Polo et al. 2004). This BCL6 peptide inhibitor (BPI) reactivated BCL6 endogenous target genes, stripped corepressors off of endogenous BCL6 target promoters, and phenocopied the BCL6-null phenotype when injected into mice (Polo et al. 2004). By exposing B cell lymphomas to BPI, we showed that BCL6 is a true oncogene, required for maintenance of the malignant phenotype of these tumors. Accordingly, BPI selectively killed diffuse large-cell lymphoma cells that express BCL6, without affecting other types of cells (Polo et al. 2004), so that BPI might be an effective targeted therapy agent for B cell lymphomas.

2.5
Could PTD Peptides Be Administered to Human Subjects?

Ideally, a peptide drug for cancer should be as short as possible, be non- or minimally toxic, be active in the nanomolar range, achieve levels in tumors, have a long half-life, and be nonimmunogenic. Animal data indicate that therapeutic cell-permeable peptides administered at effective anticancer doses are not toxic to mice, suggesting that clinical translation might be feasible (Polo et al. 2004; Snyder et al. 2004). Pharmacokinetic studies in humans, ability to establish therapeutic levels within tumors, and potential for immunogenicity

Table 3 Some examples of PTDs and cargos used to target cancer cells

PTD	Cargo	Target tumors or cells	Dose range in vitro	Tested in vivo	Reference
TAT	N-CoR fragments	APL, t(8;21) AML	0.2 µM	No	Racanicchi et al. 2005
TAT	BCL6 inhibitor peptide	DLBCL	0.1–2 µM	Yes	Polo et al. 2004
TAT	p53C/ retro-inverso	Ovarian cancer peritoneal carcinomatosis	5–30 µM	Yes	Snyder et al. 2004
TAT	NF2/Merlin	Human primary Schwannomas	60 µM	No	Bashour et al. 2002
TAT	E2F cyclin A binding peptide	Osteosarcoma and breast cancer cell lines	5–90 µM	No	Chen et al. 1999
TAT	Von Hippel Landau	786-O renal carcinoma cells	10–40 µM	Yes	Datta et al. 2001
TAT	RasGAP cleavage fragment	HeLa, U2OS, MCF7, meso1	20 µM	No	Michod et al. 2004
TAT	Smac5/DIABLO peptide that blocks IAPs	Glioblastoma	200–500 µM	Yes	Fulda et al. 2002
PolyArginine		Lung cancer cell line	20 µM	Yes	Yang et al. 2003
PolyArginine	BH3 domain	Leukemia cell lines	10–30 µM	No	Letai et al. 2002
Hydrocarbon Stapled BH3	BH3 domain helix	Leukemia cell lines	5 µM	Yes	Walensky et al. 2004
Penetratin	NEMO oligomerization blocking peptide	Retinoblastoma cells	5–10 µM	No	Agou et al. 2004
Penetratin	Plk1 Polo-box domain	MCF7, HeLa	5 uM	No	Yuan et al. 2002
Penetratin	P16$^{84-103}$	Pancreatic cancer cell lines	10–20 µM	Yes	Hosotani et al. 2002; Fujimoto et al. 2000
Penetratin	Retro-inverso Myc peptide	MCF7 cells	5–10 µM	No	Pescarolo et al. 2001

all require close attention, but do not seem insurmountable barriers given the mouse in vivo data and clinical experience with extracellular peptide or protein drugs. A critical consideration is the dose requirement. This is a function of peptide affinity to its target, its mechanism of action, and pharmacokinetics. Peptides that are only active at high micromolar concentrations are unlikely to be practical in the clinical setting. However, peptides (such as BPI) that are active in the nanomolar range might be more immediately amenable to therapeutic application (Polo and Melnick 2004). Investigators interested in developing cell-permeable peptides need to consider modifications such as engineering super-binding peptides, incorporating HA2, using D-amino acids, and including ligands that specifically direct peptides to their target cells. PTD-based drugs are currently in clinical trials using both topical and parenteral routes, though there is no public data yet on their kinetics and toxicity. Overall, it seems the time has come for this class of drug to be tested in the clinical setting. Therefore, it is appropriate to consider how cell-permeable peptide drugs might be developed as targeted therapy for APL.

3
Identifying Molecular Targets for Therapeutic Peptides

The first step in generating therapeutic peptides is to identify the molecular target. Ideally, the target should be a critical mediator of the malignant phenotype. This includes "primary" targets, such as mutant or constitutively expressed oncogenes (i.e., the RARα fusion proteins and Flt3 receptor-activating mutations in APL) or "secondary" targets, such as cellular machinery required for the activity of the oncogene and downstream mediators of oncogene effects. Examples of secondary targets include but are not limited to (1) proteins such as N-CoR and SMRT that are required for transcriptional repression by PML/RARα (Lin et al. 1998), (2) proteins that become deregulated by interference of PML/RARα with the normal functions of PML [such as p53 (Ferbeyre et al. 2000; Pearson et al. 2000)], or (3) downstream target genes of PML/RARα [such as C/EBPβ and PU.1 (Duprez et al. 2003; Mueller et al. 2006)]. Directly targeting primary oncogenes would generally be predicted to be more effective and cell type-specific than hitting secondary targets.

3.1
Transcription Factors as Therapeutic Targets

APL fusion proteins are transcription factors that mediate aberrant repression. Although transcription factors have not traditionally been exploited as therapeutic targets, the success of ATRA demonstrates that such proteins can be effectively targeted. The fact that many oncogenes and tumor suppressors are transcription factors, and that such proteins are typically upstream of an extensive network of downstream mediators is consistent with the prediction that these are worthy of consideration as therapeutic targets (Melnick 2005). Transcription factors often lack enzymatic activities and are dependent on protein–protein interactions for their functions. Since a typical transcription factor may recruit many different partners, several different components could be targeted. The fact that PML/RARα can recruit N-CoR, SMRT, histone deacetylases (HDACs), and DNA methyltransferases (DNMTs) suggests that targeting the recruitment or activity of any of these components could be useful in APL (Fazi et al. 2005; Grignani et al. 1998; Lin et al. 1998). Given the complexity of transcriptional regulation, it is safe to assume that APL fusion proteins recruit multiple cofactors, so that many potential targets exist. A general predictive model of the effect of targeting APL fusion protein complexes and their associated pathways and target genes can be conceived whereby the more proximal the peptide or drug is to the X-RARα fusion, the greater the specificity, therapeutic window, and efficacy (Fig. 1; Melnick 2005). That is, the closer one is to the oncogene directly controlling the APL genetic program, the more profound the biological impact will be, and conversely, targeting X-RARα partner proteins that are involved in many other cellular processes might have many off-target effects. Accordingly, ATRA therapy is highly effective and specific for APL, while HDAC inhibitor therapy is less effective and specific (Melnick 2005; Melnick et al. 2005).

From the *biochemical* standpoint, therapeutic peptides are well suited for disrupting protein–protein interactions or inducing conformational changes in target proteins. For protein interfaces or motifs that have large or highly complex surface areas, peptides may indeed be more specific and effective than small molecules. These properties could be very important in targeting APL-related proteins. Peptides can be designed to block enzymatic activities, although it is unclear in this case whether they would be superior to small-molecule targeting. To generate a therapeutic peptide it is useful to obtain as much structural information as possible regarding the biochemical features of the target. Ideally, X-ray crystallography or nuclear magnetic resonance of the protein interface should be performed to determine folding requirements for binding and identify the critical intermolecular contacts. Moreover, careful comparative studies of the target interface with other related proteins should be considered and tested to determine the likely specificity of the therapeutic peptide. An example of this approach is the BCL6 inhibitor peptide BPI, which was based on the crystal structure of the BCL6–SMRT complex (Polo et al.

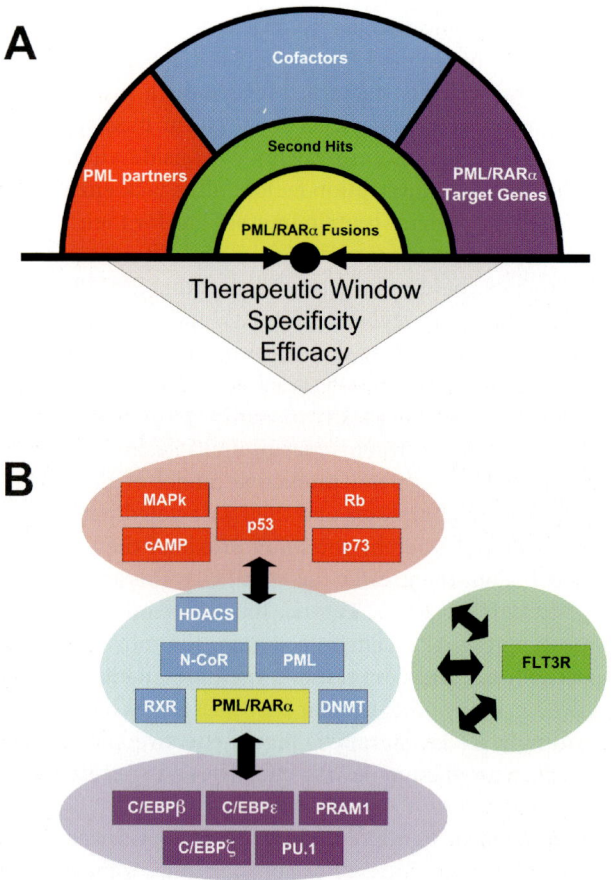

2004). The residues that mediate intermolecular contacts are unique to BCL6 among the family of BTB/POZ transcription factors, and as a consequence BPI is highly specific for BCL6 but not other proteins (Polo et al. 2004).

The most straightforward peptide-targeting strategy would utilize linear, unstructured sequences that are free of proline residues so that retro-inverso residues can be substituted for natural amino acids (the stereochemistry of proline is altered in a retro-inverso configuration and might abolish binding). If secondary structure is required, more sophisticated techniques such as is exemplified by hydrocarbon stapling of α-helical BH3 domains for inhibition of BCL2 may be required to stabilize the proper folding configuration (Walensky et al. 2004). To disrupt large protein complexes or proteins with multiple contacts, linking of several peptide motifs might be required with

Fig. 1a, b Finding therapeutic targets in t(15;17) APL. **a** Schematic representation of the kinds of therapeutic targets including, from the center toward the periphery, the PML/RARα fusion proteins, second oncogenic hits, and then PML/RARα partner proteins, PML/RARα target genes, and PML/RARα cofactors. Since PML/RARα is the central oncogene in APL, therapeutic targeting closer to the center (i.e., PML/RARα) will generally be more specific and effective, and have a greater therapeutic window. Targeting more distally is likely to affect a number of other mechanisms other than those directly involved in APL pathogenesis. **b** Some examples of possible therapeutic targets in these different compartments—color-coded to match *panel a*. *MAPk*, mitogen activated protein kinase (Hayakawa and Privalsky 2004); *cAMP*, cyclic adenosine mono phosphate pathway (Kamashev et al. 2004); *p53* (Ferbeyre et al. 2000); *p73* (Bernassola et al. 2004); *Rb*, retinoblastoma protein (Alcalay et al. 1998; Mallette et al. 2004); *HDACs*, histone deacetylases (Grignani et al. 1998; Lin et al. 1998); *RXR*, retinoid X receptor (Dong et al. 2004; Kamashev et al. 2004); *N-CoR*, nuclear receptor corepressor (Grignani et al. 1998; Lin et al. 1998); *DNMT*, DNA methyltransferase (Di Croce et al. 2002); *Flt3 receptor* (Kiyoi et al. 1997); *PU.1* (Mueller et al. 2006); *C/EBPβ*, -ε, and -ζ, CCATT/enhancer binding proteins (Duprez et al. 2003; Gery et al. 2004); *PRAM1*, PML/RARα target gene encoding an adaptor molecule-1 (Moog-Lutz et al. 2001)

consideration of proper spacing and flexibility. Targeting to the proper cellular compartment should also be considered to maximize concentration of peptide near its intended targets.

Interfering peptides can be designed based on careful mapping studies of protein–protein interactions, even in the absence of structural data. However, it is important to determine whether secondary or tertiary structure is required for binding of either of the two partner proteins, since linear peptides are most amenable for incorporation into blocking peptides. PML/RARα in its basal state interacts with the N-CoR and SMRT corepressors that mediate transcriptional silencing. Transcriptional activation by PML/RARα in response to pharmacologic doses of ATRA occurs via a conformational shift that releases these corepressors and instead recruits coactivator proteins (Grignani et al. 1998; Lin et al. 1998). Mapping of the N-CoR corepressor interaction with the ligand-binding domain of nuclear hormone receptors indicated that binding occurs through two N-CoR domains (ID1 and ID2) containing an extended helical LXXI/HIXXXI/L motif (Hu and Lazar 1999). Accordingly, ID1 or ID2 peptides could block transcriptional repression by unliganded nuclear hormone receptor in reporter assays, by blocking corepressor recruitment (Hu and Lazar 1999). The same peptides induced differentiation of NB4 APL cells when fused to pTAT, consistent with the notion that PML/RARα-mediated transcriptional repression is necessary and sufficient for the differentiation block phenotype of t(15;17) APL (Racanicchi et al. 2005).

Blocking peptides can also be identified by screening methods such as phage display (Mourez and Collier 2004) or peptide aptamer libraries, which require a functional assay for the protein or protein interface of interest (Crawford et al. 2003). For example, a peptide aptamer was recently identified that disrupts the activity of signal transducer and activator of transcription 3 (STAT3) (Nagel-Wolfrum et al. 2004). PML/RARα was recently suggested to induce aberrant STAT3 activation by blocking the inhibitory actions of wildtype PML on STAT3 (Kawasaki et al. 2003). PML/RARα could thus increase sensitivity to the growth-inducing activities of the granulocyte colony-stimulating factor (G-CSF) receptor (Kawasaki et al. 2003), and the STAT3 aptamer might abrogate this activity in APL cells.

From the *biological* standpoint, the RARα fusion proteins and their downstream pathways and cellular responses should all be considered as potential targets in APL. The more "upstream" the target, the greater the spectrum of effects that can be expected. Preferentially, the target should be dispensable for survival of normal cells to minimize toxicity. In t(15;17) APL, interference of PML/RARα with the normal functions of PML (causing resistance to cell death) and RARα (causing differentiation block and aberrant self renewal) both contribute to disease (Melnick and Licht 1999). Targeting the RARα portion of the fusion protein with N-CoR peptides induces differentiation in APL cells, and eventually leads to degradation of PML/RARα (Racanicchi et al. 2005). It is therefore reasonable to question whether directly targeting the PML portion of the fusion protein might also provide antileukemia activity complementary to targeting the RARα moiety, possibly leading to greater APL cell death. All variants of the PML/RARα fusion protein retain the PML RBCC motif (consisting of a RING domain, B-boxes and coiled-coil motif). The RING and B-boxes are zinc finger variants and mediate heterodimerization with other proteins (Jensen et al. 2001). The coiled-coil (CC) motif mediates oligomerization of PML/RARα and interaction of PML/RARα with wildtype PML (Jensen et al. 2001). Oligomerization is required for the oncogenic activity of APL fusion proteins including PML/RARα (Minucci et al. 2000). Contegno et al. constructed a p53-PML CC fusion protein to generate what they termed an "oligomerization chain reaction" that biologically inactivated wildtype p53, presumably by forming large, inactive oligomers (Contegno et al. 2002). Likewise, it is conceivable that the CC could be expressed as a TAT fusion peptide, to inactivate PML/RARα oligomers, although it might also affect other proteins that contain RBCC motifs as well. Alternatively, a TAT/CC/N-CoR interacting domain hybrid peptide, by virtue of having binding sites for both parts of the t(15;17) fusion protein, might bind with greater affinity to PML/RARα than to wildtype PML or RARα, thus achieving greater selectivity.

As targeting single oncogenic proteins is generally not sufficient to eradicate human tumors, peptide targeting should be considered in the context of other methods for attacking tumor cells. In transcription therapy of APL and other cancers, sequential targeting of a primary transcription factor, followed by targeting of an important downstream effector could potentiate response with minimal effects to normal tissues. For example, PML/RARα can disrupt the ability of the wildtype PML allele to stabilize and activate p53, and can thus overcome p53-mediated senescence (Ferbeyre 2002). Since ATRA can restore the functions of wildtype PML, tandem treatment of t(15;17) APL blasts with a p53 C-terminal activating peptide after ATRA therapy might potentiate antileukemic activity. Additional PML- and PML/RARα-interacting proteins could likewise be amenable to modulation via interference in protein–protein interactions.

Peptide inhibitors of target genes regulated by APL oncoproteins could provide important insights into molecular pathogenesis and enhance the activity of existing therapeutic agents. For example, PML/RARα (but not wildtype RARα) represses expression of the leucine zipper C/EBPβ transcription factor, and reactivation of this gene by ATRA plays an important role in APL granulocytic differentiation (Duprez et al. 2003). ATRA also overcomes PML/RARα repression of C/EBPζ, which can dimerize with C/EBPβ and C/EBPε (also a PML/RARα target gene) (Gery et al. 2004). Interestingly, the leucine zipper motif of C/EBPζ is deficient in DNA binding, so that its interaction with C/EBPβ and C/EBPε can disrupt their transactivation of myeloid genes (Gery et al. 2004). The biological significance of ATRA-induced upregulation of C/EBPζ along with C/EBPβ and C/EBPε is unknown. As structural data are available for these leucine zipper domains, it is reasonable to question whether peptides could be designed that could preferentially bind C/EBPζ and block its binding to C/EBPβ and C/EBPε, to reveal the contribution of these proteins to APL blast differentiation.

4
What Would the Clinical Applications of Peptide Interference Be in APL?

Treatment of APL with combinations of ATRA, arsenic trioxide, and chemotherapy is highly effective in inducing complete remission and long-term disease-free survival (Tallman 2004). It is thus appropriate to ask whether there is a need for development of additional targeted therapy. It can be argued, however, that since APL is remarkably susceptible to interference in its molecular pathways of leukemogenesis, it is worthwhile to attempt to achieve disease-free survival without cytotoxic drugs as a long-term scientific and medical goal. Given the facility of targeting molecular pathways by peptide interference, this approach is likely to be informative in validating molecular targets and potential therapeutic agents. Moreover, significant therapeutic challenges remain in the case of patients with acquired retinoid resistance or retinoid refractory disease.

4.1
Peptide Interference for Frontline Therapy of APL

Although current frontline therapy for t(15;17) APL it is highly effective, there is a rationale for seeking cure of the disease via targeted therapy. A remaining barrier to this goal is that with the exception of the frequent mutations of the FLT3 receptor (Callens et al. 2005), little is known about additional oncogenic hits occurring in APL. Nonetheless, recent data indicating the potential impact of cyclic adenosine monophosphate (cAMP) signaling for overcoming differentiation block in APL (Kamashev et al. 2004), the contribution of DNA methyltransferase recruitment by PML/RARα to mediate stable silencing of target genes (Di Croce et al. 2002), the impact of PML/RARα on the retinoblastoma (Rb) and p53 pathways (Ferbeyre et al. 2000; Mallette et al. 2004), etc., suggest that additional molecular targeting of PML/RARα and its downstream pathways is feasible. Potential applications of peptide interference in frontline disease could be to target downstream pathways, such as (1) enhancing the activity of wildtype PML, for example by stimulating p53 activity (e.g., by using p53C peptides), (2) enhancing differentiation by modulating the activity of downstream mediators such as CEBPβ and PU.1 (e.g., by blocking CEBPζ), or (3) targeting cooperating oncogenic hits as they are discovered.

4.2
Peptides Interference for Retinoid Resistant APL

Primary retinoid resistance in t(15:17) APL is extremely rare (Gallagher 2002), but secondary retinoid resistance is common, especially in patients with two or more relapses (Gallagher 2002). Resistance occurs through both pharmacokinetic and pharmacodynamic mechanisms (Gallagher 2002). Among the latter, mutations of PML/RARα that reduce its affinity or responsiveness to ATRA are common (Gallagher 2002). At the molecular level, patients that fail to achieve therapeutic concentrations of ATRA in APL cells, or that harbor PML/RARα mutants insensitive to ATRA, are unable to undergo the retinoid-induced release of corepressors that releases fusion protein target genes from aberrant transcriptional silencing (Gallagher 2002; Melnick and Licht 1999). However, corepressor exchange can be achieved by blocking PML/RARα with

TAT–N-CoR peptides, leading to myeloid differentiation even in retinoid-resistant APL cells (Racanicchi et al. 2005). Since TAT–N-CoR peptides also induced PML/RARα degradation, it is possible that peptide interference of PML/RARα could be clinically useful. This peptide or a combined N-CoR motif/PML CC peptide together with other agents such as arsenic trioxide might overcome most cases of acquired retinoid resistance and improve the therapeutic outcome of salvage therapy.

4.3
Peptides Interference for Retinoid Refractory APL

The t(11;17) APL variant that harbors the PLZF/RARα fusion protein is refractory to ATRA therapy. The PLZF moiety of the fusion protein contains a BTB/POZ repression domain that binds the N-CoR and SMRT corepressors in a retinoid-independent manner so that transcriptional repression is not relieved by ATRA (Grignani et al. 1998; Lin et al. 1998). The structure of the PLZF BTB domain was solved by X-ray crystallography (Ahmad et al. 1998). The BTB domain contains a charged pocket motif that is required for its transcriptional repression activity and for recruitment of N-CoR and SMRT (Melnick et al. 2000, 2002). This interface is different from that of BCL6, which recruits N-CoR and SMRT to a region of its BTB domain distinct from the charged pocket that is not conserved in PLZF (Ahmad et al. 2003). The PLZF BTB charged pocket was also required for oncogenic activities of the PLZF/RARα fusion protein (Puccetti et al. 2005). Therefore, the PLZF BTB charged pocket appears to be an excellent molecular target for development of a therapeutic agent that might synergize with ATRA to induce differentiation in t(11;17) APL cells. As the structure of the corepressor fragment that binds the PLZF–BTB charged pocket is not yet known, identification of potential binding peptides will require careful mapping of corepressor surfaces or a peptide screening approach.

In summary, specific blockade of protein–protein interactions by cell-permeable peptides is feasible and effective in vitro and in vivo. Such peptides are powerful research tools since they allow the contribution of specific proteins for maintenance of the malignant phenotype to be precisely determined. Moreover, these peptides may have therapeutic activity against APL cells that could warrant their translation into clinical trials. Given recent advances in the biochemistry of cell-permeable peptide drugs, it seems that the time for testing peptides as cancer therapeutic drugs has come. It is hoped that this review will inspire and encourage investigators in the field to take advantage of these tools to further expand the horizons of scientific progress in understanding APL fusion proteins and their normal counterparts.

Acknowledgements AMM is supported by NCI R01 CA104348, the G&P Foundation, Chemotherapy Foundation, and the Leukemia and Lymphoma Society of America.

References

Agou F, Courtois G, Chiaravalli J, Baleux F, Coic YM, Traincard F, Israel A, Veron M (2004) Inhibition of NF-kappa B activation by peptides targeting NF-kappa B essential modulator (nemo) oligomerization. J Biol Chem 279:54248–54257

Ahmad KF, Engel CK, Prive GG (1998) Crystal structure of the BTB domain from PLZF. Proc Natl Acad Sci U S A 95:12123–12128

Ahmad KF, Melnick A, Lax S, Bouchard D, Liu J, Kiang CL, Mayer S, Takahashi S, Licht JD, Prive GG (2003) Mechanism of SMRT corepressor recruitment by the BCL6 BTB domain. Mol Cell 12:1551–1564

Alcalay M, Tomassoni L, Colombo E, Stoldt S, Grignani F, Fagioli M, Szekely L, Helin K, Pelicci PG (1998) The promyelocytic leukemia gene product (PML) forms stable complexes with the retinoblastoma protein. Mol Cell Biol 18:1084–1093

Barka T, Gresik EW, van Der Noen H (2000) Transduction of TAT-HA-beta-galactosidase fusion protein into salivary gland-derived cells and organ cultures of the developing gland, and into rat submandibular gland in vivo. J Histochem Cytochem 48:1453–1460

Barka T, Gresik ES, Henderson SC (2004) Production of cell lines secreting TAT fusion proteins. J Histochem Cytochem 52:469–477

Bashour AM, Meng JJ, Ip W, MacCollin M, Ratner N (2002) The neurofibromatosis type 2 gene product, merlin, reverses the F-actin cytoskeletal defects in primary human Schwannoma cells. Mol Cell Biol 22:1150–1157

Belting M, Sandgren S, Wittrup A (2005) Nuclear delivery of macromolecules: barriers and carriers. Adv Drug Deliv Rev 57:505–527

Bernassola F, Salomoni P, Oberst A, Di Como CJ, Pagano M, Melino G, Pandolfi PP (2004) Ubiquitin-dependent degradation of p73 is inhibited by PML. J Exp Med 199:1545–1557

Brooks H, Lebleu B, Vives E (2005) Tat peptide-mediated cellular delivery: back to basics. Adv Drug Deliv Rev 57:559–577

Callens C, Chevret S, Cayuela JM, Cassinat B, Raffoux E, de Botton S, Thomas X, Guerci A, Fegueux N, Pigneux A, Stoppa AM, Lamy T, Rigal-Huguet F, Vekhoff A, Meyer-Monard S, Ferrand A, Sanz M, Chomienne C, Fenaux P, Dombret H (2005) Prognostic implication of FLT3 and Ras gene mutations in patients with acute promyelocytic leukemia (APL): a retrospective study from the European APL Group. Leukemia 19:1153–1160

Chen YN, Sharma SK, Ramsey TM, Jiang L, Martin MS, Baker K, Adams PD, Bair KW, Kaelin WG Jr (1999) Selective killing of transformed cells by cyclin/cyclin-dependent kinase 2 antagonists. Proc Natl Acad Sci U S A 96:4325–4329

Console S, Marty C, Garcia-Echeverria C, Schwendener R, Ballmer-Hofer K (2003) Antennapedia and HIV transactivator of transcription (TAT) "protein transduction domains" promote endocytosis of high molecular weight cargo upon binding to cell surface glycosaminoglycans. J Biol Chem 278:35109–35114

Contegno F, Cioce M, Pelicci PG, Minucci S (2002) Targeting protein inactivation through an oligomerization chain reaction. Proc Natl Acad Sci U S A 99:1865–1869

Crawford M, Woodman R, Ko Ferrigno P (2003) Peptide aptamers: tools for biology and drug discovery. Brief Funct Genomic Proteomic 2:72–79

Datta K, Sundberg C, Karumanchi SA, Mukhopadhyay D (2001) The 104-123 amino acid sequence of the beta-domain of von Hippel-Lindau gene product is sufficient to inhibit renal tumor growth and invasion. Cancer Res 61:1768–1775

Derossi D, Joliot AH, Chassaing G, Prochiantz A (1994) The third helix of the Antennapedia homeodomain translocates through biological membranes. J Biol Chem 269:10444–10450

Di Croce L, Raker VA, Corsaro M, Fazi F, Fanelli M, Faretta M, Fuks F, Lo Coco F, Kouzarides T, Nervi C, Minucci S, Pelicci PG (2002) Identification of a zinc finger domain in the human NEIL2 (Nei-like-2) protein. Science 295:1079–1082

Dong S, Stenoien DL, Qiu J, Mancini MA, Tweardy DJ (2004) Reduced intranuclear mobility of APL fusion proteins accompanies their mislocalization and results in sequestration and decreased mobility of retinoid X receptor alpha. Mol Cell Biol 24:4465–4475

Duprez E, Wagner K, Koch H, Tenen DG (2003) C/EBPbeta: a major PML-RARA-responsive gene in retinoic acid-induced differentiation of APL cells. EMBO J 22:5806–5816

Elliott G, O'Hare P (1997) Intercellular trafficking and protein delivery by a herpesvirus structural protein. Cell 88:223–233

Fazi F, Travaglini L, Carotti D, Palitti F, Diverio D, Alcalay M, McNamara S, Miller W HJr, Lo Coco F, Pelicci PG, Nervi C (2005) Retinoic acid targets DNA-methyltransferases and histone deacetylases during APL blast differentiation in vitro and in vivo. Oncogene 24:1820–1830

Ferbeyre G (2002) PML a target of translocations in APL is a regulator of cellular senescence. Leukemia 16:1918–1926

Ferbeyre G, de Stanchina E, Querido E, Baptiste N, Prives C, Lowe SW (2000) PML is induced by oncogenic ras and promotes premature senescence. Genes Dev 14:2015–2027

Ferrari A, Pellegrini V, Arcangeli C, Fittipaldi A, Giacca M, Beltram F (2003) Caveolae-mediated internalization of extracellular HIV-1 tat fusion proteins visualized in real time. Mol Ther 8:284–294

Fischer R, Kohler K, Fotin-Mleczek M, Brock R (2004) A stepwise dissection of the intracellular fate of cationic cell-penetrating peptides. J Biol Chem 279:12625–12635

Fittipaldi A, Ferrari A, Zoppe M, Arcangeli C, Pellegrini V, Beltram F, Giacca M (2003) Cell membrane lipid rafts mediate caveolar endocytosis of HIV-1 Tat fusion proteins. J Biol Chem 278:34141–34149

Frankel AD, Pabo CO (1988) Cellular uptake of the tat protein from human immunodeficiency virus. Cell 55:1189–1193

Fujimoto K, Hosotani R, Miyamoto Y, Doi R, Koshiba T, Otaka A, Fujii N, Beauchamp RD, Imamura M (2000) Inhibition of pRb phosphorylation and cell cycle progression by an antennapedia-p16(INK4A) fusion peptide in pancreatic cancer cells. Cancer Lett 159:151–158

Fulda S, Wick W, Weller M, Debatin KM (2002) Smac agonists sensitize for Apo2L/TRAIL- or anticancer drug-induced apoptosis and induce regression of malignant glioma in vivo. Nat Med 8:808–815

Futaki S, Suzuki T, Ohashi W, Yagami T, Tanaka S, Ueda K, Sugiura Y (2001) Arginine-rich peptides. An abundant source of membrane-permeable peptides having potential as carriers for intracellular protein delivery. J Biol Chem 276:5836–5840

Gallagher RE (2002) Retinoic acid resistance in acute promyelocytic leukemia. Leukemia 16:1940–1958

Gery S, Park DJ, Vuong PT, Chih DY, Lemp N, Koeffler HP (2004) Retinoic acid regulates C/EBP homologous protein expression (CHOP), which negatively regulates myeloid target genes. Blood 104:3911–3917

Green M, Loewenstein PM (1988) Autonomous functional domains of chemically synthesized human immunodeficiency virus tat trans-activator protein. Cell 55:1179–1188

Grignani F, De Matteis S, Nervi C, Tomassoni L, Gelmetti V, Cioce M, Fanelli M, Ruthardt M, Ferrara FF, Zamir I, Seiser C, Lazar MA, Minucci S, Pelicci PG (1998) Cloning and characterization of a novel human histone deacetylase, HDAC8. Nature 391:815–818

Hayakawa F, Privalsky ML (2004) Phosphorylation of PML by mitogen-activated protein kinases plays a key role in arsenic trioxide-mediated apoptosis. Cancer Cell 5:389–401

Hosotani R, Miyamoto Y, Fujimoto K, Doi R, Otaka A, Fujii N, Imamura M (2002) Trojan p16 peptide suppresses pancreatic cancer growth and prolongs survival in mice. Clin Cancer Res 8:1271–1276

Hu X, Lazar MA (1999) The CoRNR motif controls the recruitment of corepressors by nuclear hormone receptors. Nature 402:93–96

Jensen K, Shiels C, Freemont PS (2001) PML protein isoforms and the RBCC/TRIM motif. Oncogene 20:7223–7233

Joliot A, Prochiantz A (2004) Transduction peptides: from technology to physiology. Nat Cell Biol 6:189–196

Kamashev D, Vitoux D, De The H (2004) PML-RARA-RXR oligomers mediate retinoid and rexinoid/cAMP cross-talk in acute promyelocytic leukemia cell differentiation. J Exp Med 199:1163–1174

Kawasaki A, Matsumura I, Kataoka Y, Takigawa E, Nakajima K, Kanakura Y (2003) Opposing effects of PML and PML/RAR alpha on STAT3 activity. Blood 101:3668–3673

Kiyoi H, Naoe T, Yokota S, Nakao M, Minami S, Kuriyama K, Takeshita A, Saito K, Hasegawa S, Shimodaira S, Tamura J, Shimazaki C, Matsue K, Kobayashi H, Arima N, Suzuki R, Morishita H, Saito H, Ueda R, Ohno R (1997) Internal tandem duplication of FLT3 associated with leukocytosis in acute promyelocytic leukemia. Leukemia Study Group of the Ministry of Health and Welfare (Kohseisho). Leukemia 11:1447–1452

Letai A, Bassik MC, Walensky LD, Sorcinelli MD, Weiler S, Korsmeyer SJ (2002) Distinct BH3 domains either sensitize or activate mitochondrial apoptosis, serving as prototype cancer therapeutics. Cancer Cell 2:183–192

Letoha T, Gaal S, Somlai C, Venkei Z, Glavinas H, Kusz E, Duda E, Czajlik A, Petak F, Penke B (2005) Investigation of penetratin peptides. Part 2 In vitro uptake of penetratin and two of its derivatives. J Pept Sci 11:805–811

Lin RJ, Nagy L, Inoue S, Shao W, Miller W HJr, Evans RM (1998) Role of the histone deacetylase complex in acute promyelocytic leukaemia. Nature 391:811–814

Lin YZ, Yao SY, Veach RA, Torgerson TR, Hawiger J (1995) Inhibition of nuclear translocation of transcription factor NF-kappa B by a synthetic peptide containing a cell membrane-permeable motif and nuclear localization sequence. J Biol Chem 270:14255–14258

Mallette FA, Goumard S, Gaumont-Leclerc MF, Moiseeva O, Ferbeyre G (2004) Human fibroblasts require the Rb family of tumor suppressors, but not p53, for PML-induced senescence. Oncogene 23:91–99

Melnick A (2005) Predicting the effect of transcription therapy in hematologic malignancies. Leukemia 19:1109–1117

Melnick A, Licht JD (1999) Deconstructing a disease: RARalpha, its fusion partners, and their roles in the pathogenesis of acute promyelocytic leukemia. Blood 93:3167–3215

Melnick A, Ahmad KF, Arai S, Polinger A, Ball H, Borden KL, Carlile GW, Prive GG, Licht JD (2000) In-depth mutational analysis of the promyelocytic leukemia zinc finger BTB/POZ domain reveals motifs and residues required for biological and transcriptional functions. Mol Cell Biol 20:6550–6567

Melnick A, Carlile G, Ahmad KF, Kiang CL, Corcoran C, Bardwell V, Prive GG, Licht JD (2002) Critical residues within the BTB domain of PLZF and Bcl-6 modulate interaction with corepressors. Mol Cell Biol 22:1804–1818

Melnick AM, Adelson K, Licht JD (2005) The theoretical basis of transcriptional therapy of cancer: can it be put into practice? J Clin Oncol 23:3957–3970

Michod D, Yang JY, Chen J, Bonny C, Widmann C (2004) A RasGAP-derived cell permeable peptide potently enhances genotoxin-induced cytotoxicity in tumor cells. Oncogene 23:8971–8978

Minucci S, Maccarana M, Cioce M, De Luca P, Gelmetti V, Segalla S, Di Croce L, Giavara S, Matteucci C, Gobbi A, Bianchini A, Colombo E, Schiavoni I, Badaracco G, Hu X, Lazar MA, Landsberger N, Nervi C, Pelicci PG (2000) Oligomerization of RAR and AML1 transcription factors as a novel mechanism of oncogenic activation. Mol Cell 5:811–820

Moog-Lutz C, Peterson EJ, Lutz PG, Eliason S, Cave-Riant F, Singer A, Di Gioia Y, Dmowski S, Kamens J, Cayre YE, Koretzky G (2001) PRAM-1 is a novel adaptor protein regulated by retinoic acid (RA) and promyelocytic leukemia (PML)-RA receptor alpha in acute promyelocytic leukemia cells. J Biol Chem 276:22375–22381

Morris MC, Depollier J, Mery J, Heitz F, Divita G (2001) A peptide carrier for the delivery of biologically active proteins into mammalian cells. Nat Biotechnol 19:1173–1176

Mourez M, Collier RJ (2004) Use of phage display and polyvalency to design inhibitors of protein-protein interactions. Methods Mol Biol 261:213–228

Mueller BU, Pabst T, Fos J, Petkovic V, Fey MF, Asou N, Buergi U, Tenen DG (2006) ATRA resolves the differentiation block in t(15;17) acute myeloid leukemia by restoring PU.1 expression. Blood 107:3330–3338

Nagahara H, Vocero-Akbani AM, Snyder EL, Ho A, Latham DG, Lissy NA, Becker-Hapak M, Ezhevsky SA, Dowdy SF (1998) Transduction of full-length TAT fusion proteins into mammalian cells: TAT-p27Kip1 induces cell migration. Nat Med 4:1449–1452

Nagel-Wolfrum K, Buerger C, Wittig I, Butz K, Hoppe-Seyler F, Groner B (2004) The interaction of specific peptide aptamers with the DNA binding domain and the dimerization domain of the transcription factor Stat3 inhibits transactivation and induces apoptosis in tumor cells. Mol Cancer Res 2:170–182

Oehlke J, Scheller A, Wiesner B, Krause E, Beyermann M, Klauschenz E, Melzig M, Bienert M (1998) Cellular uptake of an alpha-helical amphipathic model peptide with the potential to deliver polar compounds into the cell interior non-endocytically. Biochim Biophys Acta 1414:127–139

Olsnes S, Klingenberg O, Wiedlocha A (2003) Transport of exogenous growth factors and cytokines to the cytosol and to the nucleus. Physiol Rev 83:163–182

Pearson M, Carbone R, Sebastiani C, Cioce M, Fagioli M, Saito S, Higashimoto Y, Appella E, Minucci S, Pandolfi PP, Pelicci PG (2000) PML regulates p53 acetylation and premature senescence induced by oncogenic Ras. Nature 406:207–210

Pescarolo MP, Bagnasco L, Malacarne D, Melchiori A, Valente P, Millo E, Bruno S, Basso S, Parodi S (2001) A retro-inverso peptide homologous to helix 1 of c-Myc is a potent and specific inhibitor of proliferation in different cellular systems. FASEB J 15:31–33

Polo JM, Dell'oso T, Ranuncolo SM, Cerchietti L, Beck D, Da Silva GF, Prive GG, Licht JD, Melnick A (2004) Specific peptide interference reveals BCL6 transcriptional and oncogenic mechanisms in B-cell lymphoma cells. Nat Med 10:1329–1335

Pooga M, Hallbrink M, Zorko M, Langel U (1998) Cell penetration by transportan. FASEB J 12:67–77

Potocky TB, Menon AK, Gellman SH (2003) Cytoplasmic and nuclear delivery of a TAT-derived peptide and a beta-peptide after endocytic uptake into HeLa cells. J Biol Chem 278:50188–50194

Prochiantz A, Joliot A (2003) Can transcription factors function as cell-cell signalling molecules? Nat Rev Mol Cell Biol 4:814–819

Puccetti E, Zheng X, Brambilla D, Seshire A, Beissert T, Boehrer S, Nurnberger H, Hoelzer D, Ottmann OG, Nervi C, Ruthardt M (2005) The integrity of the charged pocket in the BTB/POZ domain is essential for the phenotype induced by the leukemia-associated t(11;17) fusion protein PLZF/RARalpha. Cancer Res 65:6080–6088

Racanicchi S, Maccherani C, Liberatore C, Billi M, Gelmetti V, Panigada M, Rizzo G, Nervi C, Grignani F (2005) Targeting fusion protein/corepressor contact restores differentiation response in leukemia cells. EMBO J 24:1232–1242

Richard JP, Melikov K, Vives E, Ramos C, Verbeure B, Gait MJ, Chernomordik LV, Lebleu B (2003) Cell-penetrating peptides. A reevaluation of the mechanism of cellular uptake. J Biol Chem 278:585–590

Richard JP, Melikov K, Brooks H, Prevot P, Lebleu B, Chernomordik LV (2005) Cellular uptake of unconjugated TAT peptide involves clathrin-dependent endocytosis and heparan sulfate receptors. J Biol Chem 280:15300–15306

Schwarze SR, Ho A, Vocero-Akbani A, Dowdy SF (1999) In vivo protein transduction: delivery of a biologically active protein into the mouse. Science 285:1569–1572

Shen ZX, Shi ZZ, Fang J, Gu BW, Li JM, Zhu YM, Shi JY, Zheng PZ, Yan H, Liu YF, Chen Y, Shen Y, Wu W, Tang W, Waxman S, De The H, Wang ZY, Chen SJ, Chen Z (2004) All-trans retinoic acid/As2O3 combination yields a high quality remission and survival in newly diagnosed acute promyelocytic leukemia. Proc Natl Acad Sci U S A 101:5328–5335

Snowden AW, Zhang L, Urnov F, Dent C, Jouvenot Y, Zhong X, Rebar EJ, Jamieson AC, Zhang HS, Tan S, Case CC, Pabo CO, Wolffe AP, Gregory PD (2003) Repression of vascular endothelial growth factor A in glioblastoma cells using engineered zinc finger transcription factors. Cancer Res 63:8968–8976

Snyder EL, Meade BR, Saenz CC, Dowdy SF (2004) Treatment of terminal peritoneal carcinomatosis by a transducible p53-activating peptide. PLoS Biol 2:E36

Tallman MS (2004) Acute promyelocytic leukemia as a paradigm for targeted therapy. Semin Hematol 41:27–32

Tyagi M, Rusnati M, Presta M, Giacca M (2001) Internalization of HIV-1 tat requires cell surface heparan sulfate proteoglycans. J Biol Chem 276:3254–3261

Vives E, Brodin P, Lebleu B (1997) A truncated HIV-1 Tat protein basic domain rapidly translocates through the plasma membrane and accumulates in the cell nucleus. J Biol Chem 272:16010–16017

Wade PA, Gegonne A, Jones PL, Ballestar E, Aubry F, Wolffe AP (1999) Mi-2 complex couples DNA methylation to chromatin remodelling and histone deacetylation. Nat Genet 23:62–66

Wadia JS, Dowdy SF (2005) Transmembrane delivery of protein and peptide drugs by TAT-mediated transduction in the treatment of cancer. Adv Drug Deliv Rev 57:579–596

Wadia JS, Stan RV, Dowdy SF (2004) Transducible TAT-HA fusogenic peptide enhances escape of TAT-fusion proteins after lipid raft macropinocytosis. Nat Med 10:310–315

Walensky LD, Kung AL, Escher I, Malia TJ, Barbuto S, Wright RD, Wagner G, Verdine GL, Korsmeyer SJ (2004) Experimental fat embolism induces urine 2,3-dinor-6-ketoprostaglandin F1alpha and 11-dehydrothromboxane B2 excretion in pigs. Science 305:1466–1470

Yang L, Mashima T, Sato S, Mochizuki M, Sakamoto H, Yamori T, Oh-Hara T, Tsuruo T (2003) Predominant suppression of apoptosome by inhibitor of apoptosis protein in non-small cell lung cancer H460 cells: therapeutic effect of a novel polyarginine-conjugated Smac peptide. Cancer Res 63:831–837

Yuan J, Kramer A, Eckerdt F, Kaufmann M, Strebhardt K (2002) Efficient internalization of the polo-box of polo-like kinase 1 fused to an Antennapedia peptide results in inhibition of cancer cell proliferation. Cancer Res 62:4186–4190

The Design of Selective and Non-selective Combination Therapy for Acute Promyelocytic Leukemia

Y. Jing · S. Waxman (✉)

Division of Hematology/Oncology, Department of Medicine,
Mount Sinai School of Medicine, One Gustave L. Levy Place, Box 1178,
New York, NY 10029-6547, USA
samuel.waxman@mssm.edu

1	ATRA Induces APL Cell Differentiation by Overcoming PML-RARα Transcriptional Repression	247
2	As$_2$O$_3$ Induces Differentiation of APL Cells Through a PML-RARα Degradation-Dependent Pathway	249
3	As$_2$O$_3$ Induces Apoptosis of APL Cells Through a PML-RARα Degradation-Independent Pathway	250
4	Anthracycline Induces Cell Death of APL Cells	251
5	Effects of a Combination of As$_2$O$_3$ and ATRA on APL Cells	252
6	The Effects of ATRA Combined with Daunorubicin on APL Cells	254
7	Effects of As$_2$O$_3$ and Anthracyclines in Combination on APL Cells	255
8	Histone Deacetylase Inhibitors Enhance ATRA-Induced Differentiation in APL Cells	255
9	Novel Agents That Enhance ATRA-Induced Differentiation in APL Cells	257
10	Design of Combination Selective and Non-selective Therapy of APL	258
References		260

Abstract Acute promyelocytic leukemia (APL) is an unique subtype of acute myeloid leukemia typically carrying a specific reciprocal chromosome translocation, t(15;17), leading to the expression of a leukemia-generating fusion protein, PML-RARα. APL patients are responsive to APL-selective reagents such as all-*trans* retinoic acid (ATRA) or arsenic trioxide and non-selective cytotoxic chemotherapy. Nearly all de novo APL patients undergo clinical remission when treated with ATRA plus chemotherapy or with the combinational selective therapy, ATRA plus As$_2$O$_3$. Combining ATRA with As$_2$O$_3$ as an induction followed by chemotherapy consolidation results in more profound clinical remissions compared to treatment with any agent alone or any of the other possible combinations. The mechanism of action of each of these agents differs. ATRA induces APL cell differentiation and PML-RARα proteolysis. As_2O_3 induces APL cell partial differentiation, PML-RARα proteolysis, and apoptosis. Chemotherapy, mainly using anthracyclines, induces APL cell death. The combined effects of selective APL therapy (ATRA and As_2O_3) and/or non-selective chemotherapy in APL cells in vitro and their mechanisms in relation to clinical protocol design are discussed.

Acute promyelocytic leukemia (APL) accounts for approximately 10% of acute myeloid leukemia cases [1]. Molecular studies have revealed that most APL cases are characterized by a t(15;17) translocation that fuses the PML gene on chromosome 15 to the retinoic acid receptor α (RARα) gene on chromosome 17, resulting in the formation of the PML-RARα fusion protein [2, 3]. PML-RARα occurs in most APL patients and binds to retinoic acid response elements (RAREs) of DNA as a homodimer or a heterodimer with RXR and recruits the corepressors SMRT and N-CoR. PML-RARα binds these repressors more tightly than does wild type RARα, such that physiological levels of all-*trans* retinoic acid (ATRA) are not sufficient to release them from the PML-RARα protein [4-9]. Based on these findings, it has been suggested that recruitment of corepressors, SMRT/N-CoR, with subsequent repression of ATRA target genes is critical for the oncogenic function of PML-RARα (see reviews in [10, 11]). Intensive cytoreductive non-selective chemotherapy, usually combining an anthracycline and cytosine arabinoside (Ara-C), was used as the standard of treatment for APL until 1992. This anthracycline/Ara-C combination yielded complete remission rates (CR) of 50%-60% in APL patients, but less than 25% 5-year survival [12, 13]. Since then, the novel discovery that ATRA induces APL cell differentiation has modified the therapeutic approach to APL [14-16]. Complete clinical, but not molecular (residual PML-RARα transcripts), remission was induced by ATRA treatment in 90% of newly diagnosed or first-relapse chemotherapy-refractory patients with t(15;17) APL. However, relapse frequently occurred within months in patients that were initially sensitive to ATRA; therefore, chemotherapy was added to ATRA therapy. The combination of ATRA with chemotherapy cured more than 70% of these APL patients [14, 17]. However, some APL patients experienced relapse that was resistant to further treatment with ATRA plus chemotherapy. These patients frequently responded to subsequent As_2O_3 treatment with a complete clinic remission [18, 19]. Recently, it was shown that ATRA plus As_2O_3 induction followed by chemotherapy consolidation is more effective than treatment with either agent alone. Additional studies have shown that ATRA plus As_2O_3 induction followed by chemotherapy is the most effective treatment of APL [20]. Although the mechanisms of action of both ATRA and As_2O_3 in APL are still not understood completely, since APL patients expressing the PML-RARα fusion protein respond clinically to both ATRA and As_2O_3 treatment, and both agents induce PML-RARα proteolysis, it appears that PML-RARα is a major, if not the only, target of both ATRA and As_2O_3 therapy [16, 18, 19, 21–24]. Since chemotherapy is as effective in myeloid leukemia with other gene translocations such as t(8;21) and inv(16) as that in APL patients [25], it suggests that PML-RARα is not the target of anthracycline/Ara-C chemotherapy.

1
ATRA Induces APL Cell Differentiation by Overcoming PML-RARα Transcriptional Repression

ATRA induces APL blasts to undergo differentiation to the neutrophil stage leading to progressive replacement of malignant leukocytes by normal myelopoiesis. It has been reported that APL cells are induced to undergo granulocytic differentiation in vitro at a pharmacological concentration of ATRA (10^{-6} M), but not at a physiological one (10^{-9} M) [2, 3, 26]. PML-RARα binds to the nuclear receptor corepressors SMRT and N-CoR with higher affinity than wild type RARα such that a higher than physiological concentration of ATRA is required to release these corepressors from in vitro-translated PML-RARα [5–8]. This observation suggests that pharmacological, but not physiological, levels of ATRA act by overcoming PML-RARα-mediated transcriptional repression, which allows ATRA to induce its target genes and subsequent morphological differentiation [27–31]. In support of this suggestion, gene profiles that have been generated by several groups using differential display and DNA microarray assays show that many genes are induced in NB4 cells (a well-studied APL cell line) after ATRA treatment in vitro [32–35]. CCAAT/enhancer-binding protein ε (C/EBPε), a transcription factor that mediates granulocytic differentiation, is induced by ATRA in ATRA-sensitive NB4 cells, but not in an ATRA-resistant APL cell line, R4 cells [26, 36, 37]. C/EBPε is an ATRA-target gene. The induced expression of C/EBPε probably results from the ability of pharmacological concentrations of ATRA to overcome PML-RARα transcriptional repression on the RARE present in C/EBPε promoter [37]. Induction of other gene products, such as C/EBPβ and Bfl-1/A1, may also be mediated by overcoming PML-RARα transcriptional repression indirectly since they are not ATRA-target genes [26, 33, 38].

Another potential explanation for the ATRA induction of APL cell differentiation is that ATRA may overcome PML-RARα transcriptional repression by inducing PML-RARα proteolysis. PML-RARα protein undergoes complete degradation as well as partial cleavage with formation of an approximately 85-kDa truncated product, termed △PML-RARα, with suspected deletion of its N-terminus [21, 26, 39–47]. ATRA initiates PML-RARα proteolysis after only 12 h of treatment [48]. It is conceivable that this event rather than corepressor release might be the key step whereby ATRA treatment overcomes the block of cellular differentiation due to PML-RARα [42]. The activity of C/EBPα (another important transcription factor of the C/EBP family required for normal granulocytic cell differentiation) has been found to be directly inhibited by binding to PML-RARα protein; therefore, PML-RARα proteolysis, in addition to overcoming transcriptional repression, also restores the activity of C/EBPα [49, 50]. Thus, PML-RARα proteolysis appears to be important for ATRA induction of APL cell differentiation. However, several ATRA-resistant NB4 subclones do not contain PML-RARα protein, and NB4 cells treated with As_2O_3 with subsequent degradation of PML-RARα protein did not undergo differentiation [26, 51–53]. This suggests that PML-RARα proteolysis alone

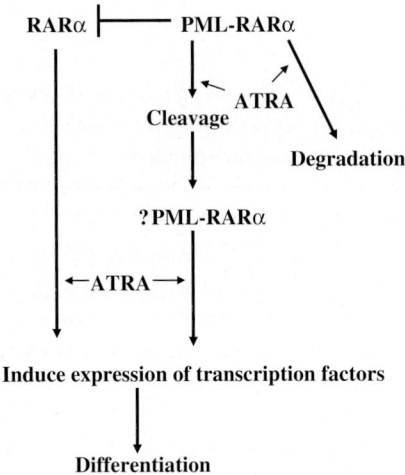

Fig. 1 Hypothetic pathways of ATRA-induced differentiation of APL cells. PML-RARα blocks ATRA-activated RARα transcriptional induction of target transcription factors. ATRA at pharmacological concentrations induces PML-RARα proteolysis leading to partial cleavage and complete degradation, which releases repression of RARα as well as other transcription factors. ATRA also induces target gene expression through RARα and the PML-RARα cleavage product (△*PML-RAR*α) which then induces granulocytic differentiation of APL cells

is insufficient to induce APL cell differentiation. Downstream gene induction due to ATRA treatment through normal RARα and/or the ΔPML-RARα cleavage product (which has PML-RARα-like activity) may be needed for granulocytic differentiation [48]. Therefore, multiple pathways as diagramed in Fig. 1 might be involved in ATRA-induced APL cell differentiation. A defect in one or more these pathways may be responsible for ATRA resistance.

2
As_2O_3 Induces Differentiation of APL Cells Through a PML-RARα Degradation-Dependent Pathway

Of APL patients that are resistant to treatment with ATRA plus chemotherapy, 90% respond to As_2O_3 treatment. Current data indicate that As_2O_3 induces remission of APL through partial differentiation and apoptosis [18, 54–56]. Pharmacokinetic studies indicate that a plasma concentration of less than 1 µM As_2O_3 mediates therapeutic effects without severe toxicity [56, 57]. More recent clinical data indicate that as little as approximately 0.5 µM As_2O_3 is an effective plasma concentration in APL patients [58]. Since As_2O_3 at 0.5 µM rarely induces apoptosis in cultured APL cells, As_2O_3 therapeutic effects in APL may occur in part through differentiation induction. This has been demonstrated in clinical studies [56].

Non-terminally differentiated APL cells have been observed in As_2O_3-treated patients and in primary APL cells treated in vitro with 0.1–1 µM As_2O_3. PML-RARα protein was degraded following As_2O_3 treatment at these concentrations [18, 19, 23, 26, 59, 60]. As_2O_3 treatment leads to complete degradation of PML-RARα without degradation of RARα in in vitro-cultured cell lines, but cell differentiation is observed only in long-term cell cultures or following the addition of ATRA. These data suggest that the cell differentiation observed in APL patients may result from restored physiological ATRA function after removal of the PML-RARα fusion protein (Fig. 2). It is possible that other physiological factors may also be involved in As_2O_3-mediated differentiation. For example, treatment with As_2O_3 plus granulocyte-macrophage colony-stimulating factor (GM-CSF) or cyclic adenosine monophosphate (cAMP) induced granulocytic differentiation in some APL clones even though each agent alone did not [61–63]. In addition, treatment with As_2O_3 plus 8-Cl-cAMP has a significant life-prolonging effect in mice bearing ATRA-resistant APL cells [64]. The arsenic metabolite, monomethylarsonous acid, did not induce PML-RARα degradation and failed to overcome ATRA-differentiation resistance [65]. This suggests that by inducing PML-RARα protein degradation and thereby eliminating its transcriptional repression effect, As_2O_3

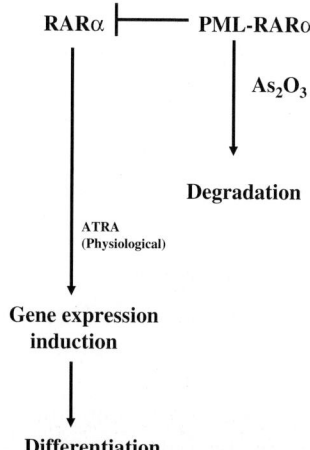

Fig. 2 Potential pathways of As_2O_3 treatment-induced differentiation of APL cells. As_2O_3 treatment induces PML-RARα degradation, which allows physiological concentrations of ATRA to induce target gene expression through RARα, which leads to cell differentiation

allows the physiological levels of ATRA, cAMP, and/or GM-CSF present in vivo to induce partial cell differentiation.

3
As_2O_3 Induces Apoptosis of APL Cells Through a PML-RARα Degradation-Independent Pathway

Although the remarkable sensitivity of APL cells to As_2O_3-induced apoptosis seems to correlate with PML-RARα degradation [23, 53, 66–68], it appears from the following observations that As_2O_3 induces apoptosis in APL cells through a PML-RARα degradation-independent pathway. As_2O_3 at 0.5–1 µM induces apoptosis in APL-derived NB4 cells, whereas other leukemia cells are resistant to As_2O_3 treatment or undergo apoptosis only in response to higher concentrations [67, 69]. The higher sensitivity of APL cells to As_2O_3-induced apoptosis is dependent on the activity of the enzymes that regulate cellular H_2O_2 content. NB4 cells have relatively low levels of glutathione peroxidase (GPx) and catalase and have a constitutively higher H_2O_2 level than U937 monocytic leukemia cells [67]. The levels of glutathione-S-transferase π (GSTπ), which is important for cellular efflux of As_2O_3, are also low in NB4 cells [67]. Treatment with 1 µM/l As_2O_3, a clinically relevant concentration, inhibits GPx activity and increases cellular H_2O_2 content in NB4 cells, but

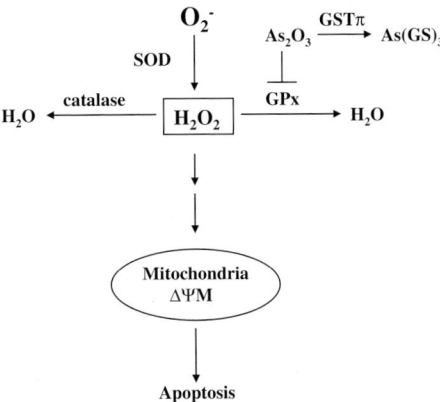

Fig. 3 As_2O_3 at low concentrations induces apoptosis of APL cells by increasing their H_2O_2 content. H_2O_2 was formed in cells from O_2^- with the action of superoxide dismutase (*SOD*) activity. H_2O_2 levels are diminished by glutathione peroxidase (*GPx*) and catalase activities. As_2O_3 increases intracellular H_2O_2 levels by inhibiting GPx activity. The increased amount of H_2O_2 decreases mitochondrial membrane potential ($\triangle\psi M$) and induced apoptosis. Glutathione-*S*-transferase π (*GST*π) detoxifies As_2O_3 by catalyzing glutathione conjugated arsenic [*As(GS)*$_3$] formation. The cellular levels of GSTπ, GPx, and catalase determine the cell sensitivity to As_2O_3-induced apoptosis

not in U937 cells [67]. In NB4 cells, antioxidants—*N*-acetylcysteine, and α-lipoic acid—block apoptosis induction, but not PML-RARα degradation, due to As_2O_3 treatment [66]. In addition, low concentrations of As_2O_3 induce PML-RARα degradation, but do not induce apoptosis [26]. Furthermore, monomethylarsonous acid is more effective than As_2O_3 in inducing apoptosis in NB4 cells. It does this without inducing PML-RARα degradation [65]. In summary, As_2O_3 induces apoptosis in APL cells through an H_2O_2-mediated pathway. The levels of GPx, catalase, GSTπ, and other enzymes might be parameters for determining cell sensitivity to As_2O_3 treatment (Fig. 3). However, it is also possible that the presence of the PML-RARα protein may inhibit the expression of these enzymes and thereby sensitize APL cells to As_2O_3-induced apoptosis.

4
Anthracycline Induces Cell Death of APL Cells

APL cells are more sensitive to anthracyclines, and anthracycline plus Ara-C was used as induction therapy of APL until 1992 [71]. Anthracyclines (daunorubicin or idarubicin) as monotherapy induces CR in 55%–90% of

APL patients, but with toxic side effects [71]. The cytotoxicity of high-dose anthracyclines was originally believed to result from DNA damage. The damage has been thought to be due to quinone-generated redox activity, intercalation-induced distortion of the double helix, or stabilization of the cleavable complex formed between DNA and topoisomerase II [72]. However, the relationship between the DNA damage and cell death after anthracycline treatment is not clear. Apoptosis induction by anthracyclines in AML cells is considered to be the mechanism of anthracycline-induced cell death [73, 74]. Anthracyclines have variable abilities to induce apoptosis in AML cells [73]. APL NB4 cells are more sensitive than U937 cells to daunorubicin treatment-induced apoptosis (Y.K. Jing and S. Waxman, unpublished data). Although it has been found that multiple pathways, such as ceramide production, Akt activation, and nuclear factor (NF)-κB activation, are involved in anthracycline-induced apoptosis, radical oxygen species (ROS) seem to play an important role [74].

The induction of clinical remission by anthracycline/Ara-C treatment in APL is often slow, without total bone marrow aplasia and with evidence of minimal differentiation of APL blasts [75]. This is consistent with the report that anthracyclines at low concentrations weakly induce differentiation of HL-60 cells [76, 77]. Anthracyclines do not induce PML-RARα degradation (Y.K. Jing and S. Waxman, unpublished data) and are effective in several types of myeloid leukemia other than APL [25]. Thus, anthracyclines induce predominantly non-selective APL cell death through a pathway independent of the PML-RARα protein, with minimal differentiation as single agent.

5
Effects of a Combination of As_2O_3 and ATRA on APL Cells

Several clinical reports indicate that ATRA in combination with As_2O_3 was more effective than either agent alone in APL patients [20, 56]. These observations and those noted above suggest a rationale for combination therapy utilizing these two agents. ATRA and As_2O_3 induce non-cross-resistant complete clinical remission in APL patients and appear to target PML-RARα by different pathways. To evaluate the effect of this combination, several studies have examined the effect of As_2O_3 on ATRA-induced differentiation and, conversely, the effect of ATRA on As_2O_3-induced apoptosis. As_2O_3 at a subapoptotic-inducing concentration (0.5 μM) decreased ATRA-induced differentiation in NB4 cells, but synergized with ATRA to induce differentiation in ATRA-resistant NB4 subclones MR-2 and R4 as measured by nitroblue tetrazolium reduction and ATRA-inducible gene expression [26]. The inhibitory effect of As_2O_3 on ATRA-induced differentiation in NB4 cells may result from its induction of complete degradation of PML-RARα, which prevents the formation of △PML-RARα, which seems to have RARα activity.

The synergistic effect of ATRA with As$_2$O$_3$ in ATRA-resistant cell lines may result from As$_2$O$_3$-induced PML-RARα degradation in cells that were resistant to ATRA-induced PML-RARα proteolysis (Fig. 4). ATRA does not induce apoptosis in APL cells after a brief culture period [26]. It has been shown that an increase in apoptosis occurs in APL cells simultaneously treated with ATRA and As$_2$O$_3$ [44]. However, As$_2$O$_3$-induced apoptosis was decreased by ATRA pretreatment of differentiation-responsive NB4 cells, but not in differentiation-resistant R4 cells, and was associated with a rapid induction of Bfl-1/A1 expression, a Bcl-2 protein family member that has antiapoptotic activity [26]. Immunodeficient mice bearing NB4 cells demonstrated "additive" survival due to treatment with these two agents together compared to treatment with either agent alone [26]. More intriguing, treatment with

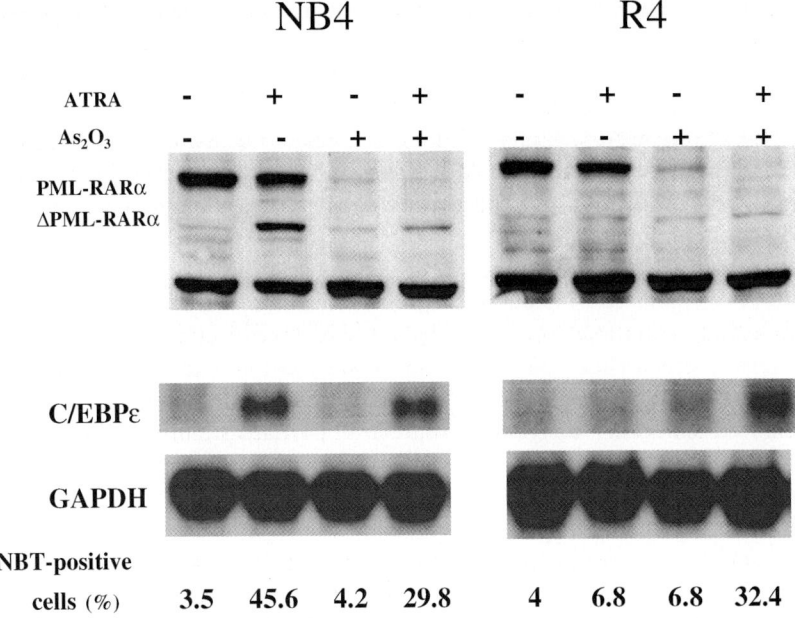

Fig.4 As$_2$O$_3$ decreases ATRA-induced differentiation in NB4 cells, but increases ATRA-induced differentiation in R4 cells. NB4 and ATRA-resistant R4 cells were treated with 1 μM ATRA, 0.5 μM As$_2$O$_3$ or their combination for 4 days. PML-RARα protein levels were determined by Western blot analysis. C/EBPε RNA levels were determined by Northern blot analysis. Cell differentiation was measured using an NBT reduction assay

ATRA plus As$_2$O$_3$ at lower concentrations significantly increased the survival time of PML-RARα transgenic mice compared to treatment with either each agent alone [60]. Since this combination did not increase the survival time of the PLZF-RARα-bearing transgenic mice [79], the combined effect of ATRA and As$_2$O$_3$ in vivo seems to result from a synergistic decrease of PML-RARα protein levels.

6
The Effects of ATRA Combined with Daunorubicin on APL Cells

ATRA induced complete remission in most APL patients, but the leukemic clone was not eliminated without addition of a chemotherapeutic agent [80]. ATRA and anthracyclines seem to act in APL patients through different mechanisms (differentiation and apoptosis). Schedule-dependent synergism and antagonism of both differentiation and apoptosis have been observed with different combinations of differentiation and apoptosis inducers [26, 44, 81]. This appears to be schedule-dependent since enhanced cell death and growth inhibition occurs in several malignant cell lines, including leukemic cells, when treated with cytotoxic agents followed by differentiation inducers or when simultaneously treated with both types of agents [82, 83]. Although there was no difference in remission rates of APL patients treated simultaneously with ATRA plus chemotherapy and with ATRA treatment followed by chemotherapy, the duration of remission was longer in patients treated simultaneously with both agents [17, 84]. These observations predict that during the ATRA-induced differentiation process there may be an induction of the expression of antiapoptotic proteins that inhibit cell death due to treatment with a cytotoxic chemotherapeutic agent. We have found that pretreatment of NB4 cells with ATRA induced Bfl-1/A1 expression and decreased doxorubicin-induced cell death [70]. Silencing of Bfl-1/A1 partially restored the sensitivity of APL cells to doxorubicin-induced apoptosis. Similarly, it has been found that upregulated Bfl-1/A1 inhibited tumour necrosis factor-related apoptosis inducing ligand (TRAIL)-induced apoptosis in NB4 cells [85]. These data suggest that differentiated APL cells with increased antiapoptotic protein expression might become resistant to chemotherapy. The therapeutic benefit of combined ATRA and an anthracycline in APL patients may result from preventing antagonism and enhancing independent activities.

7
Effects of As$_2$O$_3$ and Anthracyclines in Combination on APL Cells

As$_2$O$_3$ alone is an effective therapy for APL patients [18, 19]. Although the use of As$_2$O$_3$ plus ATRA and ATRA plus anthracycline have been tested in APL patients [20, 86], As$_2$O$_3$ plus an anthracycline has not been used for induction therapy. However, there is a report that describes that As$_2$O$_3$ treatment followed by anthracycline consolidation is more effective than As$_2$O$_3$ alone [87]. More recently it has been shown that As$_2$O$_3$ induction followed by chemotherapy is more effective than ATRA induction followed by chemotherapy in APL patients [20]. The combined effect of As$_2$O$_3$ with anthracyclines has not been tested in APL cell lines. Since As$_2$O$_3$ and anthracyclines have been used in different stages of APL therapy, it is probable that the combined beneficial effect of As$_2$O$_3$ with anthracyclines in APL patients may result from additive independent activities of each agent.

8
Histone Deacetylase Inhibitors Enhance ATRA-Induced Differentiation in APL Cells

Both RARα and PML-RARα in the absence of ligand repress transcription by recruiting the histone deacetylase (HDAC) complex through direct interaction with the nuclear corepressors N-CoR and SMRT [27, 28, 88]. HDAC activity is thought to mediate the establishment of a chromatin structure in which DNA cannot be transcribed.

It has been reported that HDAC inhibitors, sodium butyrate (NaB) and trichostatin A (TSA), enhance ATRA-induced differentiation in NB4 cells. The mechanism underlying this effect of HDAC inhibitors is thought to be the abrogation of N-CoR and SMRT association with PML-RARα [6, 7, 89, 90]. Since PML-RARα protein undergoes proteolysis in APL cells upon ATRA treatment, it is possible that HDAC inhibitors may facilitate PML-RARα proteolysis, thereby enhancing ATRA-induced differentiation. This seems to be the case, since NaB treatment of NB4 cells not only enhanced ATRA-induced gene expression, but also enhanced ATRA-mediated PML-RARα proteolysis [91]. In addition, we have found that butyrate analogs such as iodide phenylacetate and iodide phenylbutyrate do not increase acetylated H3 and H4 in NB4 cells, but have a similar stimulatory effect as that of phenylbutyrate on ATRA-induced NB4 cell differentiation (Fig. 5).

Few studies have been performed to test whether HDAC inhibitors can overcome ATRA resistance in APL cells or in patients. One report described

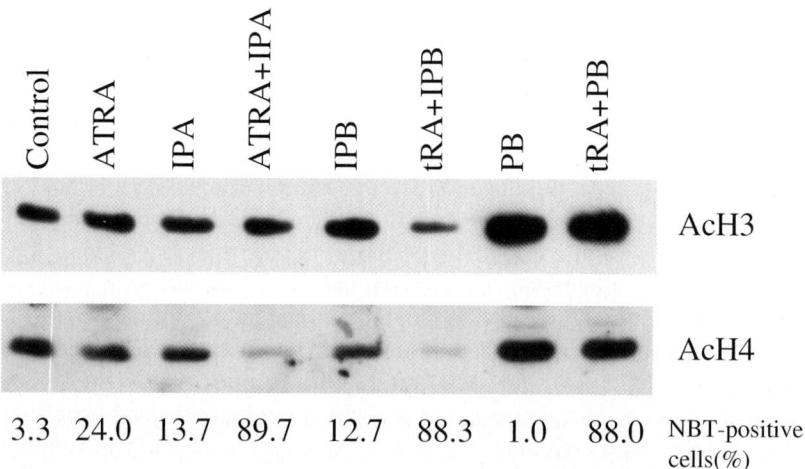

Fig. 5 Phenylbutyrate derivatives-enhanced ATRA-induced differentiation does not correlate with increases of acetylated histone 3 (*AcH3*) and 4 (*AcH4*). NB4 cells were treated with 10^{-7} M ATRA, 0.5 mM iodide phenylacetate (*IPA*),1 mM iodide phenylbutyrate (*IPB*), or 2 mM phenylbutyrate (*PB*) alone or in the indicated combinations for 3 days. AcH3 and AcH4 were measured by Western blot analysis and cell differentiation was measured using an NBT reduction assay

a patient with relapsed APL following ATRA treatment that responded to subsequent ATRA treatment when combined with phenylbutyrate [92]. However, several other APL cases failed to respond to this combination treatment [93]. We have found that butyrate and its derivatives did not overcome differentiation-resistance (or only weakly did so) in ATRA-resistant R4 cells [91] and that a similar result in the same cell line was observed using ATRA in combination with TSA [6]. Moreover, it has been found that in another ATRA-resistant NB4 subclone, NB4/RA, trapoxin A (a more potent HDAC inhibitor than NaB) failed to overcome ATRA resistance [90]. However, it has been reported that the HDAC inhibitor TSA overcame ATRA-differentiation resistance in APL cells expressing promyelocytic leukemia zinc finger (PLZF)-RARα, the t(11;17) translocation product [8, 94, 95]. In addition, a synergistic effect on leukemia remission has been obtained in PLZF-RARα transgenic mice using ATRA in combination with a new powerful HDAC inhibitor, suberoylanilide hydroxamic acid [96]. Although differentiation and clinical remission have not been obtained in t(11;17) APL cells and patients, respectively, after treatment with ATRA alone, the PLZF-RARα protein is highly sensitive to ATRA-mediated degradation [79, 97–98]. Thus, it suggests that degraded PML-RARα may be needed for an HDAC inhibitor to enhance ATRA-induced cell differentiation in ATRA-resistant APL cells. To support this, we have found that NaB enhanced As_2O_3 plus ATRA-induced differentiation in resistant APL cells [91]. The As_2O_3 treatment led to PML-RARα degradation (which allows the ATRA to induce its target genes) and the NaB treatment increased the level of acetylated histones [91]. These results suggest that elimination of the dominant-negative PML-RARα protein is required prior to inhibition of HDAC activity to fully overcome ATRA-differentiation resistance in APL cells. This provides a rationale for using a combination of ATRA, As_2O_3, and HDAC inhibitors in the treatment of ATRA-resistant APL patients. However, induction of apoptosis without differentiation can be obtained by a retinoid/butyrate prodrug in ATRA-differentiation resistant NB4 cells [100]. Recently, it has been found that HDAC inhibitors alone induced apoptosis of leukemic blasts and myeloid cell lines through activation of the death receptor pathway (TRAIL and Fas signaling pathways) [101]. It was found that TRAIL, DR5, FasL, and Fas were upregulated by an HDAC inhibitor in the leukemia cells, but not in normal hematopoietic progenitors. However, this effect is not limited to APL. A similar effect has been observed in non-APL acute myeloid leukemia [102].

9
Novel Agents That Enhance ATRA-Induced Differentiation in APL Cells

Since ATRA selectively induces clinical remission in APL patients through differentiation induction, agents that can enhance ATRA-induced differentiation have been sought. We established a screening system using NB4 cells primed with ATRA followed by treatment with other potential differentiation inducers after 48 h treatment [103]. Over 300 cytostatic agents selected from the National Cancer Institute library were screened using this method. Three compounds, NSC656243, NSC625748, and NSC144168 were found to amplify ATRA-induced differentiation with acceptable cytotoxicity. NSC656243, a benzodithiophene compound, and its derivatives were selected for the study of their mechanism of action. During ATRA-induced differentiation, these compounds did not alter global histone acetylation. The expression of some, but not all, ATRA target genes was enhanced [104]. Benzodithiophenes enhanced ATRA-mediated dissociation of the corepressor N-CoR and the association of coactivator p300 acetyltransferase with RARα proteins. These data suggest that benzodithiophenes act at a level of receptor activation, possibly by affecting posttranslational modification of the receptor (and/or co-regulators), thus leading to an enhancement in ATRA-mediated effects on gene expression and subsequent APL cell differentiation. It is possible that these compounds enhance ATRA-induced differentiation by increased ATRA-induced PML-RARα proteolysis.

It has been reported that CDDO-Im, a triterpenoid, selectively downregulated expression of the PML-RARα fusion protein and sensitized APL cells to the differentiating effects of ATRA [105]. Similarly, STI571, a tyrosine kinase inhibitor used to treat chronic myelogenous leukemia (CML), did not induce APL cell differentiation alone, but it enhanced ATRA-induced differentiation in NB4 cells [106]. In addition, STI571 relieved the cytodifferentiation block observed in the ATRA-resistant APL cell lines through retardation of the ATRA-induced degradation of PML-RARα and RARα [106]. Platelet-activating factor receptor antagonists, WEB-2086 and WEB-2170 (WEBs), have been found to induce apoptosis of ATRA-sensitive and resistant APL cells alone and enhanced ATRA-induced differentiation in ATRA-sensitive APL cells at subapoptotic concentrations [107]. Activating mutations of the FMS-like tyrosine kinase 3 (FLT3) receptor are frequently present in human APL [108]. Activated FLT3 cooperates with PML-RARα to induce leukemias [109]. SU11657, a selective, oral, multitargeted tyrosine kinase inhibitor that targets FLT3, cooperates with ATRA to rapidly cause regression of APL [110]. Although all of these compounds have been shown to enhance ATRA-induced differentiation of APL cells in vitro, the in vivo effect has not been tested.

APL cells express a considerable level of cell surface antigen CD33, which is a target of gemtuzumab ozogamicin (Mylotarg, a humanized anti-CD33 antibody-targeted chemotherapeutic agent). Gemtuzumab ozogamicin is effective against ATRA- or ATO-resistant APL cells [111] and is highly effective as a single treatment for relapsed APL [112]. There is a reported resistant case successfully treated with combination of ATRA, As_2O_3, and gemtuzumab ozogamicin [113]. Thus gemtuzumab ozogamicin may be a new agent to add to APL therapy [114].

10
Design of Combination Selective and Non-selective Therapy of APL

The laboratory and clinical data thus far presented demonstrate an enormous breakthrough in the treatment of leukemia and could be a paradigm for the treatment of all leukemias due to oncogenic fusion proteins. APL is considered a curable disease in 85%–90% of patients. This is best explained by the APL-selective therapy of three drugs: ATRA, As_2O_3, and gemtuzumab ozogamicin. In addition, APL cells are induced to apoptosis and perhaps partial differentiation by non-selective anthracyclines. The clinical problems that

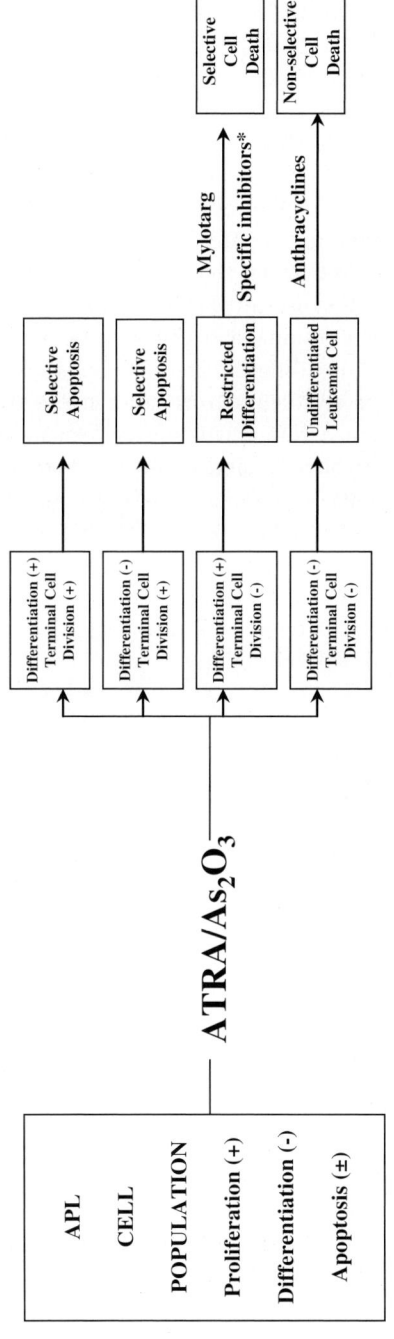

Fig. 6 The design of selective and non-selective combination therapy of APL. *, Inhibitors include: HDAC, FLT3, and tyrosine kinases

remain to be addressed include the treatment of elderly patients or those with cardiovascular disease and APL-coagulopathy. Moreover, there is the concern that secondary hematologic damage due to anthracyclines may result in a myelodysplastic syndrome and/or secondary leukemias. Thus, designing future protocols should be directed to test whether anthracycline treatment can be reduced or eliminated. A design of a combination APL-selective treatment is demonstrated in Fig. 6. The combination of ATRA and As_2O_3 may give maximal APL-selective induction of differentiation and apoptosis and clinical remission [20]. It is possible that this may result in less coagulopathy, since there is a more rapid recovery in the platelet count compared to treatment with either agent alone. The residual APL cells may be differentiated and restricted in growth or remain undifferentiated. The subsequent use of another APL-selective agent such as gemtuzumab ozogamicin may kill this population of APL cells. Thereafter, consolidation with one cycle of anthracycline may or may not be necessary to treat residual disease. Alternatively, a second cycle with the APL-selective agents (a combination of ATRA and As_2O_3 followed by gemtuzumab ozogamicin) might be effective. It is highly probable that this regimen of APL-selective agents would diminish or eliminate the need for anthracyclines in the treatment of APL. This approach should be tested in elderly high-risk patients or patients with cardiovascular disease presenting with low peripheral blood APL cell counts.

Acknowledgements The critical reading of this manuscript by Willam Scher is appreciated. This work was supported the NIH CA93533, American Institute for Cancer Research and Samuel Waxman Cancer Research Foundation.

References

1. Look AT (1997) Oncogenic transcription factors in the human acute leukemias. Science 278:1059–1064
2. de The H, Lavau C, Marchio A, Chomienne C, Degos L, Dejean A (1991) The PML-RAR alpha fusion mRNA generated by the t(15;17) translocation in acute promyelocytic leukemia encodes a functionally altered RAR. Cell 66:675–684
3. Kakizuka A, Miller WH Jr, Umesono K, Warrell RP Jr, Frankel SR, Murty VV, Dmitrovsky E, Evans RM (1991) Chromosomal translocation t(15;17) in human acute promyelocytic leukemia fuses RAR alpha with a novel putative transcription factor, PML. Cell 66:663–674
4. Koken MH, Linares Cruz G, Quignon F, Viron A, Chelbi Alix MK, Sobczak Thepot J, Juhlin L, Degos L, Calvo F, de The H (1995) The PML growth-suppressor has an altered expression in human oncogenesis. Oncogene 10:1315–1324

5. Hong SH, David G, Wong CW, Dejean A, Privalsky ML (1997) SMRT corepressor interacts with PLZF and with the PML-retinoic acid receptor alpha (RARalpha) and PLZF-RARalpha oncoproteins associated with acute promyelocytic leukemia. Proc Natl Acad Sci U S A 94:9028–9033
6. Lin RJ, Nagy L, Inoue S, Shao W, Miller WH Jr, Evans RM (1998) Role of the histone deacetylase complex in acute promyelocytic leukaemia. Nature 391:811–814
7. Guidez F, Ivins S, Zhu J, Soderstrom M, Waxman S, Zelent A (1998) Reduced retinoic acid-sensitivities of nuclear receptor corepressor binding to PML- and PLZF-RARalpha underlie molecular pathogenesis and treatment of acute promyelocytic leukemia. Blood 91:2634–2642
8. He LZ, Guidez F, Tribioli C, Peruzzi D, Ruthardt M, Zelent A, Pandolfi PP (1998) Distinct interactions of PML-RARalpha and PLZF-RARalpha with co-repressors determine differential responses to RA in APL. Nat Genet 18:126–135
9. Lin RJ, Evans RM (2000) Acquisition of oncogenic potential by RAR chimeras in acute promyelocytic leukemia through formation of homodimers. Mol Cell 5:821–830
10. Melnick A, Licht JD (1999) Deconstructing a disease: RARalpha, its fusion partners, and their roles in the pathogenesis of acute promyelocytic leukemia. Blood 93:3167–3215
11. Piazza F, Gurrieri C, Pandolfi PP (2001) The theory of APL. Oncogene 20:7216–7222
12. Thomas W, Archimbaud E, Treille-Ritouet D, Fiere D (1991) Prognostic factors in acute promyelocytic leukemia: a retrospective study of 67 cases. Leuk Lymphoma 4:249
13. Head D, Kopecky KJ, Weick J, Files JC, Ryan D, Foucar K, Montiel M, Bickers J, Fishleder A, Miller M, et al (1995) Effect of aggressive daunomycin therapy on survival in acute promyelocytic leukemia. Blood 86:1717–1728
14. Degos L, Dombret H, Chomienne C, Daniel MT, Miclea JM, Chastang C, Castaigne S, Fenaux P (1995) All-trans-retinoic acid as a differentiating agent in the treatment of acute promyelocytic leukemia [see comments]. Blood 85:2643–2653
15. Huang ME, Ye YC, Chen SR, Chai JR, Lu JX, Zhoa L, Gu LJ, Wang ZY (1988) Use of all-trans retinoic acid in the treatment of acute promyelocytic leukemia. Blood 72:567–572
16. Warrell RP Jr, Frankel SR, Miller WH Jr, Scheinberg DA, Itri LM, Hittelman WN, Vyas R, Andreeff M, Tafuri A, Jakubowski A, et al (1991) Differentiation therapy of acute promyelocytic leukemia with tretinoin (all-trans-retinoic acid). N Engl J Med 324:1385–1393
17. Fenaux P, Chastang C, Chevret S, Sanz M, Dombret H, Archimbaud E, Fey M, Rayon C, Huguet F, Sotto JJ, Gardin C, Makhoul PC, Travade P, Solary E, Fegueux N, Bordessoule D, Miguel JS, Link H, Desablens B, Stamatoullas A, Deconinck E, Maloisel F, Castaigne S, Preudhomme C, Degos L (1999) A randomized comparison of all transretinoic acid (ATRA) followed by chemotherapy and ATRA plus chemotherapy and the role of maintenance therapy in newly diagnosed acute promyelocytic leukemia. The European APL Group. Blood 94:1192–1200

18. Niu C, Yan H, Yu T, Sun HP, Liu JX, Li XS, Wu W, Zhang FQ, Chen Y, Zhou L, Li JM, Zeng XY, Yang RR, Yuan MM, Ren MY, Gu FY, Cao Q, Gu BW, Su XY, Chen GQ, Xiong SM, Zhang T, Waxman S, Wang ZY, Chen SJ, et al (1999) Studies on treatment of acute promyelocytic leukemia with arsenic trioxide: remission induction, follow-up, and molecular monitoring in 11 newly diagnosed and 47 relapsed acute promyelocytic leukemia patients. Blood 94:3315–3324
19. Soignet SL, Maslak P, Wang ZG, Jhanwar S, Calleja E, Dardashti LJ, Corso D, DeBlasio A, Gabrilove J, Scheinberg DA, Pandolfi PP, Warrell RP Jr (1998) Complete remission after treatment of acute promyelocytic leukemia with arsenic trioxide. N Engl J Med 339:1341–1348
20. Shen ZX, Shi ZZ, Fang J, Gu BW, Li JM, Zhu YM, Shi JY, Zheng PZ, Yan H, Liu YF, Chen Y, Shen Y, Wu W, Tang W, Waxman S, De The H, Wang ZY, Chen SJ, Chen Z (2004) All-trans retinoic acid/As_2O_3 combination yields a high quality remission and survival in newly diagnosed acute promyelocytic leukemia. Proc Natl Acad Sci U S A 101:5328–5335
21. Raelson JV, Nervi C, Rosenauer A, Benedetti L, Monczak Y, Pearson M, Pelicci PG, Miller WH Jr (1996) The PML/RAR alpha oncoprotein is a direct molecular target of retinoic acid in acute promyelocytic leukemia cells. Blood 88:2826–2832
22. Chomienne C, Balitrand N, Ballerini P, Castaigne S, de The H, Degos L (1991) All-trans retinoic acid modulates the retinoic acid receptor-alpha in promyelocytic cells. J Clin Invest 88:2150–2154
23. Chen GQ, Zhu J, Shi XG, Ni JH, Zhong HJ, Si GY, Jin XL, Tang W, Li XS, Xong SM, Shen ZX, Sun GL, Ma J, Zhang P, Zhang TD, Gazin C, Naoe T, Chen SJ, Wang ZY, Chen Z (1996) In vitro studies on cellular and molecular mechanisms of arsenic trioxide (As_2O_3) in the treatment of acute promyelocytic leukemia: As_2O_3 induces NB4 cell apoptosis with downregulation of Bcl-2 expression and modulation of PML-RAR alpha/PML proteins. Blood 88:1052–1061
24. Zhu J, Koken MH, Quignon F, Chelbi Alix MK, Degos L, Wang ZY, Chen Z, de The H (1997) Arsenic-induced PML targeting onto nuclear bodies: implications for the treatment of acute promyelocytic leukemia. Proc Natl Acad Sci U S A 94:3978–3983
25. Tallman MS (2001) Therapy of acute myeloid leukemia. Cancer Control 8:62–78
26. Jing Y, Wang L, Xia LJ, Chen GQ, Chen Z, Miller WH, Waxman S (2001) Combined effect of all-trans retinoic acid and arsenic trioxide in acute promyelocytic leukemia cells in vitro and in vivo. Blood 97:264–269
27. Lin RJ, Sternsdorf T, Tini M, Evans RM (2001) Transcriptional regulation in acute promyelocytic leukemia. Oncogene 20:7204–7215
28. Pandolfi PP (2001) Oncogenes and tumor suppressors in the molecular pathogenesis of acute promyelocytic leukemia. Hum Mol Genet 10:769–775
29. Guidez F, Zelent A (2001) Role of nuclear receptor corepressors in leukemogenesis. Curr Top Microbiol Immunol 254:165–185
30. Zelent A, Guidez F, Melnick A, Waxman S, Licht JD (2001) Translocations of the RARalpha gene in acute promyelocytic leukemia. Oncogene 20:7186–7203
31. Miller WH Jr, Schipper HM, Lee JS, Singer J, Waxman S (2002) Mechanisms of action of arsenic trioxide. Cancer Res 62:3893–3903

32. Benoit GR, Tong JH, Balajthy Z, Lanotte M (2001) Exploring (novel) gene expression during retinoid-induced maturation and cell death of acute promyelocytic leukemia. Semin Hematol 38:71–85
33. Liu TX, Zhang JW, Tao J, Zhang RB, Zhang QH, Zhao CJ, Tong JH, Lanotte M, Waxman S, Chen SJ, Mao M, Hu GX, Chen Z (2000) Gene expression networks underlying retinoic acid-induced differentiation of acute promyelocytic leukemia cells. Blood 96:1496–1504
34. Hughes TR, Mao M, Jones AR, et al (2001) Expression profiling using microarrays fabricated by an ink-jet oligonucleotide synthesizer. Nat Biotechnol 19:342–347
35. Morosetti R, Park DJ, Chumakov AM, Grillier I, Shiohara M, Gombart AF, Nakamaki T, Weinberg K, Koeffler HP (1997) A novel, myeloid transcription factor, C/EBP epsilon, is upregulated during granulocytic, but not monocytic, differentiation. Blood 90:2591–2600
36. Chumakov AM, Grillier I, Chumakova E, Chih D, Slater J, Koeffler HP (1997) Cloning of the novel human myeloid-cell-specific C/EBP-epsilon transcription factor. Mol Cell Biol 17:1375–1386
37. Park DJ, Chumakov AM, Vuong PT, Chih DY, Gombart AF, Miller W HJ, Koeffler HP (1999) CCAAT/enhancer binding protein epsilon is a potential retinoid target gene in acute promyelocytic leukemia treatment. J Clin Invest 103:1399–1408
38. Duprez E, Wagner K, Koch H, Tenen DG (2003) C/EBPbeta: a major PML-RARA-responsive gene in retinoic acid-induced differentiation of APL cells. EMBO J 22:5806–5816
39. Dyck JA, Maul GG, Miller WH Jr, Chen JD, Kakizuka A, Evans RM (1994) A novel macromolecular structure is a target of the promyelocyte-retinoic acid receptor oncoprotein. Cell 76:333–343
40. Yoshida H, Kitamura K, Tanaka K, Omura S, Miyazaki T, Hachiya T, Ohno R, Naoe T (1996) Accelerated degradation of PML-retinoic acid receptor alpha (PML-RARA) oncoprotein by all-trans-retinoic acid in acute promyelocytic leukemia: possible role of the proteasome pathway. Cancer Res 56:2945–2948
41. Duprez E, Lillehaug JR, Naoe T, Lanotte M (1996) cAMP signalling is decisive for recovery of nuclear bodies (PODs) during maturation of RA-resistant t(15;17) promyelocytic leukemia NB4 cells expressing PML-RAR alpha. Oncogene 12:2451–2459
42. Zhu J, Gianni M, Kopf E, Honore N, Chelbi-Alix M, Koken M, Quignon F, Rochette-Egly C, de The H (2000) Retinoic acid induces proteasome-dependent degradation of retinoic acid receptor alpha (RARalpha) and oncogenic RARalpha fusion proteins. Proc Natl Acad Sci U S A 96:14807–14812
43. Nervi C, Ferrara FF, Fanelli M, Rippo MR, Tomassini B, Ferrucci PF, Ruthardt M, Gelmetti V, Gambacorti-Passerini C, Diverio D, Grignani F, Pelicci PG, Testi R (1998) Caspases mediate retinoic acid-induced degradation of the acute promyelocytic leukemia PML/RARalpha fusion protein. Blood 92:2244–2251
44. Gianni M, Koken MH, Chelbi-Alix MK, Benoit G, Lanotte M, Chen Z, de The H (1998) Combined arsenic and retinoic acid treatment enhances differentiation and apoptosis in arsenic-resistant NB4 cells. Blood 91:4300–4310

45. Fanelli M, Nervi C, Pelicci G, Gambacorti-Passerini C (1997) Constitutive degradation of the PML/RARa protein is present in retinoic acid (RA)-resistant acute promyelocytic leukemia cells and involves the proteasome proteolytic pathway. Blood 90[Suppl]:70a
46. Idres N, Benoit G, Flexor MA, Lanotte M, Chabot GG (2001) Granulocytic differentiation of human NB4 promyelocytic leukemia cells induced by all-trans retinoic acid metabolites. Cancer Res 61:700–705
47. Benoit G, Altucci L, Flexor M, Ruchaud S, Lillehaug J, Raffelsberger W, Gronemeyer H, Lanotte M (1999) RAR-independent RXR signaling induces t(15;17) leukemia cell maturation. EMBO J 18:7011–7018
48. Jing Y, Xia L, Lu M, Waxman S (2003) The cleavage product deltaPML-RARalpha contributes to all-trans retinoic acid-mediated differentiation in acute promyelocytic leukemia cells. Oncogene 22:4083–4091
49. Lodie TA, Behre G, Zhang P, Pelicci PG, Tenen DG (1998) Expression of the leukemic fusion protein, PML/RARa inhibits C/EBPalpha DNA binding and blocks granulocytic differentiation. Blood 92:211a
50. Tenen DG (2003) Disruption of differentiation in human cancer: AML shows the way. Nat Rev Cancer 3:89–101
51. Dermime S, Grignani F, Clerici M, Nervi C, Sozzi G, Talamo GP, Marchesi E, Formelli F, Parmiani G, Pelicci PG, et al (1993) Occurrence of resistance to retinoic acid in the acute promyelocytic leukemia cell line NB4 is associated with altered expression of the pml/RAR alpha protein. Blood 82:1573–1577
52. Dermime S, Grignani F, Rogaia D, Liberatore C, Marchesi E, Gambacorti Passerini C (1995) Acute promyelocytic leukaemia cells resistant to retinoic acid show further perturbation of the RAR alpha signal transduction system. Leuk Lymphoma 16:289–295
53. Shao W, Fanelli M, Ferrara FF, Riccioni R, Rosenauer A, Davison K, Lamph WW, Waxman S, Pelicci PG, Lo Coco F, Avvisati G, Testa U, Peschle C, Gambacorti Passerini C, Nervi C, Miller WH Jr (1998) Arsenic trioxide as an inducer of apoptosis and loss of PML/RAR alpha protein in acute promyelocytic leukemia cells [see comments]. J Natl Cancer Inst 90:124–133
54. Soignet SL, Maslak P, Chen YW, Calleja E, Pandolfi DA, Scheinberg DA, Warrell RP (1998) Complete remission after clinically induced differentiation and apoptosis in acute promyelocytic leukemia by arsenic trioxide. Br J Haematol 102:225
55. Calleja EM, Warrell RP Jr (2000) Differentiating agents in pediatric malignancies: all-trans-retinoic acid and arsenic in acute promyelocytic leukemia. Curr Oncol Rep 2:519–523
56. Raffoux E, Rousselot P, Poupon J, Daniel MT, Cassinat B, Delarue R, Taksin AL, Rea D, Buzyn A, Tibi A, Lebbe G, Cimerman P, Chomienne C, Fermand JP, de The H, Degos L, Hermine O, Dombret H (2003) Combined treatment with arsenic trioxide and all-trans-retinoic acid in patients with relapsed acute promyelocytic leukemia. J Clin Oncol 21:2326–2334
57. Shen ZX, Chen GQ, Ni JH, Li XS, Xiong SM, Qiu QY, Zhu J, Tang W, Sun GL, Yang KQ, Chen Y, Zhou L, Fang ZW, Wang YT, Ma J, Zhang P, Zhang TD, Chen SJ, Chen Z, Wang ZY (1997) Use of arsenic trioxide (As_2O_3) in the treatment of acute promyelocytic leukemia (APL). II. Clinical efficacy and pharmacokinetics in relapsed patients. Blood 89:3354–3360

58. Shen Y, Shen ZX, Yan H, Chen J, Zeng XY, Li JM, Li XS, Wu W, Xiong SM, Zhao WL, Tang W, Wu F, Liu YF, Niu C, Wang ZY, Chen SJ, Chen Z (2001) Studies on the clinical efficacy and pharmacokinetics of low-dose arsenic trioxide in the treatment of relapsed acute promyelocytic leukemia: a comparison with conventional dosage. Leukemia 15:735–741
59. Cai X, Shen YL, Zhu Q, Jia PM, Yu Y, Zhou L, Huang Y, Zhang JW, Xiong SM, Chen SJ, Wang ZY, Chen Z, Chen GQ (2000) Arsenic trioxide-induced apoptosis and differentiation are associated respectively with mitochondrial transmembrane potential collapse and retinoic acid signaling pathways in acute promyelocytic leukemia. Leukemia 14:262–270
60. Lallemand-Breitenbach V, Guillemin MC, Janin A, Daniel MT, Degos L, Kogan SC, Bishop JM, de The H (1999) Retinoic acid and arsenic synergize to eradicate leukemic cells in a mouse model of acute promyelocytic leukemia. J Exp Med 189:1043–1052
61. Muto A, Kizaki M, Kawamura C, Matsushita H, Fukuchi Y, Umezawa A, Yamada T, Hata J, Hozumi N, Yamato K, Ito M, Ueyama Y, Ikeda Y (2001) A novel differentiation-inducing therapy for acute promyelocytic leukemia with a combination of arsenic trioxide and GM-CSF. Leukemia 15:1176–1184
62. Kizaki M, Muto A, Kinjo K, Ueno H, Ikeda Y (1998) Application of heavy metal and cytokine for differentiation-inducing therapy in acute promyelocytic leukemia. J Natl Cancer Inst 90:1906–1907
63. Zhu J, Chen Z, Lallemand-Breitenbach V, de The H (2002) How acute promyelocytic leukaemia revived arsenic. Nat Rev Cancer 2:705–713
64. Guillemin MC, Raffoux E, Vitoux D, Kogan S, Soilihi H, Lallemand-Breitenbach V, Zhu J, Janin A, Daniel MT, Gourmel B, Degos L, Dombret H, Lanotte M, De The H (2002) In vivo activation of cAMP signaling induces growth arrest and differentiation in acute promyelocytic leukemia. J Exp Med 196:1373–1380
65. Chen GQ, Zhou L, Styblo M, Walton F, Jing Y, Weinberg R, Chen Z, Waxman S (2003) Methylated metabolites of arsenic trioxide are more potent than arsenic trioxide as apoptotic but not differentiation inducers in leukemia and lymphoma cells. Cancer Res 63:1853–1859
66. Dai J, Weinberg RS, Waxman S, Jing Y (1999) Malignant cells can be sensitized to undergo growth inhibition and apoptosis by arsenic trioxide through modulation of the glutathione redox system. Blood 93:268–277
67. Jing Y, Dai J, Chalmers-Redman RM, Tatton WG, Waxman S (1999) Arsenic trioxide selectively induces acute promyelocytic leukemia cell apoptosis via a hydrogen peroxide-dependent pathway. Blood 94:2102–2111
68. Wang ZG, Rivi R, Delva L, Konig A, Scheinberg DA, Gambacorti-Passerini C, Gabrilove JL, Warrell RP Jr, Pandolfi PP (1998) Arsenic trioxide and melarsoprol induce programmed cell death in myeloid leukemia cell lines and function in a PML and PML-RARalpha independent manner. Blood 92:1497–1504
69. Shao W, Fanelli M, Ferrara FF, Riccioni R, Rosenauer A, Davison K, Lamph WW, Waxman S, Pelicci PG, Lo Coco F, Avvisati G, Testa U, Peschle C, Gambacorti-Passerini C, Nervi C, Miller WH Jr (1998) Arsenic trioxide as an inducer of apoptosis and loss of PML/RAR alpha protein in acute promyelocytic leukemia cells. J Natl Cancer Inst 90:124–133

70. Xia L, Wurmbach E, Waxman S, Jing YK (2006) Upregulation of Bfl-1/A1 in leukemia cells undergoing differentiation by all trans retinoic acid treatment attenuates chemotherapeutic agent-induced apoptosis. Leukemia 20:1009–1016
71. Tallman MS, Nabhan C, Feusner JH, Rowe JM (2002) Acute promyelocytic leukemia: evolving therapeutic strategies. Blood 99:759–767
72. Myers CE, Chabner BA (1990) Anthracyclines In: Chabner BA, Collins JM (eds) Cancer chemotherapy. Principles and practice. JB Lippincott, Philadelphia
73. Quillet-Mary A, Mansat V, Duchayne E, Come MG, Allouche M, Bailly JD, Bordier C, Laurent G (1996) Daunorubicin-induced internucleosomal DNA fragmentation in acute myeloid cell lines. Leukemia 10:417–425
74. Laurent G, Jaffrezou JP (2001) Signaling pathways activated by daunorubicin. Blood 98:913–924
75. Stone RM, Maguire M, Goldberg MA, Antin JH, Rosenthal DS, Mayer RJ (1988) Complete remission in acute promyelocytic leukemia despite persistence of abnormal bone marrow promyelocytes during induction therapy: experience in 34 patients. Blood 71:690–696
76. Schwartz EL, Sartorelli AC (1982) Structure-activity relationships for the induction of differentiation of HL-60 human acute promyelocytic leukemia cells by anthracyclines. Cancer Res 42:2651–2655
77. Niitsu N, Higashihara M, Honma Y (2002) The catalytic DNA topoisomerase II inhibitor ICRF-193 and all-trans retinoic acid cooperatively induce granulocytic differentiation of acute promyelocytic leukemia cells: candidate drugs for chemo-differentiation therapy against acute promyelocytic leukemia. Exp Hematol 30:1273–1282
78. Reference deleted in proof
79. Rego EM, He LZ, Warrell RP Jr, Wang ZG, Pandolfi PP (2000) Retinoic acid (RA) and As_2O_3 treatment in transgenic models of acute promyelocytic leukemia (APL) unravel the distinct nature of the leukemogenic process induced by the PML-RARalpha and PLZF-RARalpha oncoproteins. Proc Natl Acad Sci U S A 97:10173–10178
80. Fenaux P, Chomienne C, Degos L (2001) All-trans retinoic acid and chemotherapy in the treatment of acute promyelocytic leukemia. Semin Hematol 38:13–25
81. Niitsu N, Ishii Y, Matsuda A, Honma Y (2001) Induction of differentiation of acute promyelocytic leukemia cells by a cytidine deaminase-resistant analogue of 1-beta-D-arabinofuranosylcytosine, 1-(2-deoxy-2-methylene-beta-D-erythro-pentofuranosyl)cytidine. Cancer Res 61:178–185
82. Waxman S, Scher BM, Hellinger N, Scher W (1990) Combination cytotoxic-differentiation therapy of mouse erythroleukemia cells with 5-fluorouracil and hexamethylene bisacetamide. Cancer Res 50:3878–3887
83. Huang Y, Waxman S (1998) Enhanced growth inhibition and differentiation offluorodeoxyuridine-treated human colon carcinoma cells by phenylbutyrate. Clin Cancer Res 4:2503–2509
84. Dombret H, Fenaux P, Soignet SL, Tallman MS (2002) Established practice in the treatment of patients with acute promyelocytic leukemia and the introduction of arsenic trioxide as a novel therapy. Semin Hematol 39:8–13

85. Yin W, Raffelsberger W, Gronemeyer H (2005) Retinoic acid determines life span of leukemic cells by inducing antagonistic apoptosis-regulatory programs. Int J Biochem Cell Biol 37:1696–1708
86. Dombret H, Sutton L, Duarte M, Daniel MT, Leblond V, Castaigne S, Degos L (1992) Combined therapy with all-trans-retinoic acid and high-dose chemotherapy in patients with hyperleukocytic acute promyelocytic leukemia and severe visceral hemorrhage. Leukemia 6:1237–1242
87. Kwong YL, Au WY, Chim CS, Pang A, Suen C, Liang R (2001) Arsenic trioxide- and idarubicin-induced remissions in relapsed acute promyelocytic leukaemia: clinicopathological and molecular features of a pilot study. Am J Hematol 66:274–279
88. Pandolfi PP (2001) Histone deacetylases and transcriptional therapy with their inhibitors. Cancer Chemother Pharmacol 48[Suppl 1]:S17–19
89. Chen A, Licht JD, Wu Y, Hellinger N, Scher W, Waxman S (1994) Retinoic acid is required for and potentiates differentiation of acute promyelocytic leukemia cells by nonretinoid agents. Blood 84:2122–2129
90. Kosugi H, Towatari M, Hatano S, Kitamura K, Kiyoi H, Kinoshita T, Tanimoto M, Murate T, Kawashima K, Saito H, Naoe T (1999) Histone deacetylase inhibitors are the potent inducer/enhancer of differentiation in acute myeloid leukemia: a new approach to anti-leukemia therapy. Leukemia 13:1316–1324
91. Jing Y, Xia L, Waxman S (2002) Targeted removal of PML-RARalpha protein is required prior to inhibition of histone deacetylase for overcoming all-trans retinoic acid differentiation resistance in acute promyelocytic leukemia. Blood 100:1008–1013
92. Warrell R PJ, He LZ, Richon V, Calleja E, Pandolfi PP (1998) Therapeutic targeting of transcription in acute promyelocytic leukemia by use of an inhibitor of histone deacetylase. J Natl Cancer Inst 90:1621–1625
93. Novick S, Camacho L, Gallagher R, Chanel S, et al (1999) Initial clinical evaluation of 'transcription therapy' for cancer: all-trans retinoic acid plus phenylbutyrate. Blood 94[Suppl1]:60a
94. Kitamura K, Hoshi S, Koike M, Kiyoi H, Saito H, Naoe T (2000) Histone deacetylase inhibitor but not arsenic trioxide differentiates acute promyelocytic leukaemia cells with t(11;17) in combination with all-trans retinoic acid. Br J Haematol 108:696–702
95. Grignani F, De Matteis S, Nervi C, Tomassoni L, Gelmetti V, Cioce M, Fanelli M, Ruthardt M, Ferrara FF, Zamir I, Seiser C, Grignani F, Lazar MA, Minucci S, Pelicci PG (1998) Fusion proteins of the retinoic acid receptor-alpha recruit histone deacetylase in promyelocytic leukaemia. Nature 391:815–818
96. He LZ, Tolentino T, Grayson P, Zhong S, Warrell RP Jr, Rifkind RA, Marks PA, Richon VM, Pandolfi PP (2001) Histone deacetylase inhibitors induce remission in transgenic models of therapy-resistant acute promyelocytic leukemia. J Clin Invest 108:1321–1330
97. Licht JD, Chomienne C, Goy A, Chen A, Scott AA, Head DR, Michaux JL, Wu Y, DeBlasio A, Miller WH Jr, et al (1995) Clinical and molecular characterization of a rare syndrome of acute promyelocytic leukemia associated with translocation (11;17). Blood 85:1083–1094

98. Koken MH, Daniel MT, Gianni M, Zelent A, Licht J, Buzyn A, Minard P, Degos L, Varet B, de The H (1999) Retinoic acid, but not arsenic trioxide, degrades the PLZF/RARalpha fusion protein, without inducing terminal differentiation or apoptosis, in a RA-therapy resistant t(11;17)(q23;q21) APL patient. Oncogene 18:1113–1118
99. Reference deleted in proof
100. Mann KK, Rephaeli A, Colosimo AL, Diaz Z, Nudelman A, Levovich I, Jing Y, Waxman S, Miller WH Jr (2003) A retinoid/butyric acid prodrug overcomes retinoic acid resistance in leukemias by induction of apoptosis. Mol Cancer Res 1:903–912
101. Insinga A, Monestiroli S, Ronzoni S, Gelmetti V, Marchesi F, Viale A, Altucci L, Nervi C, Minucci S, Pelicci PG (2005) Inhibitors of histone deacetylases induce tumor-selective apoptosis through activation of the death receptor pathway. Nat Med 11:71–76
102. Nebbioso A, Clarke N, Voltz E, Germain E, Ambrosino C, Bontempo P, Alvarez R, Schiavone EM, Ferrara F, Bresciani F, Weisz A, de Lera AR, Gronemeyer H, Altucci L (2005) Tumor-selective action of HDAC inhibitors involves TRAIL induction in acute myeloid leukemia cells. Nat Med 11:77–84
103. Jing Y, Hellinger N, Xia L, Monks A, Sausville EA, Zelent A, Waxman S (2005) Benzodithiophenes induce differentiation and apoptosis in human leukemia cells. Cancer Res 65:7847–7855
104. Xu K, Guidez F, Glasow A, Chung D, Petrie K, Stegmaier K, Wang KK, Zhang J, Jing Y, Zelent A, Waxman S (2005) Benzodithiophenes potentiate differentiation of APL cells by lowering the threshold for ligand mediated co-repressor/co-activator exchange with RARa and enhancing changes in ATRA regulated gene expression. Cancer Res 65:7856–7865
105. Ikeda T, Kimura F, Nakata Y, Sato K, Ogura K, Motoyoshi K, Sporn M, Kufe D (2005) Triterpenoid CDDO-Im downregulates PML/RARalpha expression in acute promyelocytic leukemia cells. Cell Death Differ 12:523–531
106. Gianni M, Kalac Y, Ponzanelli I, Rambaldi A, Terao M, Garattini E (2001) Tyrosine kinase inhibitor STI571 potentiates the pharmacologic activity of retinoic acid in acute promyelocytic leukemia cells: effects on the degradation of RARalpha and PML-RARalpha. Blood 97:3234–3243
107. Laurenzana A, Cellai C, Vannucchi AM, Pancrazzi A, Romanelli MN, Paoletti F (2005) WEB-2086 and WEB-2170 trigger apoptosis in both ATRA-sensitive and -resistant promyelocytic leukemia cells and greatly enhance ATRA differentiation potential. Leukemia 19:390–395
108. Au WY, Fung A, Chim CS, Lie AK, Liang R, Ma ES, Chan CH, Wong KF, Kwong YL (2004) FLT-3 aberrations in acute promyelocytic leukaemia: clinicopathological associations and prognostic impact. Br J Haematol 125:463–469
109. Kelly LM, Kutok JL, Williams IR, Boulton CL, Amaral SM, Curley DP, Ley TJ, Gilliland DG (2002) PML/RARalpha and FLT3-ITD induce an APL-like disease in a mouse model. Proc Natl Acad Sci U S A 99:8283–8288
110. Sohal J, Phan VT, Chan PV, Davis EM, Patel B, Kelly LM, Abrams TJ, O'Farrell AM, Gilliland DG, Le Beau MM, Kogan SC (2003) A model of APL with FLT3 mutation is responsive to retinoic acid and a receptor tyrosine kinase inhibitor, SU11657. Blood 101:3188–3197

111. Takeshita A, Shinjo K, Naito K, Matsui H, Sahara N, Shigeno K, Horii T, Shirai N, Maekawa M, Ohnishi K, Naoe T, Ohno R (2005) Efficacy of gemtuzumab ozogamicin on ATRA- and arsenic-resistant acute promyelocytic leukemia (APL) cells. Leukemia 19:1306–1311
112. Lo-Coco F, Cimino G, Breccia M, Noguera NI, Diverio D, Finolezzi E, Pogliani EM, Di Bona E, Micalizzi C, Kropp M, Venditti A, Tafuri A, Mandelli F (2004) Gemtuzumab ozogamicin (Mylotarg) as a single agent for molecularly relapsed acute promyelocytic leukemia. Blood 104:1995–1999
113. Tsimberidou AM, Estey E, Whitman GJ, Dryden MJ, Ratnam S, Pierce S, Faderl S, Giles F, Kantarjian HM, Garcia-Manero G (2004) Extramedullary relapse in a patient with acute promyelocytic leukemia: successful treatment with arsenic trioxide, all-trans retinoic acid and gemtuzumab ozogamicin therapies. Leuk Res 28:991–994
114. Estey EH (2003) Treatment options for relapsed acute promyelocytic leukaemia. Best Pract Res Clin Haematol 16:521–534

Subject Index

acetylation
- of PLZF   38
acute promyelocytic leukemia (APL)   129, 245
- all-*trans* retinoic acid (ATRA)   245
- arsenic trioxide   245
all-*trans* retinoic acid (ATRA)   129, 207
alternative lengthening of telomeres (ALT)   63
D-amino acid   228
anthracycline   252
- apoptosis   252
- ROS   252
anti-CD33 antibody   150
anti-PML antibody   146
AOS1   52
APL   246, 247, 254, 255
- ATRA   246, 247, 254
- daunorubicin   254
- differentiation   247, 255
- histone deacetylase inhibitor   255
- PML-RARα   246
apoptosis   60, 251
- As_2O_3 251
- H_2O_2 251
- induced by PLZF   41
arsenic trioxide   129, 150, 213, 214
- adverse effects   134
- dosage   130
- pharmacokinetics   130
artifacts   227
As_2O_3 253

ATRA   150, 210, 211, 253, 256, 257
- differentiation   256, 258
- HDAC inhibitor   257
- Mylotarg   258
- novel agent   257
- phenylbutyrate   256

base excision repair (BER)   59
Bloom (BLM) helicase   60
BTB/POZ   228

c-myc
- repression of PLZF   40
caretakers   60
CD33   208, 211
CD56   31
cell-permeable peptides   222
cellular senescence   60
charged pocket motif   237
chromosome cohesion   51
condensin   56
corepressor   228
cyclin A2
- repression of PLZF   40
cytosine arabinoside (Ara-C)   209

DNA methyltransferases   231
double-strand breaks (DSBs)   57

ETO
- interaction with PLZF   36
export
- of PLZF to cytoplpasm   38

FAZF   34
FISH   146

Subject Index

Flt3
- action on PLZF 39
fluorescence in situ hybridization (FISH) 206
fusogenic HA2 motif 226

GATA2
- interaction with PLZF 40
gatekeepers 60
gemtuzumab ozogamicin (GO) 213
glucocorticoids
- induction of PLZF 35
GO 214

hematopoietic stem cells
- role of PLZF in 33
histone deacetylases 231
- interaction with PLZF 35
homologous recombination (HR) 56
Hoxb2 34
HuM195 212, 213
hydrocarbon stapling 232

idarubicin 213
inclusion bodies 227
isoform 206

leucine zipper 235
LIM domain
- interaction with PLZF 37
linear peptides 233
LXXI/HIXXXI/L motif 233

macropinocytosis 226
maintenance therapy 211
megakaryocyte
- role of PLZF in 33
molecular relapse 149

nested RT-PCR 150
non-homologous end-joining (NHEJ) 57

p53 62
p53 C-terminal activating peptide 235

PCNA 58
penetratin 224
peptide aptamer 234
phage display 234
phosphorylation
- of PLZF 38
PIASy 62
PLZF-RARα 207
PLZF/RAR variant 208
PLZF/RARα 237
PML 63
PML-RARα 248, 249, 253
- apoptosis 250
- As_2O_3 249, 250
- differentiation 248, 249
- proteolysis 248
pRB 62
primary retinoid resistance 236
protein transduction domains (PTDs) 224
pTAT 224

RA or differentiation syndrome 210
RAD6 58
RBCC motif 234
real-time PCR 150
RecQ-like helicase 61
- BLM 61
- RecQ 61
- WRN 61
retro-inverso configuration 228
ribosomal DNA (rDNA) loci 55
RT-PCR 146, 210, 212, 213

senescence 57
SMC proteins 51
SMT3 52
SP100 63
spermatogonia
- role of PLZF 41
SUMO
- modification of PLZF 39
SUMO E3 ligase 49
- gei-1 53
- gei-17 49
- Mms21 59

Subject Index

- Mms21/Nse2   49
- Nse2   59
- Pc2   49, 50
- Pli1   49, 56
- Ran BP2   49
- RanBP1   50
- SIZ/PIAS   49, 50
- Su(var)2–10   49, 55
SUMO protease   49
- SENPs   49
- SMT4   49
- Smt4p   55
- SUSP1   54
- SUSPs   49
- Ulp2p   55
- Ulps   49
sumoylation   137
sumoylation motif (ψKxE/D)   50

telomerase   57
telomere maintenance   63
therapeutic window   231
thymine DNA glycosylase
    (TDG)   59

topoisomerase   55, 60, 61
- TOP3   60
- Topo-I   60
- Topo-II   60
transcription-therapy   222
transcriptional activator
- PLZF as   37
translesion synthesis (TLS)   58
tumour-suppressor   62
tyrosine phosphorylation
- of PLZF   36

UBA2   52
UBC9   52

variant   207
VDUP1
- interaction with PLZF   37
venoocclusive disease
    (VOD)   213
vitamin D3 receptor
- interaction with PLZF   40

Werner (WRN) helicase   60

Current Topics in Microbiology and Immunology

Volumes published since 1989 (and still available)

Vol. 269: **Koszinowski, Ulrich H.; Hengel, Hartmut (Eds.):** Viral Proteins Counteracting Host Defenses. 2002. 47 figs. XII, 325 pp. ISBN 3-540-43261-2

Vol. 270: **Beutler, Bruce; Wagner, Hermann (Eds.):** Toll-Like Receptor Family Members and Their Ligands. 2002. 31 figs. X, 192 pp. ISBN 3-540-43560-3

Vol. 271: **Koehler, Theresa M. (Ed.):** Anthrax. 2002. 14 figs. X, 169 pp. ISBN 3-540-43497-6

Vol. 272: **Doerfler, Walter; Böhm, Petra (Eds.):** Adenoviruses: Model and Vectors in Virus-Host Interactions. Virion and Structure, Viral Replication, Host Cell Interactions. 2003. 63 figs., approx. 280 pp. ISBN 3-540-00154-9

Vol. 273: **Doerfler, Walter; Böhm, Petra (Eds.):** Adenoviruses: Model and Vectors in VirusHost Interactions. Immune System, Oncogenesis, Gene Therapy. 2004. 35 figs., approx. 280 pp. ISBN 3-540-06851-1

Vol. 274: **Workman, Jerry L. (Ed.):** Protein Complexes that Modify Chromatin. 2003. 38 figs., XII, 296 pp. ISBN 3-540-44208-1

Vol. 275: **Fan, Hung (Ed.):** Jaagsiekte Sheep Retrovirus and Lung Cancer. 2003. 63 figs., XII, 252 pp. ISBN 3-540-44096-3

Vol. 276: **Steinkasserer, Alexander (Ed.):** Dendritic Cells and Virus Infection. 2003. 24 figs., X, 296 pp. ISBN 3-540-44290-1

Vol. 277: **Rethwilm, Axel (Ed.):** Foamy Viruses. 2003. 40 figs., X, 214 pp. ISBN 3-540-44388-6

Vol. 278: **Salomon, Daniel R.; Wilson, Carolyn (Eds.):** Xenotransplantation. 2003. 22 figs., IX, 254 pp. ISBN 3-540-00210-3

Vol. 279: **Thomas, George; Sabatini, David; Hall, Michael N. (Eds.):** TOR. 2004. 49 figs., X, 364 pp. ISBN 3-540-00534X

Vol. 280: **Heber-Katz, Ellen (Ed.):** Regeneration: Stem Cells and Beyond. 2004. 42 figs., XII, 194 pp. ISBN 3-540-02238-4

Vol. 281: **Young, John A. T. (Ed.):** Cellular Factors Involved in Early Steps of Retroviral Replication. 2003. 21 figs., IX, 240 pp. ISBN 3-540-00844-6

Vol. 282: **Stenmark, Harald (Ed.):** Phosphoinositides in Subcellular Targeting and Enzyme Activation. 2003. 20 figs., X, 210 pp. ISBN 3-540-00950-7

Vol. 283: **Kawaoka, Yoshihiro (Ed.):** Biology of Negative Strand RNA Viruses: The Power of Reverse Genetics. 2004. 24 figs., IX, 350 pp. ISBN 3-540-40661-1

Vol. 284: **Harris, David (Ed.):** Mad Cow Disease and Related Spongiform Encephalopathies. 2004. 34 figs., IX, 219 pp. ISBN 3-540-20107-6

Vol. 285: **Marsh, Mark (Ed.):** Membrane Trafficking in Viral Replication. 2004. 19 figs., IX, 259 pp. ISBN 3-540-21430-5

Vol. 286: **Madshus, Inger H. (Ed.):** Signalling from Internalized Growth Factor Receptors. 2004. 19 figs., IX, 187 pp. ISBN 3-540-21038-5

Vol. 287: **Enjuanes, Luis (Ed.):** Coronavirus Replication and Reverse Genetics. 2005. 49 figs., XI, 257 pp. ISBN 3-540-21494-1

Vol. 288: **Mahy, Brain W. J. (Ed.):** Foot-and-Mouth-Disease Virus. 2005. 16 figs., IX, 178 pp. ISBN 3-540-22419X

Vol. 289: **Griffin, Diane E. (Ed.):** Role of Apoptosis in Infection. 2005. 40 figs., IX, 294 pp. ISBN 3-540-23006-8

Vol. 290: **Singh, Harinder; Grosschedl, Rudolf (Eds.):** Molecular Analysis of B Lymphocyte Development and Activation. 2005. 28 figs., XI, 255 pp. ISBN 3-540-23090-4

Vol. 291: **Boquet, Patrice; Lemichez Emmanuel (Eds.)** Bacterial Virulence Factors and Rho GTPases. 2005. 28 figs., IX, 196 pp. ISBN 3-540-23865-4

Vol. 292: **Fu, Zhen F (Ed.):** The World of Rhabdoviruses. 2005. 27 figs., X, 210 pp. ISBN 3-540-24011-X

Vol. 293: **Kyewski, Bruno; Suri-Payer, Elisabeth (Eds.):** CD4+CD25+ Regulatory T Cells: Origin, Function and Therapeutic Potential. 2005. 22 figs., XII, 332 pp. ISBN 3-540-24444-1

Vol. 294: **Caligaris-Cappio, Federico, Dalla Favera, Ricardo (Eds.):** Chronic Lymphocytic Leukemia. 2005. 25 figs., VIII, 187 pp. ISBN 3-540-25279-7

Vol. 295: **Sullivan, David J.; Krishna Sanjeew (Eds.):** Malaria: Drugs, Disease and Post-genomic Biology. 2005. 40 figs., XI, 446 pp. ISBN 3-540-25363-7

Vol. 296: **Oldstone, Michael B. A. (Ed.):** Molecular Mimicry: Infection Induced Autoimmune Disease. 2005. 28 figs., VIII, 167 pp. ISBN 3-540-25597-4

Vol. 297: **Langhorne, Jean (Ed.):** Immunology and Immunopathogenesis of Malaria. 2005. 8 figs., XII, 236 pp. ISBN 3-540-25718-7

Vol. 298: **Vivier, Eric; Colonna, Marco (Eds.):** Immunobiology of Natural Killer Cell Receptors. 2005. 27 figs., VIII, 286 pp. ISBN 3-540-26083-8

Vol. 299: **Domingo, Esteban (Ed.):** Quasispecies: Concept and Implications. 2006. 44 figs., XII, 401 pp. ISBN 3-540-26395-0

Vol. 300: **Wiertz, Emmanuel J.H.J.; Kikkert, Marjolein (Eds.):** Dislocation and Degradation of Proteins from the Endoplasmic Reticulum. 2006. 19 figs., VIII, 168 pp. ISBN 3-540-28006-5

Vol. 301: **Doerfler, Walter; Böhm, Petra (Eds.):** DNA Methylation: Basic Mechanisms. 2006. 24 figs., VIII, 324 pp. ISBN 3-540-29114-8

Vol. 302: **Robert N. Eisenman (Ed.):** The Myc/Max/Mad Transcription Factor Network. 2006. 28 figs. XII, 278 pp. ISBN 3-540-23968-5

Vol. 303: **Thomas E. Lane (Ed.):** Chemokines and Viral Infection. 2006. 14 figs. XII, 154 pp. ISBN 3-540-29207-1

Vol. 304: **Stanley A. Plotkin (Ed.):** Mass Vaccination: Global Aspects -- Progress and Obstacles. 2006. 40 figs. X, 270 pp. ISBN 3-540-29382-5

Vol. 305: **Radbruch, Andreas; Lipsky, Peter E. (Eds.):** Current Concepts in Autoimmunity. 2006. 29 figs. IIX, 276 pp. ISBN 3-540-29713-8

Vol. 306: **William M. Shafer (Ed.):** Antimicrobial Peptides and Human Disease. 2006. 12 figs. XII, 262 pp. ISBN 3-540-29915-7

Vol. 307: **John L. Casey (Ed.):** Hepatitis Delta Virus. 2006. 22 figs. XII, 228 pp. ISBN 3-540-29801-0

Vol. 308: **Honjo, Tasuku; Melchers, Fritz (Eds.):** Gut-Associated Lymphoid Tissues. 2006. 24 figs. XII, 204 pp. ISBN 3-540-30656-0

Vol. 309: **Polly Roy (Ed.):** Reoviruses: Entry, Assembly and Morphogenesis. 2006. 43 figs. XX, 261 pp. ISBN 3-540-30772-9

Vol. 310: **Doerfler, Walter; Böhm, Petra (Eds.):** DNA Methylation: Development, Genetic Disease and Cancer. 2006. 25 figs. X, 284 pp. ISBN 3-540-31180-7

Vol. 311: **Pulendran, Bali; Ahmed, Rafi (Eds.):** From Innate Immunity to Immunological Memory. 2006. 13 figs. X, 177 pp. ISBN 3-540-32635-9

Vol. 312: **Boshoff, Chris; Weiss, Robin A. (Eds.):** Kaposi Sarcoma Herpesvirus: New Perspectives. 2006. 29 figs. XVI, 330 pp. ISBN 3-540-34343-1

Printing: Krips bv, Meppel
Binding: Stürtz, Würzburg